Descriptions and Prescriptions

Descriptions and Prescriptions

Values, Mental Disorders, and the DSMs

EDITED BY

JOHN Z. SADLER, M.D.
Professor, Department of Psychiatry
University of Texas Southwestern Medical Center at Dallas
Dallas, Texas

The Johns Hopkins University Press ▪▪ Baltimore and London

© 2002 The Johns Hopkins University Press
All rights reserved. Published 2002
Printed in the United States of America on acid-free paper
9 8 7 6 5 4 3 2 1

The Johns Hopkins University Press
2715 North Charles Street
Baltimore, Maryland 21218-4363
www.press.jhu.edu

LIBRARY OF CONGRESS CATALOGING-IN-PUBLICATION DATA

Descriptions and prescriptions : values, mental disorders, and the DSMs
/ edited by John Z. Sadler.
p.   cm.
Includes bibliographical references and index.
ISBN 0-8018-6840-8 (hardcover : alk. paper)
1. Mental illness—Classification—Social aspects.   2. Mental illness—
Classification—Moral and ethical aspects.   3. Diagnostic and statistical
manual of mental disorders.   I. Sadler, John Z., 1953–   .
[DNLM: 1.   Mental Disorders—classification.   2.   Social Values.
WM 15 D449 2002]
RC455.2.C4D47 2002
616.89′001′2—dc21

2001002186

A catalog record for this book is available from the British Library.

Contents

Contributors

GEORGE J. AGICH, Ph.D., F. J. O'Neill Chairman, Department of Bioethics, Cleveland Clinic Foundation, Cleveland, Ohio

CAROL BERKENKOTTER, Ph.D., Professor of Rhetoric, Department of Humanities, Michigan Technological University, Houghton, Michigan

LEE ANNA CLARK, Ph.D., Professor, Department of Psychology, University of Iowa, Iowa City, Iowa

K. W. M. FULFORD, D.Phil., F.R.C.Psych., Professor of Philosophy and Mental Health, Department of Philosophy, University of Warwick, Coventry; and Honorary Consultant Psychiatrist, Department of Psychiatry, University of Oxford, Oxford, United Kingdom

IRVING I. GOTTESMAN, Ph.D., Sherrell J. Aston Professor of Psychology and Professor of Medical Genetics (Pediatrics), Department of Psychology, University of Virginia, Charlottesville, Virginia

LAURA LEE HALL, Ph.D., former Director of Research, NAMI (National Alliance for the Mentally Ill); biomedical and health care analyst and writer.

CATHY LEAKER, Ph.D., Visiting Instructor of English and Women's Studies, Empire State College, State University of New York, Rochester, New York

CHRIS MACE, M.D., M.R.C.Psych., Senior Lecturer in Psychotherapy, Department of Psychology, University of Warwick, Coventry, United Kingdom

LAURIE McQUEEN, M.S.S.W., DSM Project Manager, American Psychiatric Association, Washington, D.C.

CHRISTIAN PERRING, Ph.D., Assistant Professor, Department of Philosophy and Religious Studies, Dowling College, Oakdale, New York

JAMES PHILLIPS, M.D., Clinical Associate Professor, Department of Psychiatry, Yale University School of Medicine, New Haven, Connecticut

HAROLD ALAN PINCUS, M.D., Professor and Executive Vice Chairman, University of Pittsburgh School of Medicine; and RAND Senior Scientist and Director, RAND–University of Pittsburgh Health Institute, Pittsburgh, Pennsylvania

JENNIFER H. RADDEN, D.Phil., Professor, Department of Philosophy, University of Massachusetts at Boston, Boston, Massachusetts

DORIS J. RAVOTAS, M.A., L.L.P., Instructor of Psychology, Department of Education, Michigan Technological University, Houghton, Michigan

PATRICIA A. ROSS, Ph.D., Assistant Professor, Department of Philosophy, and Resident Fellow, Minnesota Center for Philosophy of Science, University of Minnesota, Minneapolis, Minnesota

JOHN Z. SADLER, M.D., Professor and Director of Undergraduate Psychiatric Education, University of Texas Southwestern Medical Center at Dallas, Dallas, Texas

KENNETH F. SCHAFFNER, M.D., Ph.D., University Professor of Medical Humanities and Professor of Philosophy, George Washington University, Washington, D.C.

MICHAEL ALAN SCHWARTZ, M.D., Professor, Department of Psychiatry, Tufts University School of Medicine, New England Medical Center, Boston, Massachusetts

DANIEL W. SHUMAN, J.D., Professor of Law, Southern Methodist University, Dallas, Texas

ALLYSON SKENE, Ph.D., Department of Philosophy, York University, Toronto, Ontario, Canada

JEROME C. WAKEFIELD, D.S.W., Professor, School of Social Work and Institute for Health, Health Care Policy, and Aging Research, Rutgers University, New Brunswick, New Jersey

THOMAS A. WIDIGER, Ph.D., Professor, Department of Psychology, University of Kentucky, Lexington, Kentucky

OSBORNE P. WIGGINS, Ph.D., Professor, Department of Philosophy, University of Louisville, Louisville, Kentucky

Acknowledgments

LIKE MANY edited scholarly books, this one was conceived in concert with a conference. I am grateful to the people and institutions that contributed funds to support a large and diverse meeting. John W. Burnside, associate dean at the University of Texas Southwestern Medical Center at the time, conveyed, as always, unabashed enthusiasm for this project and managed to scrape up some money from here and there for it. William F. May, then the Maguire Professor of Ethics at Southern Methodist University, was a personal inspiration as well as essential in helping me secure grant funding for the meeting and, ultimately, this book. William Stubing and the Greenwall Foundation were essential sources of support as well as encouragement about the importance of values in mental disorder classification. My colleagues in the Association for the Advancement of Philosophy and Psychiatry were generous as well, both in checkbook and in spirit—and, of course, ideas. Danny and the anonymous others who, in large part, supported the conference deserve great thanks; without them it could not have happened, at least not in the grand manner in which it did. My chairman, Kenneth Z. Altshuler, as always, was a significant source of encouragement and support as well. I'm aware, and therefore doubly appreciative to all, of the novel, perhaps idiosyncratic vision of the conference at the time. Partly because of all the individuals who were involved, the whole "values" matter is less novel and considerably less idiosyncratic at the time of this book's completion.

Showing her characteristic enthusiasm and tenacity, Linda Muncy, my assistant, deserves much of the credit for pulling this off, from the initial exploration of the idea, to the preparation of proposals, letters of invitation, and reports, hosting visitors, and, ultimately, this book's manuscript. I salute her flexibility and commitment and am ever grateful.

Who could ask for a more congenial, constructive, and thoughtful group of contributors? The positive attitudes and active listening of all, especially in the face of often substantial disagreement, were key outcomes of the conference, and ones that I hope this volume can perpetuate as we consider the future of mental disorder classification. A key element in the success of the conference was the contribution of the numerous other authors and commentators, people who had substantial pieces but for space considerations had to be left out of this book. To recognize their unpublished contributions in modest measure, let me name them: Lee Anna Clark, Irving I. Gottesman, Patricia S. Greenspan, Robert John Hamm, Loretta Kopelman, Jerome Kroll, James Phillips, Robert L. Spitzer, George Agich, K. W. M. Fulford, Harold Pincus, Louis A. Sass, Kenneth F. Schaffner, Jerome C. Wakefield, Thomas Widiger, and J. Melvin Woody. Kenneth Z. Altshuler, Elena Bezzubova, Pat Greenspan, Jerry Kroll, Bill May, James Phillips, and Mel Woody chaired sessions and introduced speakers with grace and aplomb.

On the publishing end, Wendy Harris has stewarded this publication with the kindness and patience she exhibited the last time around. You'd think she would learn! I'm grateful to the Journals staff at the Johns Hopkins University Press and to K. W. M. Fulford for the publicity and support generated through our journal, *Philosophy, Psychiatry, and Psychology.*

Abbie, Evan, and Cole deserve special thanks for putting up with an often frazzled husband and occasionally grumpy daddy. They all are the wellspring of love, satisfaction, and contentment that generates creative and productive work.

Part One

. . . .

Introduction and Background

1

· ·

Introduction

JOHN Z. SADLER, M.D.

WESTERN CULTURE is wary of values. Such wariness can be recognized through considering our ordinary talk. For instance, when we are in the position of meeting new people, we often introduce ourselves by describing what we do. In my case, I introduce myself through various descriptive functions: psychiatrist, husband, father, gardener, taxpayer, photographer, and so on. Were I to introduce myself instead with the language of evaluation rather than description, I would be seen as pretentious, idiosyncratic, or downright weird: "Hi, I'm John Sadler, and I'm loyal, stubborn, and bright." But the wariness of values is not limited to social intercourse. If I were to look for "values" in my local newspaper, it would be in the "Religion and Values" section, not on the front page. Newspapers are where (we hope) the facts are, not the values. Indeed, Western society seems stratified according to places where one can consider or discuss values with comfort. As far as days of the week go, Sundays (and other holy days) seem reserved for reflection about the good, the right, and the sacred. This Balkanization of the evaluative, however, is not limited to the calendar. In particular, those with scientific or technical backgrounds (e.g., people likely to read this book) find themselves amazed by the rich vocabulary of values in common parlance in other settings: for instance, listening to the talk of art dealers, artists, and connoisseurs at an opening for a gallery show. From where do these people come up with these wellsprings of evaluation?

Values in matters scientific have been suspect for at least the past two hundred years. Enlightenment rationalism permitted reason little of anything smacking of emotivism or the passions, and from Francis Bacon to Max Weber (and indeed, the present day), the wish of science has been to eliminate values in true science (Proctor, 1991). Value considerations in science, in sum, are often considered pollutants. But this aversion to values is changing, and such change is evident from diverse social strands.

Perhaps most obvious has been the bioethics "movement." Emerging from well-publicized legal cases of medical battery, horrific exploitations of biomedical research subjects, and struggles over the "good death," bioethics established the value ladenness of medical practices. But what about medical and scientific concepts? Are they value laden too? The historical culminations of the Enlightenment ethos of rationality, logical positivism and logical empiricism, ran into insoluble problems in the 1950s and 1960s when the strict rules governing the relations between theory and observation failed to appear or to be found. Hanson (1958), Feyerabend (1978), and especially Kuhn (1970, 1977) sealed the fate of just-so rationalistic science through their studies of discovery, irrationalism, and values in science. Kuhn (1977), in particular, argued that the only way reasonable scientists could disagree, given the same facts and different theories, was through different evaluations of theory: some theories were simpler, others more comprehensive, some had more predictive power, and so on. Indeed, he led the way to the recognition that scientific concepts (including values), framed by theory and background knowledge, contributed to the recognition, interpretation, and even the "shape" of the facts. After all, to establish knowledge required an evaluation of the knowledge claim: some theories or explanations were better than others, which meant that judgments of good and bad were indispensable to knowledge. Value theory had grabbed science by the genitals.

Psychiatry, as always, marched in step with the culture that generated such rethinking of the role of values in science, knowledge, and human action. In 1973, about the time the reviews of the second edition of Kuhn's *The Structure of Scientific Revolutions* were emerging in the history, philosophy, science, and medical journals, the American Psychiatric Association had decided by member vote to declassify homosexuality as a mental disorder (Bayer, 1981, 1987). Robert Spitzer, an acknowledged leader of the move to depathologize the gay, articulated the issue around homosexuality to be more of an issue of value judgments than science (Spitzer, 1981). The whole controversial mess around this change brought to popular awareness the notion that psychopathology involved value judgments, an idea that, up to that time, was a trope for academics and intellectuals only. Spitzer went on to spearhead the third revision of the *Diagnostic and Statistical Manual of Mental Disorders* (DSM), which sought a scientific rigor to mental disorder diagnosis which had theretofore not been attempted. Spitzer and his colleagues on the DSM-III committee wished to make diagnosis more reliable, and ultimately more valid, by augmenting the descriptive rigor of psychiatry's diagnostic manual. Such efforts bring us to this volume, which, as K. W. M. Fulford has noted in his summative fantasy at the end of the book, reflects an intent to augment the *evaluative* rigor of classification efforts in psychiatry. The parallel between descriptive and evaluative rigor warrants some further discussion.

Through operationalizing diagnostic concepts into specific criteria, the DSM-III group attempted to diminish ambiguities in psychiatric diagnostic concepts in DSM-I and -II. Instead of the cryptic and general descriptions of the earlier manuals, the DSM-III specified, as much as practicable, the operations required for a patient to qualify for a particular diagnosis. Numerous advantages were expected with such a move; clinicians could discuss similarly diagnosed patients with a greater confidence that their patients were truly similar in salient ways; researchers could have more homogeneous populations of subjects in which to develop general explanations and treatments; psychiatry in general could be more "medical" through a more explicit modeling of mental disorder after disease concepts and disease language. With a "postvalues" awareness, we might say that the DSM-III made mental disorder diagnosis more *accountable;* one could not label a patient with a diagnosis in just any way or without reference to a method, a system, and indeed, a professional organization, the American Psychiatric Association. What was initially intended as a purely "scientific" enterprise nevertheless brought in a set of relatively novel moral elements to psychiatric practice, with "accountability" only one of the many values involved.

This book might be construed as an effort to extend this "accountability thesis" of the post–DSM-III era. What the DSM-III did was add an explicit emphasis and method to approximately half of the experiential universe of mental disorder, that is, the descriptive/factual elements of clinical experience. This book, building on earlier groundwork (Sadler, Schwartz, and Wiggins, 1994b), attempts to raise explicit awareness of the other half of the experiential universe, that of value and evaluation in mental disorders. For every delusion there is a complementary jealousy, fear, or family member's tears; for every addiction there is tragedy; for every depression there is at least one lament. Psychiatry has always had its evaluations; indeed, without them, it would be an impoverished field. This book moves values from the background of psychiatric diagnosis to the foreground, where, I believe, they belong.

The awareness of values in diagnostic classification is not limited to just the negative values of suffering from symptoms and their consequences. As we shall see in the chapters to follow, values shape what is clinically relevant (what the clinician sees or doesn't see); what clinical evidence is salient, useful, or otherwise important; the criteria of pathology; the credibility of the diagnostic process, even the priorities in designing a classification.

■ ■ Why Psychiatric Classification?

A prospective reader might wonder why the focus on psychiatric classification, nosology, and diagnosis in a book that might well have focused on the "values of psychiatry" instead. Perhaps the most obvious, and least interesting, reason is simply one of focus. As can be seen from the rest of this book, a project that aims to make substantive comments about the values in psychiatric classification is already a large enterprise. An enterprise that aspires to address values in psychiatry in general (e.g., diagnosis, therapies, social-professional roles) will be a truly colossal project.

Psychiatric classification, however, has good reasons to be nominated for careful attention to value commitments. First, the DSMs and ICDs (the World Health Organization's *International Classification of Diseases*) are commonly used, nearly universal anchor points for clinical practice, research, education, and administration of mental health care. The categories of these diagnostic manuals are the common language, for better or for worse, of mental health practitioners around the world. As Michael Schwartz and Osborne Wiggins note in their chapter, the DSMs, at least in the United States, dominate the field of clinical research, in essence serving as a checkpoint, even a "pass" requirement for research funding and publication. Administratively, the DSM/ICD code is found in epidemiological records, insurance billing, hospital statistics—essentially, at every level of mental health administration. Educationally, the DSM and ICD categories frame the structure of curricula in mental health care: textbooks are organized around groups of DSM/ICD disorders, diagnostic criteria are the core reference for recognizing and diagnosing psychopathology, and educational media are built around DSM/ICD categories. Such universality of the DSM/ICD influence means that these manuals broker the thinking that is turned into public policy concerning mental health.

Perhaps most important from the public perspective, the DSM/ICD classifications are the reference points for public understanding of mental disorders—the manuals shape lay, not to omit professional, notions of mental illness. In the context of psychiatric classification and public understanding, W. V. O. Quine's witty motto "Ontology recapitulates Philology" is particularly apt. For Quine, what something *is* is reflected in the historical unfolding of the language that speaks of it. In the case of the DSMs and ICDs, the immeasurably complex phenomenon of mental life is encapsulated and compartmentalized in particular ways; other ways of framing mental life are possible, but such alternative framings will require their own terms and linguistic conventions, as can been seen in the chapter by Berkenkotter and Ravotas in this book. Psychiatric classification warrants a "values analysis" even for those who reject such manuals—the DSM influence is nonetheless powerful, a social phenomenon to be contended with even if one disagrees with the DSM "approach" to the manifold presentations of psychopathology.

▪ ▪ Why Values?

This book takes *values* in a broad and general sense. As used here, the term reflects a range of preferences, predilections, esteems, and predispositions to act. When I think about values, I define them as concepts that (a) tend to direct action, and (b) are subject to praise or blame in reference to such actions (Sadler, 1997). Values in this sense may be in the foreground of what we wish to do and frame as goals (e.g., psychiatric classification should be "user-friendly") or may occupy a Quinian ontological background where values and "morality" shape how we think about things and choose to live our lives—as clinicians, as citizens, as spiritual beings, as scientists, as parents, as spouses, and so on. Such latter manifestations of value reflect what the layperson calls a "philosophy of life," whether carefully thought out and articulated (conscious in the Freudian sense) or simply assumed and enacted in everyday life (preconscious or unconscious in the Freudian sense). As we shall see, the values that saturate the DSM enterprise represent all levels of intention and awareness on the part of the classification's creators—some values are quite explicit, but many more are implicit. Implicit values raise the question about whether they are intentionally selected or merely a happenstance, accidental selection.

Hence a book such as this one is useful in that the evaluations (values) involved in the DSMs and ICDs become more explicit and therefore more amenable to critical thought and reconsideration. As I suggested earlier in this introduction, the role of values in classification may be Balkanized in the DSMs just like values are Balkanized in real life. But their influences, nonetheless, are powerful. The values of the DSMs are answers to the "should" questions that are the most fundamental for a diagnostic manual; such questions include: Should we have a diagnostic manual? What should it include? How should we put it together? Whom should we include in making such a manual? To whom should we direct this manual? How should we decide which methods and scientific data are meritorious and which are not?

A consideration of the values behind psychiatric classification should also help us understand the controversies and arguments concerning specific points of the manual. For instance, what are the values involved in considering whether to include premenstrual dysphoric disorder as a disorder in DSM-IV? Although a consideration of values will certainly not guarantee a resolution of conflict, making them explicit permits the distinguishing of true areas of disagreement from misunderstandings and misconceptions. Moreover, much like the field of bioethics has raised awareness of difficult ethical conflicts in general medicine and provided medicine with a language with which to articulate such conflict, so do our authors hope to raise awareness of ethical and values-related issues in classification and in so doing help provide an identity, a language, and a common ground to discuss the many difficult decisions psychiatric nosologists make.

The authors in this volume were encouraged to write their essays as a contribution to a future edition of a DSM or ICD; indeed, many have explicit recommendations for a DSM-V. As I (along with previous coeditors, in Sadler, Wiggins, and Schwartz, 1994a) have said before, a book that addresses such a relatively novel element of psychiatric classification cannot attempt to be comprehensive but rather exploratory instead, and certainly this book should be considered an exploration of the evaluative territory of the DSMs rather than a comprehensive map of said territory.

While most of the contributors here take an explicitly philosophical perspective on the question of values in psychiatric classification, I felt it important not to give philosophy the only "voice" here. Philosophers may be the theoreticians of values, but they are certainly not the arbiters of them. Indeed, there are no arbiters here but rather a collection of voices who share various interests in the outcome of psychiatric classifications such as the DSMs. I hope this collection of voices will initiate and stimulate an ongoing and lively public dialogue about values in psychiatric classification, one that will benefit the lives of the mentally ill, their families, and those who care for and about them.

The Limits of an Evidence-Based Classification of Mental Disorders

HAROLD ALAN PINCUS, M.D.,
AND LAURIE MCQUEEN, M.S.S.W.

EVIDENCE-BASED approaches to psychiatric classification are essential to assure the credibility of the field and to conform to current scientific standards. They do, however, have important limitations and are not without their own explicit and implicit set of values. This chapter reviews and describes the origin, background, and goals of the DSM-IV, the principles of evidence-based psychiatry, and how those principles were applied during the DSM-IV process. The limitations of this approach and recommendations and projections for the future are also discussed.

■ ■ Why Classify? Goals of a Classification/DSM-IV

The goals of the DSM-IV can be divided into four main categories: clinical, research, educational, and information management. The clinical goals of the DSM-IV were paramount because the book is used primarily by clinicians.

Clinical

In our view, the highest priorities in developing the DSM-IV were the clinical application of criteria to define specific mental disorders and the enhancement of the reliability of communication and assessment by clinicians. The definitions and subtypes of the DSM-IV should be of use to them as they conceptualize their treatment planning. However, as stated in the DSM-IV introduction, a DSM-IV diagnosis by itself should in no way constitute the full spectrum of the knowledge needed to develop a treatment plan. It is simply a start. Importantly, the text in the DSM-IV provides some useful collateral information that is helpful for clinicians in their work with patients.

Research

The most important research goal of the DSM-IV was to define homogeneous groups for study. In a research setting, the criteria can also enhance the reliability of assessment. We encourage researchers not to be limited by the DSM criteria, since we are rapidly learning more about psychiatric disorders and the classifications should be continually evolving. It is important to encourage research in this regard by considering alternative definitions and to promote further hypothesis testing.

Educational

The DSM-IV has served, with both good and bad effects, as a textbook of psychopathology. It has been used to teach residents in psychiatry as well as students in psychology, social work, nursing, and other disciplines. To some extent, it has been used as a teaching tool in medicine in general. In 1995, a Primary Care Version of the DSM-IV (American Psychiatric Association, 1995) was developed to provide a better link to the educational needs of primary care physicians and to aid them in making a clinical diagnosis in mental health. There are a number of important appendixes in the DSM-IV which are particularly useful for educational purposes. Among these are decision trees, a conceptual framework for a cultural assessment of individuals with a mental disorder, and a glossary of culturally related conditions. A library of educational tools has been developed for use in conjunction with the DSM-IV. These include videotapes, a casebook, a guidebook, and a CD-ROM that links the DSM-IV both to other textbooks and to the American Psychiatric Association's (APA) practice guidelines and the recent literature.

Information Management

The DSM-IV categorizes information derived from many different clinical sources and clinical practitioners for use in information management. The book was designed to be completely compatible with the codes and short glossary definitions of the *International Classification of Diseases,* 10th edition (ICD-10) (World Health Organization, 1992a), which are used internationally. It is also fully compatible with the Clinical Modification of the ICD-9, the ICD-9-CM (U.S. Department of Health and Human Services, 1997), which is the classification system used in the United States for coding. The American Psychiatric Association worked collaboratively with the American Health Information Management Association to maintain and ensure the compatibility between the ICD system and the DSM-IV. The ICD-9-CM, as the official reimbursement classification in the United States, developed and maintained by the federal government, is required for reimbursement from Medicare, Medicaid, and most third-party payers. The DSM-IV is not, and was not developed to be, a reimbursement manual for psychiatry. The DSM-IV simply selects the appropriate codes from the ICD-9-CM and attaches them to DSM definitions. To assist information managers and facilities, the DSM-IV is available in an electronic format. By and large, however, the primary purpose of the DSM-IV is as a communication tool for use among clinicians and between clinicians and researchers.

▪ ▪ Historical Context

Efforts to classify mental illness have existed for thousands of years. Egyptian and Sumerian references to senile dementia, melancholia, and hysteria date from 3000 B.C. Ancient Greeks and Romans described five categories of disorders: phrenitis, mania, melancholia, hysteria, and epilepsy (Zilboorg and Henry, 1941).

Throughout the evolution of systems to classify mental disorders, several challenging issues have persisted. For instance, some systems favored a large number of narrowly defined conditions (e.g., a system proposed by Boissier de Sauvages in the sixteenth century identified more than twenty-four hundred conditions, each of which was essentially a symptom), whereas others were based on more inclusive, broad conceptualizations (e.g., Philippe Pinel in the eighteenth century proposed a system of only four clinical types: mania, melancholia, dementia, and idiotism) (Frances, First, and Pincus 1995). Classification systems have also varied in the extent to which the categorization of disorders could be based on etiology (e.g., in the early nineteenth century William Griesinger predicted that all mental disorders would be classified according to their underlying brain lesion), the course of the illness (e.g., Benedict-Augustin Morel depicted schizophrenia solely in terms of the course of the illness in the early nineteenth century), or the description of symptom patterns (Frances, First, and Pincus, 1995).

Emil Kraepelin, in the latter half of the nineteenth century, developed a system that drew from these various approaches. Kraepelin studied groups of patients whose disorders had the same course in order to determine their shared clinical features. This overall approach was largely retained in the development of the current DSM system (Frances, First, and Pincus, 1995).

• • Early History of DSM Classifications

Long before the DSM-IV was published, during the early days of the U.S. census, the very first attempt at classifying mental disorders in this country occurred. In 1840 there was a single classification in the census for people who were hospitalized in mental institutions. Current classifications had their root in the data collection purposes of the census. Today, the ICD-9-CM and the DSM-IV are still used for data collection, and these data are used for statistical and epidemiological reporting purposes.

The first international classification system, the ICD-6, was developed by the World Health Organization in 1948. In the United States, the American Psychiatric Association developed an alternative classification, the DSM-I (American Psychiatric Association, 1952), which had short glossary definitions for the different disorders. The ICD-8 and the DSM-II (American Psychiatric Association, 1968) were, for the most part, very similar and consisted of a paragraph of general description of the different conditions. Both were fairly short volumes and did not receive the broad public and clinical attention of DSM-III and DSM-IV.

• • DSM-III Paradigm Shift

The DSM-III represented a major shift in psychiatric diagnosis. It was intended to be descriptive and have, by and large, a nonetiologic focus. It introduced diagnostic criteria to define disorders better and, importantly, to provide a way of improving reliability through these explicit definitions.

The DSM-III also introduced a multiaxial system, which acknowledged that simply having a single name attached to a diagnosis was not sufficient information to assess the treatment needs of a particular individual. In addition, it introduced the concept of multiple diagnoses, which held that there was not necessarily a single etiology or a single diagnostic class in which a patient might fit. A significant number of clinicians found the multiaxial system a useful way to describe more fully the clinical populations they saw.

DSM-III Advantages

The DSM-III had important advantages. It improved reliability and facilitated communication between clinicians and researchers. It made clear that if an article in the *American Journal of Psychiatry* and the *Archives of General Psychiatry* used DSM criteria for describing the clinical population of subjects in a study, one would have a good understanding of what those subjects were like and how they relate to one's own patients. The DSM-III was widely used by clinicians, researchers, educators, and trainees. It included important methodological and content innovations such as diagnostic criteria and the multiaxial system. The DSM-III was a success far beyond expectations, and it promoted an emphasis on empirical data. By pushing the diagnostic envelope, the DSM-III was an intellectual leap forward.

DSM-III Disadvantages

There were, however, some important disadvantages to the DSM-III. Users took the manual very seriously—much more seriously than the developers intended. Many categories were very long, complex, and user-unfriendly. In some instances, the criteria were made very specific (e.g., that the symptoms had to occur within one month or within sixty days, five out of ten symptoms had to be present) in an attempt to become more precise. This "pseudoprecision" of the diagnostic criteria was sometimes arbitrary because of limitations in the available empirical data. Communication problems among DSM-III users and international users of the ICD-9 were a result of the differences between the two classification systems. In addition, there were a number of specific controversies, for example, the elimination of neurosis and some arguments about the inclusion of homosexuality, which detracted from the DSM-III's true import.

▪ ▪ DSM-III-R

Seven years later, in 1987, the DSM-III-R was published. Like the DSM-III before it, the DSM-III-R had important advantages and disadvantages. By and large, this revision followed the same model and the same architecture of the DSM-III, but it was intended to identify and correct inconsistencies. It also demonstrated that the DSM system was self-correcting—that it was not a static process but a system that responds to new empirical data and information. The DSM-III-R introduced new diagnostic categories and criteria based on the accumulation of data, reduced diagnostic hierarchies, and heightened the issue of comorbidity as a way to describe more accurately the clinical picture for a given individual.

The DSM-III-R also had some disadvantages. It was perceived as being too much change too soon. It went too far beyond simply correcting inconsistencies by changing criteria and was therefore a disruption to researchers and educators. Researchers had to redevelop their instruments, and many studies already under way had to be changed. An important disadvantage of the DSM-III-R was that for many of the changes no consistent rationale was provided. In some cases there was clear empirical support, but in others there may not have been empirical support, or if it existed, it was not specified or documented. In developing the DSM-IV, we took into consideration the lessons learned during both the DSM-III and the DSM-III-R processes.

▪ ▪ Evidence-Based Medicine

During the years between the DSM-III-R and the DSM-IV a sea change was going on in all of medicine, with increased calls for accountability, an increased role of evidence and empirical data, and, most critically, the increased availability of data. Information that was not previously available could now be applied to the decision-making process and inform the DSM-IV.

Sackett (1997) and proponents of evidence-based medicine, which exists in England, Canada, and now the United States, define evidence-based medicine as "the conscientious, explicit, and judicious use of the current best evidence in making decisions about the care of individual patients" (Sackett, 1997, p. 3). For the DSM-IV that definition was taken beyond individual patients and applied systematically in a broader clinical/policymaking process.

The principles of evidence-based medicine have been described by Sackett and others. A critical component of evidence-based medicine is the understanding of the rules of evidence, what are called "critical appraisal skills for the evaluation of published studies." Another important component of evidence-based medicine is that there be a comprehensive and systematic searching, extracting, arraying, documenting, assessing, and integrating of all the published literature. This is a critical issue because it must be done in an unbiased, systematic way, particularly with the availability of new information technologies, the growth of search techniques, and the development of more extensive library systems. The comprehensive review of the literature must be done explicitly. The methodologies used to conduct the literature review (e.g., the specific search terms, databases searched, criteria used to extract the literature, arraying the information) should be documented, in a fashion similar to the methodologies used in research studies, to allow for replication. The decision-making process for inclusion/exclusion of studies should be explicit and documented as well.

The stepwise process that has been applied in the DSM and other projects begins with developing systematic methods for searching the published literature, extracting the data from the literature, synthesizing and arraying the information, assessing the data, and using and integrating the data into the product being developed. Clinical perspectives must also be integrated to ensure that a diverse set of perspectives is represented. Finally, this is a feedback process in which the outcomes of the process are continually monitored and evaluated in an empirical manner. This built-in monitoring is important in improving the methodologies used throughout the process. The DSM-IV and APA practice guidelines are examples of the products that result from the application of an evidence-based process.

▪ ▪ Principles and Processes for the DSM-IV

DSM-III/DSM-III-R/ICD-10 Process

The processes to develop the DSM-III, DSM-III-R, and ICD-10 (whose development overlapped with that of the DSM-IV) were somewhat different. They were developed by limited "expert consensus" groups, or the "bogsat" method (i.e., "a bunch of guys sitting around a table"). The expert consensus or "bogsat" method involves bringing together individuals who, using their knowledge of the literature and professional experiences, make determinations about the issues at hand.

This approach has limitations. The decisions made by the consensus group are not necessarily generalizable to a broad population. The decisions reflect the group's own experience and views of the literature. The range of specialty interests may not be fully represented on the panel, and the individuals chosen may not represent all the interests of their specialty. In addition, the consensus group decision may not reflect a comprehensive review of the literature if a methodical search has not been conducted. Finally, documentation of the process and the rationale for the decisions made may not occur.

When the DSM-III and DSM-III-R were developed, the available literature had gaps and limitations, and the tools to conduct systematic and comprehensive searches of the peer-reviewed literature were not as readily available as they are today. Review and revision by expert consensus was the most viable option for the DSM-III and DSM-III-R. In fact, the major contribution of the DSM-III was that it did lead to the availability of a large amount of evidence and information that would later be applied in the DSM-IV process.

There was a major difference in the research environment at the time the DSM-III and DSM-III-R were being developed, as compared with the DSM-IV development period, when a great deal more data and more research funding were available. For example, in 1984, departments of psychiatry received approximately $82 million in National Institute of Health (NIH) research support. In comparison, in 1998, the NIH provided more than $400 million in research support. Psychiatry went from being the tenth-ranked department in medical schools in research funding support to the second-ranked. However, not all that research is directly relevant to the DSM-IV process.

Principles of the DSM-IV Process

One of the principles of the DSM-IV process was to involve the leaders in the field, as well as regular clinicians, from a broad array of disciplines and specialties. It was important to represent as wide a breadth and diversity of people and expertise as possible. Literally thousands of individuals participated in the DSM-IV process in one form or another. A second principle was to decentralize, so that the process was informed by the field rather than the field being informed by the process. To that end, for each work group, an expert from that area was appointed as chairperson. The work group members were also experts in that field. Fostering a completely open process was the third principle. Every piece of information about the process was made available so that one would know what decisions were being made and understand why they were made. To encourage the sharing of information, the DSM-IV Task Force published a large number of articles about the process as it developed. In addition, a newsletter about the DSM-IV development process and progress was sent to more than three thousand individuals worldwide. Many of the individuals involved in the process (i.e., work groups and members) published articles and presented papers at meetings on the progress of the work groups.

Finally, the DSM-IV Sourcebooks documented the entire process. There was also a great deal of international collaboration, especially with those developing the ICD-10. The most important principle in the DSM-IV process was that all changes should be based on systematic data collection and review. This basic principle undergirded the entire project and the functioning of each work group. At the very beginning of the project a methods workshop, attended by the work group chairpersons, the DSM-IV Task Force, and others, was held. The workshop, a seminar on how to implement evidence-based medicine, laid out very explicit instructions on what the work groups were supposed to do and how they were to do it. The specific steps and the process each work group had to follow to come to a decision were explained in detail and with examples (Frances, Widiger, and Pincus, 1989).

Types of Changes

The work groups were asked to resolve five types of issues: adding and deleting categories, subtyping disorders, revising criteria sets, considering the placement of disorders in the classification, and the updating of the text. It is important to note that the DSM-IV consists of several different elements. One is the classification itself, which lists the names of disorders and their ICD-9-CM codes; another is the diagnostic criteria. In addition to the diagnostic criteria, text information about prevalence, course, familial patterns, age, gender, and cultural issues of the disorders is provided to help clinicians and students understand how to apply the criteria.

Adding and Deleting Categories

The addition and deletion of disorders was one of the high-profile issues for the DSM-IV process, but it was not the "meat and potatoes" of the revision. More than 150 different proposals were received for adding categories to the DSM-IV. These proposals ranged from offhand ideas to very serious recommendations with a rich tradition of clinical literature and empirical support. A number of arguments were made for adding and deleting categories. The most common argument in support of adding a new category (or not deleting an old one) was that if the category was not included, there would be a large number of individuals whose treatment needs would go unmet and whose conditions would not be researchable; clinicians might also have problems communicating about the nature of the treatment for these individuals (Pincus et al., 1992). For many proposals, the generalizability of the supporting data for the proposed condition was problematic. Oftentimes the suggested additions were proposed by individuals, groups, or centers that had a great deal of experience in assessing a particular class of individuals, but it was unknown if the components of the condition they assessed would translate more broadly to the full range of persons whose disorders were diagnosed using the DSM-IV. Therefore, one of the questions asked with regard to a proposed condition was, Is there a generalizable set of information in support of including this new disorder? Another problem with some of the suggested additions was the potential for misuse. Would the condition be inappropriately used once it was disseminated more broadly? Do the data support the fact that it can be reliably assessed by average clinicians? Yet another concern was the added complexity of the system. Ultimately, there had to be a substantial amount of evidence—from peer-reviewed literature—to add something new to the DSM-IV.

Unlike the DSM-III and DSM-III-R, which included more categories so as to help stimulate research, the DSM-IV was intended to be led by research. Nevertheless, to encourage research, the DSM-IV has an appendix that includes certain conditions with a substantial research literature behind them but which are not formally included in the DSM-IV. This appendix provides a common language to encourage research on those conditions. Conditions that were considered for addition, such as mixed anxiety-depression and other subthreshold conditions, binge-eating disorder, and premenstrual dysphoric disorder, were included in the appendix. Only thirteen new disorders were added to the DSM-IV (e.g., acute stress disorder, bipolar II, Asperger's disorder). Most of these additions were simple oversights that had not been added to the DSM-III-R, such as substance-induced sexual dysfunction. Several conditions were deleted from the classification because there was no evidence base to support their continued inclusion and no literature showing ongoing research into the conditions (e.g., identity disorder). In addition, the childhood anxiety disorders were reformulated and incorporated within the adult disorders.

The subtyping of disorders was another area that was tackled by the work groups. The inclusion of subtypes was similarly based on a comprehensive review of the research and clinical utility. For example, in anorexia nervosa, two subtypes—a binge-eating subtype and a restricting subtype—were added because in the past individuals with binge eating in addition to anorexia nervosa had been given two different diagnoses, bulimia nervosa and anorexia nervosa. By adding these subtypes only one diagnosis need be given. Another example of the addition of subtypes is specific phobia. There was good evidence that the blood injection/injury type phobias were different from the other phobias, both from a family history perspective and physiologically, resulting in different treatment implications. Subtypes for depression and dementia were also added. A thorough review of the literature for the melancholic features of depression was conducted, and the condition remained in the DSM with some changes in the criteria. Dementia with behavioral disturbance as a subcategory of dementia was added because it is an important issue in nursing homes for treatment planning.

The task of revising the diagnostic criteria was the bulk of the work for the work groups, and it became a balancing act for them. For each set of criteria the work group had to weigh a number of different issues. One issue was whether to increase the relevance and the importance of core features of a particular condition in a prototypical way versus improving the capacity to discriminate features of the disorder from those of other disorders ("near neighbors") in the differential diagnosis. Another issue was balancing the complexity or simplicity criteria sets and how that would affect the validity and reliability. A great deal more reliability could be gained by very complex criteria sets, but on the other hand, the criteria could be made so complex that they would not be used. Other questions of balance concerned how specific and detailed each criterion should be in terms of its operationalization versus the level of inference that could be expected (which also affects the reliability and validity of the disorder) and how one balances operational rules versus clinical judgment. Finally, there was the issue of thresholds. Where should a fixed threshold be established, when is that threshold changed, and on what sort of evidence should the decision be based?

These questions, when applied to the criteria sets, resulted in some of the following investigations. One was an attempt to have somatization disorder defined by a much less complex set of criteria. The issue for somatoform disorder was that the DSM-III-R criteria set was rarely applied because there were thirty-five different items and the clinician had to decide whether thirteen of them would be endorsed. The literature review documented the high reliability and validity of the condition, and through an analysis of data pooled from a number of different sites, a much simpler criteria set was defined, one that identified the same group of patients. A five-site field trial of this reformulated criteria set examined the proposed criteria, assessed the set's ease of use, reliability, and generalizability, and used semistructured interviews comparing the simplified set with the DSM-III, DSM-III-R, ICD-10, and original Briquet syndrome. The field trial results found that there was virtually no change in caseness and excellent reliability for the revised criteria set (Yutzy et al., 1995).

The issue of adding more inference to antisocial personality disorder (i.e., attempting to incorporate notions of a lack of conscience) was reviewed and evaluated. Although some minor changes were made, there were insufficient data to implement this proposal. The potential for operationalizing bulimic episodes, defined as eating a large amount of food in a very short period of time, was also considered. Could the amount of food and the time period be specified? These particulars could not be operationalized in a reliable and valid manner and therefore were not added to the criteria set.

Another issue in the revision of diagnostic criteria was the pseudoprecision of some of the DSM-III-R criteria. Mood disorders offer an example. The seasonal pattern for mood disorders specifies a sixty-day window in which symptoms have to appear and disappear in a seasonal pattern. If the symptoms were present sixty-one or fifty-nine days, does it make a difference? Rather than perpetuating this pseudoprecision, the criteria set was changed to be less explicit and stated that "there has been a regular temporal relationship between the onset of Major Depressive Episodes . . . and a particular time of the year."

For schizophrenia, the issue of duration was examined because the ICD-10 required a one-month duration of active symptoms and the DSM-III-R used a two-week duration. A field trial conducted to examine this issue empirically demonstrated little change in caseness if the DSM-IV moved to a duration of one month, to be compatible with the ICD-10 (Flaum et al., 1998).

The issues of placement deal with both the overall organization of the DSM-IV and the conceptual framework for the various groupings—that is, what level of abstraction should be applied, under what name a disorder should be categorized, and finally, what the location of each specific disorder should be. Typical questions were, Should hypochondriasis be an anxiety disorder or a somatoform disorder? and Should we have a section on stress-related conditions?

Each work group formulated each of these issues as a question and established a hierarchy of evidence that could answer the question. A literature search was conducted to gather the evidence, which was ordered from most important to least important according to this a priori hierarchy. Once the literature review had been completed and the data compiled and summarized, the summary was circulated to between fifty and one hundred international and national advisors/experts in the field to determine if the work group had missed any pertinent literature or if the data had been misinterpreted. These summaries of the literature review were formulated as options for solutions to resolve the questions. Across all work groups, these options were collated into the *DSM-IV Options Book—Work in Progress* (American Psychiatric Association, 1991), which was made widely available for review and comment. A second version—the *DSM-IV Draft Criteria* (American Psychiatric Association, 1993a), developed from responses to the *Options Book*—was disseminated to another four thousand individuals. This version was then slightly modified and approved by the APA before publication.

To assist in the DSM-IV process, the work groups solicited relevant data sets that may not have been analyzed with regard to specific issues for the DSM-IV but which could be reanalyzed and which could be funded under a grant from the MacArthur Foundation. The work group formulated proposed options for making changes which were researched through the MacArthur Data Reanalysis Studies. The National Institute of Mental Health/NIDA/NIAAA (NIMH) funded field trials for the DSM-IV project. This was, in fact, one of the most complex grants that the NIH ever evaluated, involving twelve different projects with eighty-eight sites internationally and more than seven thousand patients.

Throughout the process an atmosphere of conservatism prevailed to avoid the disruption of clinical and research efforts begun with the DSM-III and DSM-III-R. Compatibility between the DSM system and the ICD-10 system was also important. Most important, the changes that resulted in the DSM-IV were driven by the data available. The evidence was also balanced with clinical judgment. Small changes that were supported by many good data and fixed big problems were favored over big changes with limited data for little problems. A commonsense judgment was used. By far the most important change in the DSM-IV was the use of a methodical, evidence-based process to develop the manual.

Probably the biggest contribution of the DSM-III, which continued with the DSM-IV, was the integration of both clinical and research criteria into one set of diagnostic criteria. The ICD currently consists of separate clinical and research criteria, and this has been proposed for the DSM. Integrated criteria sets facilitate the application of research findings in clinical practice and diagnostic reliability among clinicians. They ensure that the clinical and research communities are working with the same populations, the same definitions, and the same entities. The criteria sets can also be useful in clinical practice as a way of educating patients about the nature of their condition.

▪ ▪ Limitations of Evidence-Based Approaches

Although the DSM-IV represented a successful use of an evidence-based process, there are some problems in applying evidence-based approaches, as Ken Kendler discussed in his article "Toward a Scientific Psychiatric Nosology" (Kendler, 1990) and summarized here.

Kendler discussed these issues from the framework of an evidence-deterministic approach, in contrast to the other extreme of a more advocacy-driven model. With an evidence-deterministic model (in which there must be direct empirical testing of all nosological hypotheses), historical tradition, clinical evidence, clinical experience, and common sense have a very limited role. Some areas that are less accessible to scientific investigation (e.g., the requirement of a multicultural system) cannot be included. There are also clinical and educational needs that may not necessarily be served by a purely evidence-based process, because it could create a degree of complexity which would not be realistic or practical in application to the real world. Issues that need to be resolved should also be covered completely and thoroughly. If a very, very high standard of evidence is applied, only a very small number of conditions would be validated, and these would not meet administrative or clinical needs.

Applying strictly empirical approaches also presents a variety of specific problems. Disagreement can arise over the construct of a disorder. For example, is depression a mood disorder, a cognitive disorder, or a motor disorder? Depression can be conceptualized in any one of those three ways, and how it is conceptualized will change how it is assessed and what kind of criteria are used. There may be disagreement about the importance of different validators. For example, is family history more important for determining the criteria for schizotypal personality disorder, or is clinical course more important? The importance of varying data (e.g., reliability versus validity) can also be a source of disagreement. Obviously, in all of science there can be disagreements about the interpretation of data. The nongeneralizability of data is another problem. Most of the data collected in the empirical literature are from tertiary care medical centers. How well that translates to the average patient of the average practitioner is not always clear. Data may also be insufficient. Little or no data may be available for many areas, and many of the studies that do exist may not have been conducted with an ideal level of rigor.

▪ ▪ Suggestions for the Future

There are a number of recommendations for improving the DSM developmental process, some of which were applied in various ways for the DSM-IV. First, the database needs to be improved. More evidence, better evidence, and more relevant evidence are needed. Initial efforts have begun in collaboration with the NIMH to consider the foci and nature of data that would need to be available for the next iteration of the DSM.

Truth in advertising is also necessary. All people using the DSM-IV should read its introduction because it contains an extensive critique of the manual. It also outlines, as explicitly as possible, the process for the development of the DSM-IV—what was done, how it was done, and why it was done. The introduction points out that the DSM-IV is not to be taken too literally. This is an important message. Somebody once said during the

DSM-IV development process that subliminally emblazoned on every page of the DSM-IV should be the word "THINK!"

Although the DSM-IV process was explicit, open, and documented, the DSM process could be improved in some ways. More could be done to involve patients and families. The link with clinicians could also be made stronger by informing them of the issues so that they can participate more fully. Additional input from philosophers might also be pursued. A more effective dialogue and collaboration internationally, and specifically with the ICD-10, are needed. In some cases, explicit distinctions between the ICD-10 and the DSM-IV are helpful in promoting such dialogue and collaboration. The International Version of the DSM-IV (American Psychiatric Association, 1995) lays out these differences.

The evidence-based process can be further delineated by being more explicit about how we think about the evidence-based issues, separating out the "big picture" and "small picture" issues. As Kendler said, when working on the small picture issues, evidence plays a larger role than when working on medium and big picture issues. For both sizes of issues the subsets of these issues must be separated out. Then, in an a priori manner, the basis for making determinations on each issue can be further explicated.

A number of "big picture" issues affect both the development of the DSM and, more important, the future of psychiatric classification and nosology. Some of these issues relate to the basic nosological approach that is applied: categorical versus dimensional approaches (in particular, in the personality disorders) or cross-sectional versus longitudinal approaches. Other issues involve varying consideration of what might be termed "dependent variables and independent variables" in diagnosis, the role of symptoms versus impairments in criteria, whether to incorporate both descriptive and biological measurement into the diagnostic criteria, integration of phenotype and genotype data, and how information on internal and external experiences, behavior, treatment response, and biological mechanisms should be addressed.

"Medium picture" issues affect more directly the clinical practice of psychiatrists both diagnostically and for treatment planning. Included in this set of issues is the question of which multiaxial approaches to assessment should be included. And should there be distinct axes for syndrome, pathology/pathophysiology, genetics, course of a disorder, the level of impairment/disability, and the patient's personality and adaptive mechanisms?

For both "medium picture" and "big picture" issues, the ways of defining mental disorders may involve more than evidence. Information is drawn on which might not be clearly labeled "evidence" but which may relate to different evidentiary bases such as logic, common sense, tradition, the elegance, clarity, and utility of an idea, administrative requirements, practicality, and time.

Psychiatric classification also has an array of specific issues (i.e., "small picture" issues) related to the actual content of the DSM which were discussed earlier. Among these are decisions about what disorders are added or deleted, revisions to the criteria sets, subtyping of disorders, the organization and placement of disorders in the DSM, and, finally, text revisions.

There are many issues to address, studies to conduct, and evidence to gather, but not all of these can be done. Priorities need to be set. In addition, some "nonevidence" items are actually subject to a kind of evidentiary evaluation. For example, one can assess clinical utility in an empirical way. In short, the role and type of evidence shift, depending on the size and level of abstraction of the kinds of issues. Ultimately, however, the one need for the future in the DSM-IV or DSM-V is more and better information to guide us in our evidence-based process.

3

Values, Politics, and Science in the Construction of the DSMs

THOMAS A. WIDIGER, PH.D.

THE CONSTRUCT OF A mental disorder is no more value laden than the construct of a physical disorder. We can accept the relative validity of both physical and mental disorder constructs because the limitations to their fundamental validity would be problematic only if the world itself were fundamentally different. However, mental disorder diagnoses are more easily contaminated by cultural, professional, personal, theoretical, and other biases. The failure of the authors of the DSM to be entirely value free, unbiased, and apolitical should be recognized, acknowledged, and addressed in each edition of the DSM. Nevertheless, a scientifically based nomenclature of mental disorder diagnoses can be developed, and the DSM-IV is a productive step in this direction. I describe this tension between a scientifically based but value-laden DSM process, discuss how such a tension was addressed in the DSM-IV process, and argue that the existing DSM developmental structure represents a reasonable approach to resolving such tensions.

It is perhaps trivial to state at the outset that the DSM-IV is not a value-free, apolitical scientific classification of mental disorders. However, it is important to begin with this acknowledgment, as critics of various editions of the DSM have attributed a claim of neutrality to its authors. Such a claim would be inaccurate and rather naive. Each edition of the DSM has been constructed by people and, as such, has failed to fulfill its aspiration to be without bias. There is no disagreement with respect to this point. What is unclear are the implications of this contamination, notably whether the authors of future editions of the DSM should continue to aspire to be value free and apolitical and, if so, how best to attempt to reach this goal.

▪ ▪ Values

A mental disorder is essentially an "involuntary organismic impairment in psychological functioning" (Widiger and Trull, 1991, p. 112). This and all other definitions of mental disorder do include a fundamental value judgment (Wakefield, 1992a; Widiger, 1997). The concept of mental disorder values necessary, adequate, or optimal psychological functioning. A diagnosis of a mental disorder engenders a value judgment about inadequate psychological functioning. It is hypothetically possible for persons in this world, or in another world, not to value necessary, adequate, or optimal psychological functioning. In such a world, the construct of mental disorder might still be valid, but it would have no relevance or meaningful application.

It is indeed an interesting and informative thought experiment to consider such a world. However, we do not in fact exist in this hypothetical world (Wakefield, 1994). In our world, including virtually all societies, a value has been placed on necessary, adequate, or optimal functioning, including psychological functioning (although each of these constructs can be operationalized somewhat differently within any particular society; Rogler, 1999). Therefore, in this world, throughout its history and for all reasonable time to come, the concept of a mental disorder will likely continue to be meaningful and valid.

Because the mental disorder concept does depend in part on the social world, the concept is not truly universal or invariant. However, one should not be particularly apologetic or troubled by this constraint or limitation on its validity. The concept of physical disorder is equally arbitrary and relative to a necessary, adequate, or optimal physical functioning of a particular biological organism. Reducing the concept of mental disorder to a biological mechanism does not eliminate the need for a value judgment, contrary to the arguments of Lilienfeld and Marino (1995).

For example, Lyme disease is a disorder only from the perspective of the human host organism; from the "perspective" of the spirochete bacterium, the human is its means of survival (see Sedgwick, 1982b). Characterizing the condition of the human as disordered is comparable to characterizing the blood-sucking ectoparasite that transmits this bacterium as a pest. Nature does not care who ultimately survives in this world. The concept of physical disorder involves a value judgment reflecting human interests in physical survival.

The concept of physical disorder, however, is nevertheless universal across biological organisms, as one can identify and research the disorders of spirochetes and deer ticks, just as easily as one can identify and research the disorders of the human. There will be physical disorders that are apparently unique to the human organism and to the deer tick, just as there will be mental disorders that will appear to be unique to different cultures, but the fundamental principles of pathology and dysfunction will be largely universal. The organismic and cultural specificity of physical and mental disorders does not suggest that pathology does not exist, is illusory, or is invalid.

In a world of people who place no value on necessary, adequate, or optimal physical functioning, or in a world in which there is no impairment or threat to physical functioning, the concept of physical disorder would have no importance and perhaps no utility (except as an interesting thought experiment). However, in the world as it currently exists, and will likely continue to exist, biological organisms do interact with and harm one another, and the concept of physical disorder does have substantial meaning. Likewise, in the world as it currently exists, persons do relate to and interact with one another and do often wound and harm one another psychologically, and the concept of mental disorder has substantial meaning and validity.

The construct of a mental disorder is, then, as fundamentally arbitrary, illusory, or invalid as the construct of a physical disorder. We can live with this trivial limitation as it becomes meaningful or problematic to the fundamental validity of the construct only when (or if) our world is no longer in existence. The construct of nature is itself similarly relative to the world (or universe) as it currently exists. It is an interesting and informative thought experiment to contemplate other universes that would have a different reality and different laws of nature (Hawking, 1988; Linde, 1991), but during this time in which the world does exist, the constructs of nature, physical disorder, and mental disorder do have an actual and a substantial meaning and validity.

Points of Demarcation

However, a difficulty for the authors of a DSM in identifying (and agreeing on) the threshold of dysfunction for a diagnosis of mental disorder is that the precise boundaries of the category or construct are unclear and debatable (Clark, Watson, and Reynolds, 1995). There is probably no clear or qualitative point of demarcation between normal and abnormal psychological functioning, between mental and physical disorders, or between mental and relational disorders (Widiger, 1997). It is not surprising, then, that persons disagree on where to place the point of demarcation. If the demarcation is along a continuum of functioning, some amount of uncertainty, ambiguity, and disagreement is to be expected and should be tolerated.

The presence of a debatable point of demarcation along a continuum of functioning between normal (healthy, adequate, or optimal) functioning and abnormal (unhealthy, inadequate, or suboptimal) functioning does not render the concept of mental disorder invalid, as suggested by Carson (1996). The fact that a point of demarcation along a continuum is inherently debatable does not mean that the continuum does not exist or that a selected point of demarcation is necessarily random or meaningless. Reasonable and meaningful points of distinction can be made along distributions of continuous functioning; indeed, such points were the focus of significant deliberation for the DSM-IV work groups.

Consider, for example, the diagnosis of the mental disorder of mental retardation. There is no nonarbitrary, qualitatively distinct point along the continuum of degree of intelligence which would unambiguously and conclusively distinguish cases of adaptive (normal, healthy) intelligence from cases of maladaptive (abnormal, retarded) intelligence. Current convention places the distinction at an intelligence quotient (IQ) of 70 (American Psychiatric Association, 1994), but it is evident that this point of demarcation does not carve nature at a discrete joint. It is simply that point at which clinicians, researchers, and scientists have decided it is meaningful to characterize the dysfunctions that are secondary to the relatively more limited intelligence as constituting a clinically significant retardation to functioning. It is reasonable to disagree over which point of demarcation along the continuum best distinguishes between an inadequate (retarded, deficient, abnormal) and an adequate (sufficient, normal) intelligence. Persons with a level of intelligence above the current point of demarcation will experience significant and meaningful impairments to their functioning (e.g., success within education or career) secondary to their limited level of intelligence, but a debatable point of demarcation does not suggest or imply that the entire continuum of intelligence is not itself highly correlated with adequacy of functioning (Gottfredson, 1997). The presence of a continuum and debatable points of demarcation do not diminish the validity of the construct of mental retardation; they question only the validity of a qualitative dichotomy between normal and abnormal intelligence (Widiger, 1997).

Culturally Biased Points of Demarcation

Mental disorders are perhaps relatively more universal across different cultures than physical disorders are across different organisms. There are perhaps fewer culture-bound syndromes than there are species-specific syndromes (Guarnaccia and Rogler, 1999; Kessler, 1999). However, the selection of points of demarcation for mental disorder diagnoses are relatively more susceptible to cultural conventions and biases than physical disorders. Physical disorder diagnoses are not immune to cultural biases, but they are relatively less susceptible to them (Lilienfeld and Marino, 1995). The history of mental disorder diagnosis includes instances of obvious error, such as the diagnosis of draepetomania (the uncontrollable urge to escape slavery) in the nineteenth century and perhaps homosexuality in the twentieth century (Bayer and Spitzer, 1982; Spitzer, 1981). These errors are at times trumpeted by critics of the DSM as indications that all mental disorder diagnoses are probably equally fallacious. These prior mistakes should give serious pause to any person who presumes that no further errors are being made, but the correction of these past mistakes also suggests that progress is in fact being made.

There is no doubt that the DSM-IV continues to be contaminated by some degree of problematic cultural bias. Again, it would be naive to state otherwise. However, it is not the case that the presence of some cultural bias within DSM diagnoses means that they lack sufficient construct validity or that the perspectives of all cultures with respect to the behaviors being diagnosed are equally valid, as argued, for instance, by Kirmayer (1994) and Kleinman (1988).

The latter point is illustrated by the feminist therapist Simola (1992). She documented well the unwitting presence of paternalistic, conservative, and sexist values in traditional forms of marital and family therapy. She was also correct that "therapists are never neutral or objective" (p. 399). However, she concludes that because "neutrality is both a myth and a fallacy" (p. 399), "the question is not one of whether therapists can be neutral but rather which ideology is reflected in their work?" (p. 399). She rejects the effort to be nonsexist because it will be unsuccessful and may only contribute to a myth of neutrality. She favors instead an openly Marxist, socialist, or radical feminism. She suggests that it is better to be openly biased in favor of a Marxist feminist perspective than to be unsuccessful in an effort to be nonsexist.

Simola (1992), Kirmayer (1994), and Kleinman (1988) are to be commended for identifying the presence of problematic values that would and do contaminate optimal clinical diagnosis and treatment. However, the valid assessment of optimal psychological functioning is obtained by the reduction of these contaminating values, not by their overt, conscious, and willful embracement and promotion. One does not obtain physical health by promoting equally all forms of viral infections; nor does one obtain psychological health by promoting all forms of cultural, social biases. If we were to take Simola's relativism seriously, the overt, open promotion of racist and sexist values by racist/sexist clinicians would be as valid as the promotion of feminist values.

The optimal method for overcoming problematic cultural biases is the continued application of a critical scientific perspective. Societies that aspire to base their beliefs on an objective, dispassionate consideration of carefully designed and incisive empirical research do often fail to be successful in this effort, but it is reasonably safe to believe that a culture that makes this effort will be relatively more successful in overcoming biases, and will be relatively more successful in getting closer to the truth, than cultures that are less reliant on the principles and methods of science. There is perhaps some degree of cultural bias and misconception in the diagnosis of schizophrenia (Carson, 1996), but the explanation for hallucinatory phenomenon by Black and Andreasen (1994) is probably closer to the truth than the explanations provided by the Arctic Inuit offered by Kirmayer (1994).

This is not meant as any disrespect for or devaluation of the beliefs of another culture. Clinicians, and any members of a multicultural or international community, must and should respect alternative belief systems to function adequately and appropriately within this community. In addition, many advances in the field of psychopathology have arisen and will continue to arise from societies and cultures that do not rely on the scientific method. Being less scientific does not mean being worthless, ignorant, or wrong. On the other hand, an acceptance of and respect for alternative belief systems does not require or suggest that all belief systems are equally valid or credible. Beliefs do appear to vary in the extent of their validity, and cultures that rely on or emphasize the scientific method to develop and advance their belief systems probably experience more success (although not always) in obtaining accurate and valid knowledge. The advances in knowledge in physics, chemistry, biology, astronomy, and geology in cultures that have emphasized the scientific method compared with cultures that have not provide overwhelming prima facie evidence of the success of the scientific method (Bergner, 1997).

Our current understanding of optimal physical and psychological functioning is not entirely universal. However, the extent and implications of cultural and social diversity have been exaggerated. What is considered to be adaptive, healthy, or optimal functioning within one culture may not be considered as such within another (Rogler, 1996), but this does not reduce all constructs of optimal or healthy psychological functioning to simply cultural idioms or local folklore. On the contrary, cultural diversity in the explanation and understanding of psychological phenomena may also suggest that cultures (or societies) vary in the extent to which they are accurate or valid in their conception of mental (and physical) disorders.

For example, the perceptual experiences of persons who would be diagnosed as having DSM-IV schizophrenia could be considered within a particular culture as involving an actual religious experience (Kirmayer, 1994). Those who share this belief system may indeed be correct. A person may actually hear the voice of a god or may in fact be possessed by a demon. However, if this person also met the DSM-IV criteria for schizophrenia, including a six-month insidious deterioration in functioning (e.g., in self-care or work) and a one-month duration of disorganized speech, grossly disorganized behavior, and negative symptoms, along with hearing the voice of a god, one should be more confident in diagnosing this person with the mental disorder of schizophrenia than in concluding that he did in fact hear the voice of a god. This would not reflect a biased perspective of a culture that does not value or believe in this god; it reflects instead the substantial amount of scientific research to support the validity of the diagnosis of schizophrenia (Black and Andreasen, 1994) and the lack of comparable research to support the validity of the religious explanation.

The history of belief systems is filled with many obvious instances of error, including, for example, the belief that the sun revolves around the earth. This was a culturally biased perspective that was eventually refuted sufficiently by the critical and empirical methodology of science. Persons can be reasonably confident in the validity of the belief that the earth revolves around the sun. Continued progress in our understanding of the etiology and pathology of mental disorders will most likely also occur with the continued application of the scientific method, not by embracing any and all belief systems as being equally valid or by promoting the belief system that happens to be most consistent with one's own social or political values.

A diagnosis of a mental disorder does become particularly problematic when the disorder is due in part to the socialization of the person within a particular culture. It is unlikely that all societies are equally conducive toward optimal psychological functioning, if societies do in fact vary significantly in the psychological functioning they promote or discourage. However, judgments as to which and how societies are relatively more or less conducive to optimal psychological functioning would be very difficult and potentially highly controversial, as there are also valid differences in what constitutes acceptable, optimal, or adaptive behavior across different environments, societies, and cultures. One should not presume that what is optimal, adaptive, healthy, or ideal in one's own culture is, or should be, optimal, adaptive, healthy, or ideal in any other particular culture (Kirmayer, 1994; Kleinman, 1996; Mezzich et al., 1996). On the contrary, fully optimal psychological functioning will vary, at least to some extent, across different environments and across different cultures.

On the other hand, environments also vary in the extent to which they are conducive to an optimal psychological functioning within any particular culture, just as they vary in the extent to which they are conducive to optimal physical functioning. For example, societies, across time and national boundaries, have varied in their socialization of adequate, healthy, or optimal substance-use behavior and, likewise, in their failure to address adequately or minimize the development of the mental disorders of substance abuse and dependence. Valid differences in the cultural environments, and biases in the understanding of these differences, will complicate substantially the diagnosis of these disorders (Westermeyer, 1996), but there does appear to be sufficient research to indicate that there is such a thing as a substance dependence disorder, and societies and cultures do appear to vary in the extent to which they have contributed to its development or prevention. Scientific research into the etiology and pathology of opioid abuse (Woody and McNicholas, 1997), nicotine dependence (Fiester, 1997), caffeine dependence (Strain and Griffiths, 1997), and alcohol dependence (Kranzler, Babor, and Moore, 1997) has been (or should be) of substantial, universal benefit to all societies in which these drugs are used. The same point can be made with respect to the variation across societies in the development and prevention of other mental disorders, such as sexual dysfunctions, dissociative disorders, and personality disorders.

▪ ▪ Politics

A related and equally problematic contaminant in the development of a scientific nomenclature of mental disorders is social, professional, and personal politics. The DSM-IV was created and is controlled by the American Psychiatric Association, and it has been suggested that the DSM is largely a tool of this organization to maintain and increase its economic wealth, social influence, and political power (e.g., Caplan, 1995; Follette and Houts, 1996; Kirk and Kutchins, 1992; Rogler, 1997; Schacht, 1985; Zimmerman, 1988).

The American Psychiatric Association does have a tremendous responsibility and burden in controlling the process and outcome of the DSM. Part of this burden is to ensure that it does not exploit this power to serve its own ends. This is indeed a heavy responsibility, and one that would be difficult for any organization to fulfill, including the American Psychological Association. In my opinion, the American Psychiatric Association is to be commended for the conscientious effort it has made and for all it has done for the field of psychopathology with each edition of the DSM.

However, there is some truth to the concerns raised by Caplan (1995), Kirk and Kutchins (1992), Rogler (1997), and Schacht (1995). It would be inaccurate, perhaps even naive, to think otherwise. For example, it is not unreasonable to question the motive for defining a mental disorder as a subset of medical disorders (Schacht and Nathan, 1977) or the motive for changing the name of the construct of "mental" disorder to "psychiatric" disorder (Frances, First, and Pincus, 1995). The occasional failure to be objective or apolitical, however, is understandable. Scientists, on average, are not as political as politicians, but they are not immune to self-serving machinations, backroom dealing, self-interested advocacy, and other shenanigans (Feyerabend, 1988). The critiques by Caplan (1995), Kirk and Kutchins (1992), Rogler (1997), Schacht (1985), Schacht and Nathan (1977), and others are very helpful in alerting the consumers and the authors of various editions of the DSM when this has occurred or might be occurring.

On the other hand, these critiques are at times grossly exaggerated, overstated, and even *ad hominem* (e.g., Caplan, 1995; Kirk and Kutchins, 1992). Many of the criticisms and concerns they raise should be given serious consideration (e.g., the complex influence of the substantial financial investment by drug companies), but the authors do appear at times to compromise their own credibility by their inflammatory rhetoric and loose accusations. These critiques can have the effect of polarizing a dispute rather than helping to resolve it.

Nevertheless, the authors of the DSM should appreciate the honorable bases for their passion. The DSM aspires to be a scientific document, but it is also a social document (Widiger and Trull, 1993). Decisions to include or exclude diagnoses or to raise or lower the thresholds for a diagnosis are scientific decisions, but these decisions can also have substantial social repercussions for a large number and a wide variety of persons and groups within the society (Frances et al., 1990). Errors can be costly. A diagnosis of draepetomania was not a trivial mistake, nor is misdiagnosing a woman with a premenstrual dysphoric disorder (Caplan, McCurdy-Myers, and Gans, 1992).

This is not to say that a decision concerning premenstrual dysphoric disorder should be controlled by such social concerns (Nathan, 1994). Whether premenstrual dysphoric disorder is a mental disorder is a scientific decision, as indicated by the empirical support for its congruency with the construct of mental disorder (Blashfield and Livesley, 1991; Morey, 1991; Robins and Guze, 1970; Widiger, 1993a, 1993b). If one allows social, political, or professional concerns to govern any of the decisions for a DSM, the scientific credibility of the entire manual becomes suspect. However, it would be socially irresponsible, perhaps even unethical, not to be especially cautious or conservative when setting the threshold for a questionably valid diagnostic construct, such as premenstrual dysphoric disorder, when its misdiagnosis could actually do some harm (Ross, Frances, and Widiger, 1995).

Both sides of DSM proposals have at times contaminated the decision-making process through the use of political influence and pressure (Bayer and Spitzer, 1982, 1985; Spitzer, 1985). Some persons have in fact been quite forthright in their advocacy of political pressure. Walker, a staunch opponent of the inclusion of the diagnoses of self-defeating personality disorder and premenstrual dysphoric disorder in the DSM-III-R (Walker, 1987, 1994), acknowledged explicitly that "the political advocacy of the battered women's movement, along with the feminist mental health network, managed to force the psychiatrists . . . to place in the appendix several . . . newly proposed diagnoses" (Walker, 1989, p. 699). It is disappointing that one would feel pride rather than embarrassment in having undermined through political pressure what should be a scientific effort. However, it is difficult not to succumb to the temptation, particularly if one believes that one's opponents are using comparable tactics or if one believes strongly that one's righteous motives justify the means.

Organized political pressure, however, is perhaps less problematic than the more subtle politicking used by individuals during the course of formal and informal meetings. Again, the members of the DSM-IV work groups and Task Force were fallible humans, who would be tempted to use the power of their position to obtain a revision to a diagnosis which is more consistent with their own theoretical perspective than with the empirical research. To offset this problem, a number of formal safeguards were included in the process by which the DSM-IV was developed (Frances, Widiger, and Pincus, 1989), but they were not always successful.

Ideally, at least as the process was developed for the DSM-IV, one should not be able to predict the final decisions to be made simply on the basis of the a priori publications of the members of the respective work groups and Task Force. "The ideal is to reach the conclusions a person with no fixed preconceptions (a consensus scholar) would discover from a comprehensive overview of the entire research literature, not confined to any particular research program or theoretical orientation" (Frances, Widiger, and Pincus, 1989, p. 374). To the extent that the final decisions reflect simply the a priori viewpoints of the persons in closest proximity to the decision-making power, the process can become (or at least appear to become) more political than scientific. The decisions become based not on the scientific literature but on the amount of control, power, or influence one has over the decision-making process. An individual researcher's impact on the DSM would be a matter not of the quality of the research but of the proximity to the position of influence.

This problem, however, is endemic to all fields of science. It is a problem experienced to varying degrees by scientific journals and granting agencies, as well as by the authors of the DSM (Blashfield, 1982; Guze, 1982; Kendell, 1982b; Strauss, 1982). In addition, the final decisions made for the DSM-IV are at times consistent with the a priori publications of its authors in part because positions of power, control, and influence in science are usually provided on the basis of the quality and the compelling nature of one's research. Some persons are also appointed to editorial review boards, and to the DSM-IV, to represent a particular perspective. They are expected to be objective and fair yet also represent well the perspective for which they were appointed.

▪ ▪ Science

Despite all these problems and limitations, it is my belief that a scientifically based nomenclature of mental disorders can be developed. Others suggest, however, that a scientific nomenclature of mental disorders has not and can never be developed, owing to the apparently inconclusive nature of scientific research. For example, Lilienfeld and Marino (1995) argued that a scientific nomenclature cannot be developed until mental disorders are reduced to neurochemical mechanisms, and Kendler (1990) argued that even then the effort would still fall fundamentally short of being scientific. Each of their arguments will be discussed in turn.

▪ ▪ Psychological versus Physical Science

Lilienfeld and Marino (1995) argued that "the question of whether a given condition constitutes a mental disorder cannot be answered by means of scientific criteria" (p. 417). In a manner reminiscent of Szasz (1987), they suggested that the concept of a mental disorder would remain nonscientific until its "inner nature" was discovered and it was reduced to or defined by biological and neurochemical mechanisms rather than psychological constructs.

It is indeed the case that biological or physical constructs can be relatively more precise in their boundaries than psychological constructs (e.g., the physical disorder of Down syndrome versus the mental disorder of mental retardation), but many such constructs will also lack fully operational definitions (Moore, 1975; Rorer, 1991). The discrete joints are not always that clear even within nature (Feyerabend, 1991). In addition, physical disorder is itself a hypothetical concept. "Functional impairment or disability, not the presence of a lesion, is the essential element in the medical [physical] concept of disease" (Bergner, 1997, p. 245). A biological functional impairment is as conceptual as a psychological functional impairment.

In any case, psychological constructs do not need to be reduced to biological or neurochemical mechanisms in order to become scientifically viable. The absence of an operational definition does complicate research, often substantially, but it does not prevent informative empirical research or scientific progress. Scientific progress can be obtained with theoretical constructs that lack operational definitions (Meehl, 1986; Morey, 1991; Widiger and Trull, 1993). The question of whether a given condition constitutes a mental disorder can be answered by means of scientific criteria. One cannot define absolutely what is meant by a mental disorder, but it can be defined in a manner that is more than sufficient for informative, meaningful, and valid scientific, empirical research. Its validity is addressed by obtaining data that are consistent with a particular theory of psychopathology and which refute rival, alternative theories (Morey, 1991). The process of confirmation and refutation is fallible and imperfect, but this is inherent to other domains of scientific research in psychology, astronomy, and physics (Meehl, 1986; Rorer, 1991; Feyerabend, 1988). Such psychological constructs as schizophrenia, extraversion, and intelligence lack infallible, fully operational definitions, yet they are doing quite well as scientific constructs.

▪ ▪ Science and the Scientist

Kendler (1990), a prominent member of the DSM-IV Task Force, argued that a scientifically based nomenclature can never be developed because of the continued inadequacy and inconclusive nature of the empirical research. Indeed, no single study or sets of studies are unambiguous or conclusive in their findings. There is always room for alternative interpretations (Meehl, 1978). Kendler (1990) argued that the inconclusive nature of empirical research must then ultimately reduce the process to subjective, value-based decisions: "The fundamental problem is that the scientific method can only answer 'little' questions (e.g., what is the rate of escape from dexamethasone suppression in major depression …). By contrast, in nosology, we need answers to 'big questions' (e.g., what is the best criteria set for the diagnosis of anorexia nervosa)" (p. 972).

Kendler suggested that the big questions "are fundamentally nonempirical and cannot be addressed by the scientific method" (p. 969) because the intervening step between the empirical findings and the big questions requires subjective, nonscientific value judgments, such as which validator to emphasize when different validators provide conflicting results. "We pretend to be 'objective' and 'empirical' when, in reality, we are making informed value judgments" (p. 972).

Kendler based his conclusions, however, on an inaccurate and simplistic model of positivistic science. It is true that empirical data are subject to alternative interpretations, even the research concerning little questions (Meehl, 1978), but the ambiguity of empirical data does not render the decision making nonscientific. Science has never been a mindless accumulation of empirical data that speak for themselves. This is a narrow understanding of logical empiricism (Faust and Miner, 1986). Interpretation, discussion, disagreement, and debate concerning the relevance and ambiguity of an empirical finding are integral to the scientific method and occur in all branches of science (Feyerabend, 1988; Rorer, 1991). Empirical findings must always be interpreted with respect to their relative degree of confirmatory and disconfirmatory support, their consistency across studies, the internal validity of the experimental design, and their relevance to the constructs at issue. Kendler (1991) himself subsequently illustrated this process quite well in his systematic review of the research to address the big question of whether mood-incongruent psychotic affective illness (MICPAI) is a variant of (1) mood, (2) schizoaffective, or (3) schizophrenic disorder. He "proceeded to review the empiric literature, all published since 1979, that could attempt to answer the questions posed by these nosologists" (p. 368), and he documented well the ambiguity and inconsistency of the findings across validators for the alternative proposals. Nowhere did he suggest that his ultimate conclusion that "the accumulated evidence tends to support the decision of the framers of the DSM-III and DSM-III-R in considering MICPAI to be a subtype of affective illness" (pp. 368–69) reflected a nonscientific value judgment rather than a reasoned, appropriate interpretation of the empirical research.

Validators will at times have different implications for the construction and revision of a diagnostic criteria set. Kendler (1990) is correct that the "validation of a psychiatric disorder cannot . . . occur in a vacuum" (p. 970), but this vacuum is not filled by personal, idiosyncratic value judgments. What is often necessary for the interpretation of data is a theoretical model that guides the understanding of the relevance of alternative validators (Morey, 1991). The validation of a mental disorder is inherently the validation of a particular theoretical formulation of the diagnosis, and it cannot occur in the absence of this formulation (Follette and Houts, 1996; Widiger and Trull, 1993). The choice among competing formulations that place a different emphasis on alternative validators is a choice between competing theoretical formulations of the disorder. It is not a value judgment; it is a scientific decision with respect to the conceptual and empirical support for the alternative theoretical models.

Disagreement with respect to the degree of empirical support for proposals and alternative validators can result in part from culturally, theoretically, and personally biased misinterpretations of the research. It was for this reason that the DSM-IV literature reviews, data reanalyses, and field trials were subjected to substantial critical review by committee members, advisors, conference participants, and journal editors (Frances et al, 1990; Widiger et al., 1991).

This critical review is also inherent to the scientific method (Bartley, 1984). "To be rational in one's endorsement of a position, one must criticize it" (Weimer, 1979, p. 41). It is not difficult to provide a justification for a particular theory or for a proposed revision to the nomenclature. It is much more difficult and, most important, much more informative to survive critical review (Popper, 1963, 1972). As Faust and Miner (1986) noted, "this process [of critical review] is not 'objective' in the strict sense, but it is not irrational or 'subjective' either" (p. 965). There is no gold standard for determining which proposal or theoretical model has more verisimilitude (truth value or validity). Therefore, any proposal, like any scientific theory, must survive the test of attempted critical refutation. This is not an appeal to value judgments. It is how science proceeds.

▪▪ The Scientific Development of the DSM-IV

The development of the DSM-IV proceeded through three interactive stages of scientific, empirical input: (1) literature reviews, (2) data reanalyses, and (3) field trials (American Psychiatric Association, 1994; Frances, Widiger, and Pincus, 1989; Frances et al., 1990; Widiger et al., 1991). The first stage required that any proposed revision to the DSM-III-R be preceded by an explicit, systematic, and comprehensive review of the scientific and clinical literature. These reviews were modeled closely after the empirical, scientific meta-analytic method for literature review (Cooper, 1984). An explicit, uniform format for the report of the review was required to encourage adherence to the spirit of being systematic, objective, and comprehensive and to facilitate the identification of any failure to do so (Widiger et al., 1990). For example, introductory sections were required to state explicitly each issue or proposal being reviewed and its clinical or theoretical significance. In addition, a methods section was required in which the authors had to indicate explicitly the nature and quality of the research that would be considered and the process by which these research findings would be identified. A total of 175 such reviews were completed and published. "Those issues for which the published data were insufficient or equivocal and for which there were relevant unpublished data were submitted to a second stage of DSM review: data reanalyses" (Davis et al., 1998, p. 4).

Many researchers have unpublished data sets that can provide informative, relevant findings to address a particular issue or proposed revision. Systematically sampling a variety of unpublished data sets across different research programs was also useful in minimizing any bias that might result from confining deliberations to the findings of only one or two researchers (Widiger et al., 1991). The reports of these data reanalyses also had to adhere to a required format to facilitate critical review (e.g., failure to address all the relevant issues or a failure to solicit all relevant research sites). A total of thirty-six such data reanalysis reports were completed and published. The third stage for the consideration of empirical research consisted of field trials of proposed revisions. Emphasis was given to trials of the most substantial or controversial revisions that could be tested in the limited period of available time. A requirement of each field trial was to compare alternative proposals (including the research criteria being developed for the World Health Organization's International Classification of Diseases [World Health Organization, 1992a]) using a variety of validators across multiple sites that provided the most relevant clinical populations. Twelve such studies were conducted and published.

In addition, each of the reports from the literature reviews, data reanalyses, and field trials was widely circulated for review, including the persons who would most likely be opposed to the proposed revisions (Frances et al., 1991, "Toward a More Empirical Diagnostic System") and the fifty to one hundred advisors to each work group (which also included potential opponents to proposed revisions). The authors of the reports were also encouraged to present papers at professional conferences and to submit their reports for publication to provide further circulation and obtain additional critical review. Advisors from different professional organizations were also provided with work group and Task Force reports to keep these organizations systematically informed and to be informed by them of their concerns or objections. Special advisory committees were established to address specific issues (e.g., cross-cultural and forensic issues). Details of progress and initial conclusions were also published regularly in a DSM-IV newsletter (sent to all advisors) and in a regular column for *Hospital and Community Psychiatry* (Davis et al., 1998). Two inexpensive drafts of the DSM-IV were also made available to alert clinicians, researchers, and other interested persons to the proposals being considered for the manual and to solicit from them any further concerns, criticisms, or suggestions (Task Force on DSM-IV, 1991, 1993).

The process by which DSM-IV was developed could certainly be improved (Blashfield, Sprock, and Fuller, 1990; Nathan, 1994; Pincus et al., 1992). One specific suggestion for the DSM-V is to provide enough time and funding to field-test systematically and comprehensively all the significant proposals to all the criteria sets. Even seemingly minor revisions to a criteria set can have substantial effects on a diagnosis, many of which would not have been anticipated (Blashfield, Blum, and Pfohl, 1992). The funding for such field trials would be expensive, but the American Psychiatric Association has experienced substantial profits from the sales of the DSM-IV which could be used to fund the development of the DSM-V.

The final decisions that were made for the DSM-IV were, in any case, conscientious and well-reasoned decisions guided by the scientific literature. There were certainly instances in which a step in the process was unsuccessful in its aspiration (e.g., the literature review for factitious disorder), and there may be instances in which value judgments had an inappropriate impact on a final decision (e.g., the failure to give official recognition to the diagnosis of premenstrual dysphoric disorder), but the process was reasonably successful in maximizing the likelihood of systematically considering all the relevant empirical research and in reaching conclusions that would be consistent with the scientific literature. Critics of any particular decision that was made should address the rationale and bases for that decision published in one or more of the volumes of the *DSM-IV Sourcebook.* "The DSM-IV Sourcebook . . . is intended to provide a comprehensive and convenient record of the clinical and research support for the various decisions reached by the Work Groups and the Task Force" (American Psychiatric Association, 1994, p. xx). Any failure to be guided adequately by the scientific literature should be readily apparent through a critique of the published bases for each decision. A major purpose of the *DSM-IV Sourcebook* was precisely to facilitate critical reviews of the scientific nature of the DSM-IV decisions (Frances, Widiger, and Pincus, 1989; Widiger et al., 1991). Such critiques are now being published (e.g., Bornstein, 1997; Rogler, 1996; Sadler, 1996b), and they will be of substantial benefit to the authors of the DSM-V.

Part Two

Conceptual and Methodological Considerations

4

· ·

Values and Objectivity in Psychiatric Nosology

PATRICIA A. ROSS, PH.D.

BECAUSE OF THE nature of the classification project, nosology appears to fall outside traditional discussions of objectivity in science. Classical scientific objectivity is thought to arise from the methods of routine science. Perhaps because of the unique tasks of classification, the issue of the relations between objectivity and values in classification has been neglected. This chapter examines objectivity in order to understand the place of values in psychiatric nosology.

▪ ▪ Values, Objectivity, and Science

To address the question of values in psychiatric nosology, one must begin by examining how these values arise, where they are located, and if and how they are problematic. However, if one asks the question in this way, it quickly becomes clear that there is not simply *one* "question of values" in this context. Some authors, for example, speak of the values inherent in theories. Their claim is that since theories reflect cultural, historical, and social preferences, they are value laden. Any use that is made of such theories will be likewise affected. Other authors are concerned with how decisions are made to include or exclude criteria or categories from the DSMs. Their claim is that such decisions are value laden. Still others are simply disturbed by the presence of normative terms such as *deficit* or *subaverage,* claiming that such terms reflect unwarranted normative judgments.

In light of this, I want to begin by laying out just which question of values I address. As an aside, I must admit that if I had read only the title of the "Call for Papers" for the conference from which this book was drawn, I would not have submitted a paper. That is not because I do not find the topic of interest or think it important. Rather, when I see the word *values*, I think "ethics" or "moral philosophy," and there are many people far more qualified than I to speak on such issues. However, something in the fine print caught my attention. In talking about the debate over the virtues and liabilities of taxonomies for mental disorders, the "Call for Papers" read: "While a significant portion of this debate involves routine scientific disputes and the problems of insufficient knowledge about mental disorders and their etiologies, another portion of the debate involves values and how they drive the concept of mental disorder, particular diagnostic categories and criteria, and the development of diagnostic classifications." It was the juxtaposition of routine science on the one hand and values on the other which caught my eye, and it is from this perspective that I want to examine the question of values in psychiatric nosology.

This juxtaposition is a reflection of a larger picture that goes unexamined in our thinking about values. This picture suggests that scientific research, when done according to established methods and with strict standards, is value free. Questions of values arise outside this scientific context. Any decisions or hypotheses made without strict scientific standards guiding them are likely to be value laden. Thus, in the case of psychiatric nosology, one might argue that the scientific theories informing the classification project are value free but that values arise because of the practical considerations and compromises that must be made outside the scientific context in developing a diagnostic manual. Values are taxonomic fallout. As an example of the kind of thinking I am concerned with, here is an excerpt from the Sadler, Wiggins, and Schwartz edited volume entitled *Philosophical Perspectives on Psychiatric Diagnostic Classification* (1994b): "There is no mystery about the firmly scientific self-image of ICD and DSM. The success of these classifications is a direct result of the adoption of a descriptive approach to the definition of mental disorders, more or less consciously emulating the scientific basis of disease classification in physical medicine. . . . Given all this scientific momentum, then, it is surely the more remarkable that we should find value terms, terms expressing judgments of good and bad [*sic*], liberally distributed throughout both ICD and DSM" (Fulford, 1994, pp. 212–13). Despite the good science employed, values somehow, surprisingly, have crept in. Good science is taken to be value free, by definition.

My plan is not to deny that scientific research provides us with objective knowledge about psychiatric diseases, but I do want to question this picture. In particular, I want to examine why we believe that science is inherently value free, producing objective knowledge, while the taxonomic process is inherently value laden. I believe that such a picture is wrong on both counts and, moreover, that the elimination of values in both areas requires the same procedure. In this regard, routine science and taxonomy are not distinct sorts of projects.

To begin, I want to examine our conception of objectivity and how we have traditionally understood it to be the product of routine science. I believe the origin of values in psychiatric nosology can be explained best through reference to our traditional account of objectivity. Such an account, however, is not without its problems. I then consider an alternative account of objectivity. With this account, we get a very different understanding of how objective knowledge arises from science and the role that values play within the method for obtaining objectivity. By understanding how values function within science we can better understand how they arise in psychiatric nosology and what can be done to deal with them.

▪ ▪ The Traditional Conception of Objectivity in Science

Let us begin, then, with the traditional conception of objectivity, which promotes the view that scientific research, if done in a particular way, according to a particular method, will produce value-free, objective knowledge. The answer would be simple if we could rely on careful observation and accurate description as our scientific method. However, we long ago realized that mere observation and description, mediated by individuals with their own particular background knowledge, assumptions, and biases, often fall victim to subjective interpretation. Thus, the empirical method of science itself does not necessarily guarantee the objectivity of knowledge.

Then what does? The account of objectivity which has most strongly influenced how we answer this is most easily explained by appealing to the logical empiricists' distinction between the context of discovery and the context of justification (Salmon, 1989). The context of discovery, logical empiricists claimed, contains all the factors that make up the way in which a hypothesis is developed or obtained. So, for example, if a particular scientist finds the answer to a puzzle by gazing into a fire or having a religious experience, or if the Communist Party comes to power and a scientist finds that promoting a particular hypothesis is politically useful, these are factors that fall within the domain of the context of discovery.

Although questions of values obviously arise in this context, we need not worry that they will bear negatively on the objectivity of a hypothesis. This is because objectivity is not a product of the context of discovery but rather a product of the context of justification. Here, the proposed hypothesis, regardless of the manner by which it is obtained, is subjected to strict logical evaluation. This evaluation determines whether a particular relation obtains between a hypothesis and the evidence that is marshaled to support the hypothesis. The relation invokes abstract, universal rules whereby the hypothesis is demonstrated to follow from the evidence in an "objective" way. It is free from subjective elements and therefore values. Thus, the relationship between evidence and hypothesis is evaluated within the context of justification, and regardless of the peculiar, idiosyncratic reasons there may have been for originally proposing the hypothesis, the evaluation, which invokes logical and universal rules, determines whether the evidence supports the hypothesis so as to establish its objectivity. All the subjective elements are packed into the context of discovery, and the context of justification guarantees that they do not play a role in hypothesis acceptance.

Given this distinction, it becomes possible to see how the dichotomy introduced earlier in this chapter—that between routine science and values—arises. Routine science, committed to finding objective theories, takes place in the context of justification, in which universal, abstract rules are applied to data to establish the objectivity of a theory. Questions of values are introduced at the individual level and persist only if we remain outside this justificatory context. The abstract, universal method of justification is what factors out values; individual interpretation factors them in.

Turning to the question of how values arise in nosology, we can now derive the standard picture described above. Scientific theories and facts come to the taxonomic process value free as a result of having been evaluated in the context of justification. In contrast, the taxonomic process is concerned with synthesizing observations and facts into molar wholes, a process much closer to the discovery process than to the context of justification. Because the taxonomic process is not so much concerned with an evaluation of the fit between hypotheses and evidence, it falls outside the context of justification. As such, it is subject to values. Thus, the taxonomic process is value laden while the science informing this process is value free, resulting in a nosology that is likewise value laden, all of which is due to the taxonomic process.

▪ ▪ An Alternative Account of Objectivity

Helen Longino, in her book *Science as Social Knowledge* (1990), provides us with an alternative account of objectivity in science. I recommend her book for a complete analysis of the traditional account, as well as a fuller presentation of her alternative. For our purposes, here, I merely summarize the points she makes.

The traditional account that we have just looked at pictures objectivity as the product of the application of particular rules to data. As Longino points out, the only question that has been asked concerning this account is whether any actual science has ever met the standards of objectivity which the account proposes. As Longino puts it:

> As long as one takes the positivist analysis as providing a model to which any inquiry must conform in order to be objective and rational, then to the degree that actual science departs from the model it fails to be objective and rational. . . . Both the historians and philosophers who have attacked the old model and those who have defended it have at times taken this position. The only disagreement regarding objectivity, then, seems to be over the question of whether actual, historical science does or does not realize the epistemological ideal of objectivity. (p. 65)

However, it is obvious that another question can be asked—whether the account itself is adequate. Although evaluation of the traditional account of objectivity has focused on whether any actual science lives up to the methods proposed, Longino asks whether the method proposed could possibly be correct. Is the picture of objectivity we get from the traditional account adequate for capturing the notion of objectivity, or is there a better, more accurate way of looking at objectivity?

The source of her concern with the traditional account lies in the highly individualistic nature of objectivity it promotes. Traditionally, as we have seen, objectivity has been taken to be an attribute of a particular method, and an individual is objective if he or she follows that method. "Scientific method, on this view, is something that can be practiced by a single individual: sense organs and the capacity to reason are all that are required for conducting controlled experiments or practicing rigorous deduction" (Longino, 1990, p. 66).

The problem with this traditional account, as Longino sees it, lies in its promotion of objectivity as achievable by an individual. She maintains that science is essentially a social practice, thus requiring the participation of two or more individuals, and that objectivity is a product of this practice. It should be noted that objectivity on this account is still understood as the product of following a particular method, but now the method, rather than being abstract and universal, is supplied by the practices in which the scientific community engages. We should not think of these practices as simply a collection of individuals working on their own, following some abstract method and then compiling the results. Rather, objectivity is the product of the particular social interactions of this practice.

What, in particular, is it about the social nature of inquiry which gives us objective knowledge? Longino argues that it is the constant critical scrutiny and modification of each individual's work by other members of the community which leads to objectivity. Experiments must be repeatable, and repeatable by others. Procedures such as peer review are necessary. Here, other points of view are brought to bear on an individual's work, and revisions are suggested (and expected to be made) in light of these reviews. This social give-and-take—interacting with others in a critical way—is what produces objective knowledge, and not the demonstration of some abstract relationship between data and theory.

A number of questions may arise concerning this proposal, not the least of which is the question of why such a process does not merely reinforce a particular group's background beliefs and assumptions. Values may never be questioned and thus flourish within a community's collective work. Likewise, we might think that alternative points of view may be suppressed by this critical scrutiny. Longino maintains that the social nature of science—the process of critical scrutiny itself—allows us to avoid these problems. The possibility of intersubjective criticism promotes objectivity as long as the community meets several criteria. First, recognized avenues for criticism are needed. Second, there must be shared standards that critics can invoke. Third, the community must be responsive to this criticism. Finally, intellectual authority must be shared equally among participants in the process. A community will be objective to the degree that it satisfies these criteria.

▪ ▪ Objectivity and Values in Psychiatric Nosology

I have presented the traditional account of objectivity and Longino's alternative not to debate the merits or plausibility of either but rather to provide a framework that might stimulate dialogue about objectivity and values in psychiatric nosology. The traditional account of objectivity will not help to do this, for the taxonomic project cannot be adequately understood as falling within either the context of discovery or the context of justification. Organizing preexisting knowledge into a useful manual for purposes of diagnosing mental illness does not fall within the context of discovery, where questions of values traditionally arise. Moreover, since no theories are being tested against evidence, the project cannot be seen as falling within the context of justification. With respect to this latter point, there is the further issue that the nosological work in the DSM is atheoretical. The approach taken is descriptive with respect to etiology or pathology and does not promote any particular theory of mental health and disease. If this is the case, the project clearly falls outside the context of justification, and the traditional account of objectivity is of no use in understanding value concerns.

As an aside, I think that the DSM is actually best described as theoretically pluralistic. The claim is that no one theory takes precedence over any other in the attempt to provide the best available, or most useful, explanations. But considering that observations are theory laden and observation is the basis for the descriptions in question, theory is ever present. Moreover, the descriptions included are not just a mere collection of all those available. Rather, pragmatic considerations were employed to determine what were the best available, or most useful, explanations. Considerations such as satisfying clinical and research needs are driving forces, and concepts are considered acceptable if they are "workable." Clearly, a pragmatic sense of validity is in use here, whereby utility is driving the taxonomic process.

All of this, however, does not contradict the claim that the taxonomic process falls outside the context of justification, as traditionally conceived. None of these are questions concerning the relationship between theories and the evidence marshaled to support them. The taxonomic process, however, is not about discovery, either, and it is not clear that it can be extended to help us understand how to develop a taxonomy free of values. As we have already said, the information considered for use in the DSM comes from theories that are already in existence. Moreover, the taxonomic enterprise is a matter of organizing information into a useful classification system. No interpretation occurs. If the theories being used are free of values, compiling these theories (albeit pieces of them) does not involve any personal interpretations that might reintroduce values by way of background assumptions and so on. The content of the theories does not change.

In general, it would seem that distinctions made by the traditional account which help to locate sources of values and provide solutions for how to rid ourselves of these values are just not useful for understanding the problem in psychiatric nosology. In fact, the obvious candidates for where values might arise—in the choices that are being made concerning which explanations to include and which to ignore, and the pragmatic considerations motivating these choices—do not fit any categories provided by the traditional account.

I propose that we look at psychiatric nosological work in terms of Longino's account of objectivity. This account can address the decision-making processes that are the candidates for value introduction and thus can help us to understand how to go about eliminating values that arise in this context. Recall that Longino treats science as a social process and objectivity as one of the products of this process. It is easy enough to extend this view to nosology, for certainly, if it is anything, coming up with something like a psychiatric nosology is a highly social enterprise that involves the participation of many individuals in the scientific community and perhaps beyond. To begin to understand how values arise in this context, we need to evaluate the kinds of interaction which occur in developing classifications of psychopathology. In particular, we need to see if the kinds of interactions which give rise to something like the DSM are the sort that Longino characterizes as necessary for objectivity. Keep in mind that critical scrutiny is the hallmark of objectivity. If such scrutiny does not occur, background assumptions and values are never brought forth and addressed.

However, from what I understand about such projects as the DSM, consensus and compromise are the key elements of success. The goal is to find concepts that are "workable, generally agreed to, or the best we can do all things considered" (Agich, 1994, p. 237). Karen Ritchie tells of a debate that took place over the inclusion of several disorders in the DSM-III. The American Psychiatric Association (APA) invited seven female feminist psychologists and psychiatrists to meet with the DSM Task Force prior to the revision of the DSM-III. The purpose was to discuss several disputed diagnostic categories—categories that some mental health professionals were finding objectionable. Among these categories was paraphilic rapism, which "would have designated a group of compulsive rapists as having a mental disorder" (Ritchie, 1989, p. 698). The women were there to voice the concern that this would allow a group of rapists to plead insanity, thereby avoiding a prison term. The women, on presenting their argument, were surprised that the Task Force found this consideration persuasive enough to drop the diagnostic category entirely from the manual.

The women also expressed their concern with the category masochistic personality disorder (symptoms: remaining in exploitative relationships, sacrificing one's own interests for others, rejecting help so as not to be a burden), claiming that, given the way the disorder was defined, a behavior that is historically, culturally, and often religiously acceptable and desirable for women was being labeled "abnormal." Women are often socialized to act in the self-effacing ways described by the category. At this point the APA committee began its deliberation, reportedly creating and dispensing with revisions by having individuals shout out criteria that would make the category appear less "normal." One such revision was dropped because a committee member claimed, "I do that sometimes" (Ritchie, 1989, p. 698). "The women asked whether jogging, playing football, or wearing high heels and girdles constituted masochism. The answer they received was that sports activities are not masochistic. Nor is wearing high heels, but wearing a girdle is, unless a woman is over 70" (Ritchie, 1989, p. 698).

This is certainly an example of compromise and maybe even consensus. But I wonder whether it is a process that helps to ensure that the categories obtained are free from values. Looked at through the perspective of Longino's account of objectivity, the point where problems are introduced becomes clearer. Consensus and compromise do not provide the kind of critical scrutiny necessary to put values in check. What is essential for obtaining objectivity is the critical review of conclusions by others in the community. This process will draw attention to any values that are present and result in the revision of hypotheses.

As you will recall, regarding this critical review, Longino claims that there are four criteria that measure the degree of objectivity obtained: (1) recognized avenues for criticism must exist; (2) there must be shared standards that the critics can evoke; (3) the community must be responsive to these criticisms; and within this process, (4) intellectual authority must be shared equally. Let us think about these criteria with respect to the nosological process.

Are there recognized avenues for criticism of the DSM? We should take as our model scientific research in which findings are published and peer review occurs. One worry might be that, owing to its theoretically pluralistic nature, no recognized avenues of criticism exist as yet. For example, criticism may appear in journals or other places that represent only one particular theoretical viewpoint. Thus, such criticism is read by individuals already in agreement with that viewpoint. As a result, it never enters into the larger context of critical scrutiny that produces objectivity.

The second of Longino's criteria is that there must be shared standards that critics can evoke. This presents a problem in a theoretically pluralistic context. If there are any existing standards to appeal to, they would most likely be a part of a particular theoretical framework. Critical standards appropriate only within one particular theoretical context are not acceptable. Thus, it is most likely that other, independent critical standards need to be established for this particular task. A further concern here is that the standards that critics are currently evoking really satisfy no one. For example, a criticism against the inclusion of a symptom simply because the critic claims to "do that sometimes himself" does not seem to be satisfactory.

Longino's third criterion is that the community must be responsive to criticisms that arise through these channels. I am not sure that responsiveness has been a problem. It is more likely that it is the kind of responses and the selection of which criticisms to respond to which are the biggest sources of trouble. These issues would presumably be dealt with by setting critical standards and establishing recognized avenues of criticism.

The final criterion is that intellectual authority must be shared. I am aware of some criticism claiming that, although the DSM claims to be atheoretical, it is in fact biased in favor of one particular theory. This is due to the hierarchical classification scheme it employs. This itself might be a result of the personal biases of those involved in the project and reflect a biased distribution of authority. Obviously, if the goal is a value-free classification of psychopathology, then such bias must be eliminated. The sharing of intellectual authority is necessary for the elimination of such bias.

These are just a few examples of the ways in which the criteria for obtaining objectivity might help to identify current problems with classification; they are not necessarily suggestions for concrete changes. What I am proposing is that the process leading to classification be evaluated in the same terms that are used for other scientific work. My hope is that the criteria for objectivity will be used to look more carefully at the process to determine how best to establish the kind of critical scrutiny necessary to eliminate values from this context. This evaluation should treat this process just like any other scientific development and hold it to the same standards for obtaining objectivity to which routine science is held.

▪ ▪ Future Directions for Nosological Work

Developing a diagnostic classification system is an activity that is not typical of routine science. Traditional accounts of objectivity in science overlook the possible sources of values in this activity because such accounts focus on the scientific activities of theory discovery and theory justification. There is simply no recognition of any other type of scientific activity. Thus, the traditional account of objectivity leads one to the conclusion that values that arise by way of an activity such as psychiatric nosology cannot be understood as a product of the scientific work that is being done.

By understanding objectivity as the product of a particular kind of social activity, we gain a more useful means for looking at our nosological activity. With this understanding, the method for evaluating objectivity within routine scientific work can be extended outside that framework. By moving away from the conception of objectivity as intrinsically tied up with routine science and toward the view in which objectivity is a product of particular kinds of social interactions, we can identify a source of values which is not otherwise easily identifiable and, moreover, have at hand an understanding of how to deal with them.

5

Survival of the Fittest? Conceptual Selection in Psychiatric Nosology

CHRIS MACE, M.D.

WHAT IS A DIAGNOSIS? What sort of system is a diagnostic classification? How does study of the way classifications change reveal the values shaping them? Is it possible for psychiatric diagnosis to improve? In this chapter, psychiatric diagnosis is examined in light of Stephen Toulmin's (1972a, 1972b, 1976) analyses of (1) scientific theory as a conceptual system, and (2) change within intellectual disciplines as a selection process, acting on a "pool" of concepts. A case study of the history of hysterical disorders illustrates this analysis in understanding selection and modification of diagnostic concepts in psychiatry. The applicability of this analysis to psychiatric nosology in the era of the DSM-IV is critically considered. Toulmin's account of how intellectual disciplines uphold values that determine how their concepts are selected and modified can illuminate differences between psychiatry and other specialties. Various developments in psychiatric nosology increasingly reflect the influence of extradisciplinary values, and the chapter concludes by discussing the problems these will pose in the future.

▪ ▪ Diagnosis and Nosography

It is impossible to resolve problems of diagnostic classification in psychiatry without a clear understanding of what a diagnosis is. This chapter introduces some insights from the philosophy of science which permit diagnoses to be reevaluated and may illuminate a number of past and present classificatory difficulties. In line with recent trends in the philosophy of science, my account tries to keep description and prescription apart. I attempt to illustrate how the nature of psychiatric diagnosis (irrespective of content) has changed considerably during the present century and how failure to recognize this leads to many problems for clinicians, classifiers, and philosophers.

It is now so common for diagnosis to be discussed in the context of classification that it is possible to think of diagnoses as taxonomic labels. However, they are both more and less than this. *Diagnosis* is an ambiguous word, denoting a process and a category. Not only has diagnosis been the most characteristic activity of doctors, but diagnoses are the basic units of medical thought. An individual diagnosis embodies ontological and pragmatic understandings about the nature of the thing it labels and what can be done about that thing. Diagnostic thinking is therefore indispensable to medical practice, a situation summarized by Faber (1923, p. 211): "To the physiologist and the worker in the laboratory, morbid categories are subordinate concepts, but to the physician, to the clinician, the reverse is the case: he cannot live, cannot speak, cannot act without them."

Individual diagnoses enjoy the status of mental as well as linguistic entities, organizing the experience of clinicians who have learned to rely on them in this way. Whereas diagnoses are essential, classification, however desirable, is not. It is important to distinguish between the corresponding activities of nosography, by which individual diagnoses are consolidated in the light of clinical practice, and nosology, the study of their classification. Medical history suggests that, although nosography never stands still as new diagnostic concepts are always being introduced, developed, and discarded, nosological enthusiasm waxes and wanes. At times in medical history, interest in such formal arrangements can be so prominent as to compromise attempts to correlate diagnoses with the pathological findings. In philosophical terms, this tendency represents a triumph of nominalism (in which names have no reality beyond their constituent words) over naturalism (by which names correspond directly to distinctions between natural kinds). This was the case in eighteenth-century medicine, when many formally complete, but essentially speculative, taxonomies were attempted after the model of Linnaeus. It is a situation that has many parallels with the avid manualizing of nosographic concepts by contemporary psychiatry in the descriptions of the ICD-10 and DSM-IV which are discussed in the final section of this chapter.

Because they convey knowledge other than that of formal relations and have functions independent of the classification, psychiatric diagnoses are not merely taxonomic labels. What, then, are they? They certainly resemble taxonomic categories in that they are concepts. However, to understand what kind of concepts they may be and the implications of this, it is helpful to examine some recent contributions to the philosophy of science. Through highlighting the place of concepts in scientific thought, diagnostic concepts can be located in psychiatry, and the kind of values that influence their selection may be understood.

▪ ▪ Toulmin on Concepts and Disciplines

A philosopher-historian, Stephen Toulmin has provided an account of science that, if extended to psychiatry, calls for a reappraisal of diagnosis (Toulmin, 1953, 1972b). His analysis of the processes by which knowledge is organized and extended clarifies how a commitment to reason links a broad range of scientific, technological, and judicial activities. Moreover, it clarifies how values intrinsic to each individual discipline ensure that the discipline's thinking and practice remain distinct. Like ideas in the fields of study he describes, Toulmin's own ideas were in steady evolution and ultimately inseparable from those of like-minded contemporaries. I focus here on two key themes: the role of concepts in scientific thought and the nature of conceptual change. Each is briefly summarized, followed by a discussion of their past, present, and future implications for psychiatric nosology.

To Toulmin, the concept (rather than the proposition or the theory) is the most fundamental unit of scientific discourse. These definable abstractions, such as "energy" or "gene," are essential components of testable generalizations such as Boyle's or Mendel's laws and are in turn defined and redefined through the theories expressed in terms of them. Although the same concept may be used for a considerable period before it is displaced, it is likely to change in meaning as its permitted relations change in the course of scientific theorizing. Concepts are basic units of scientific discourse because a person's understanding of a science depends on assimilation of its current concepts and of when and how they are used, rather than individual theories. Even if theoretical propositions might be ordered in a highly systematic and possibly hierarchical fashion within a science, its concepts, found at varying levels of abstraction, are unlikely to have simple interrelationships. Because they lie beyond observation statements and theoretical propositions and are likely to be components of more than one theory at any one time, a science's core concepts are not simply proven or disproven. Conversely, as they are rarely immortal, tend-ing to be discarded, transformed, or superseded, the explanation of conceptual change becomes a critical task for philosophers of science. For Toulmin, a science's technical concepts are the key referents around which its current activity and thinking are articulated.

Within the philosophy of science, Toulmin's view opposed those of many others, such as Duhem, Hempel, and Popper, who, whatever their disagreements over matters of verification, all stressed the primacy of scientific theories and their strict logical relationship to component propositions and observation statements. In more recent times and within the era of cognitive science, the climate has changed so substantially that writers for whom the priority of concepts in scientific explanation is a given (e.g., Thagard, 1992) make scant acknowledgment to Toulmin's pioneering work. In fact, in expounding his quietly radical view on the priority of concepts, Toulmin was indebted to another philosopher-historian, R. G. Collingwood (Toulmin, 1972a). Collingwood, despite forays into the philosophy of science (Collingwood, 1945), was not a natural scientist and valued science primarily for what it taught us about ourselves rather than about nature. When he took concepts to be primary to theories in scientific thinking, this was consistent with a personal model by which all areas of intellectual activity identify themselves by the questions they ask and the concepts through which they couch their answers. The content even of a technical concept with an explicit definition cannot be reduced to the theories in which it is currently used: it inevitably carries implicit meaning from all the functions it has had. The history of any intellectual activity should therefore be summarized in terms of the questions it addressed and the concepts that were characteristic of it.

Collingwood's work fell within a Kantian tradition in which concepts had originally been viewed not only as prior to other aspects of thought but also to be fixed because they were innate. As a historian, Collingwood readily conceded that concepts could and did change, but he found it no easier than other neo-Kantians to account for how change occurred. Toulmin wished to redress this lack and was also uneasy with a further facet of Collingwood's analysis, namely, its relativism. If, in scientific enterprises at least, changes in questions and concepts occur, change should represent an improvement on the state of affairs prior to the change. In Collingwood's scheme, maintaining coherence between questions and concepts in each field of study was paramount. Should questions about the nature of progress arise, these were simply designated as the proper concern of only one discipline among others (i.e., philosophy). Profound dissatisfaction with this relativism, despite admiration for much of Collingwood's other philosophy, inspired Toulmin's own most important contribution to the philosophy of science. This was his novel account of conceptual change.

The problem of conceptual change led Toulmin to formulate what has been termed an evolutionary theory of scientific progress. Although, like Darwin, Toulmin disowned this label, there are many analogies between his account of mechanisms by which conceptual change occurs in science and Darwinian natural selection. He believed that Darwinian "fitness" in the face of objective constraints ensured that conceptual selection in science was a rational process. To reach this point, Toulmin made a move that had previously led others toward relativism—he paid attention to the social context of scientific activity. Toulmin emphasized the collective nature of human concepts and how explanatory concepts were the common property of a community of intellectuals working within a discipline. Members of a discipline share a set of common aims and values that set their discipline apart from others. However, unlike a famous fellow student of the sociology of scientific knowledge, Thomas Kuhn, Toulmin was keen to differentiate between more and less rational enterprises. Traditional scientific disciplines such as physics, whose basic aims were to explain a range of natural phenomena, embodied a high level of rationality. This would be associated with the discipline being "compact," that is, enjoying a tight consensus regarding its core aims and the standards by which new ideas were tested. At the same time, there was a continuum of disciplines, with the more diffuse, technological disciplines still enjoying a pool of concepts which was unique to them, as well as concepts they shared with a parent science. It is important to note that a discipline could serve pragmatic rather than explanatory aims and remain rational, Toulmin's preferred example here being law.

The association of concepts with specific disciplines has affinities with Collingwood's account of disciplines being identified with a specific set of questions. However, Toulmin's typical discipline is more directly embedded in human affairs and will assert characteristic aims beyond the questions that define its current lines of inquiry. The current problems of any discipline reflect the contrast between its explanatory ideals and its current capacities. For example, while the explanatory ideals that identify the emerging discipline of molecular genetics can be couched in terms of clarifying the relationship of phenotypic variation to the genome, the problem set at any instant will depend on both the discipline's achievements to date and its capabilities to pursue questions that remain unresolved. To be distinct, a discipline needs to be identified with unique values, the ideal discipline promoting what Toulmin calls a compact discipline. The examples he gives here are of well-established, explanatory disciplines such as atomic physics which not only have distinct objects of study but whose members acknowledge the same technical problems and employ a common system of reasoning in addressing them (cf. Toulmin, 1972b, p. 378 ff.).

Toulmin portrays conceptual change in science as a process of selection occurring within an established discipline. Clear, publicly sanctioned aims provide a constraint against which concepts are selected or rejected. There is a supposition that more than one concept is available to be promoted or refined within a discipline at any one time, but the selection that is made will reflect the prevailing aim within a discipline, as well as external factors such as the state of neighboring disciplines. By analogy with speciation, Toulmin thought genealogical and ecological factors each operated in conceptual selection. Genealogical factors were paramount if an ascendant concept recommended itself by virtue of its continuity with its predecessors, perhaps through a capacity to synthesize previously conflicting yet indispensable ideas. Ecological factors dominated if a novel concept was selected through a pressing need for a concept to perform a particular function, that is, to fill an already vacant niche within a framework of explanation. The ecological demands peculiar to each discipline would reflect the landscape imposed by its particular aims and values.

The cumulative effect of conceptual selection was that the pool of prominent concepts within a discipline changed as individual concepts became obsolete, divided, displaced, or subsumed by others with the passage of time. These possibilities are represented diagrammatically in figure 5.1. Time is running horizontally from left to right in the figure. The letter A marks concepts that become obsolete with the passage of time. The entry of a new concept to the pool is marked by B. Creation of new concepts by hybridization between existing ones (C in the figure) or by differentiation of existing ones (point D) are both important methods of change.

Changes in the concept pool will bring cumulative shifts in the explanatory scope of the entire discipline. Because of this, disciplines tend to change in their breadth and content over time. Figure 5.2 illustrates how changes in the conceptual population of a discipline at successive points in time are reflected in variation in an "envelope" that defines its content at each point.

The specific form of any conceptual change will reflect interaction between the current problem set of the discipline and its resources. When an ecological need for innovation is apparent, selection between more than one new concept is likely to lead to acceptance of one that fits the ex-

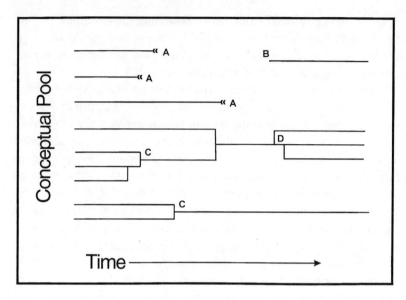

FIG. 5.1. **Typical patterns of conceptual change in an evolving discipline**
(adapted from Toulmin, 1972b)

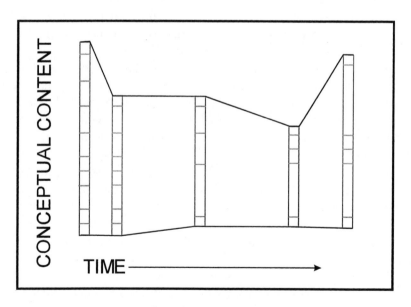

FIG. 5.2. **How disciplinary scope changes with conceptual content**
(adapted from Toulmin, 1972b)

planatory needs best. Figure 5.3, combining the previous two charts, sum-marizes this evolutionary process.

Toulmin provided an elegant model of how human understanding progressed which was not tied to content. He allowed disciplines and their concept pools to be broadly defined, ranging well beyond the pure sciences. However, despite his avowed interest in technology and his interest in the intellectual history of the law, he eschewed detailed study of medicine in general and nosology in particular. It is possible now to discuss, for the first time, the relevance of his ideas to psychiatry.

▪ ▪ Concepts and Psychiatric Diagnosis

It is startling how, despite a quarter century of discussion, Toulmin's ideas have not been applied to medical disciplines. Indeed, it can be argued that medicine in general and psychiatry in particular are more overtly concept centered than purely scientific disciplines, given the central place of diagnosis and the relatively unsystematic nature of their theory. The history of psychiatry would suggest that its conceptual core comprises words such as *delusion, paranoia, depression, dementia, psychopathy, hypochondriasis, delirium,* or *psychosis.* The meaning of each of these terms has

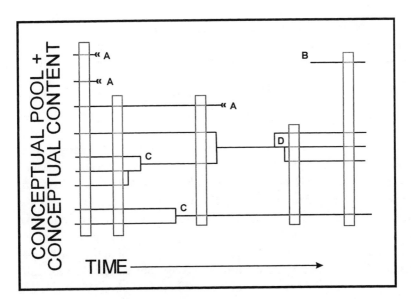

FIG. 5.3. **Evolutionary representation of disciplinary changes**
(adapted from Toulmin, 1972b)

changed with time, as have their perceived relationships. None are completely redundant, at least currently. Even for those that appear obsolete, resurrection from the diagnostic tomb remains an ever present possibility, as the career of words such as *melancholia* or *neurasthenia* indicate. These were widely used in the early decades of this century, rarely used by the 1960s, yet resurrected respectively by the authors of the DSM-III (American Psychiatric Association, 1980) and the ICD-8 (World Health Organization, 1967). What they all have in common is that they are, have been, or remain qualifiers of diagnoses. Whereas it may be professional orthodoxy to attribute very different status to some of these terms than others, for example, those designating disorders of personality against disorders of affect, in an important sense they are all equivalent. This relates to their use rather than their specific content and to their role as currency between members of a psychiatric profession.

It is one of the ironies of psychiatry that, while fiercely resisting militant attacks on the use of diagnostic concepts by people outside the discipline, considerable diffidence remains within it about acknowledging diagnoses for what they are—members of a pool of concepts developed in the light of shared professional needs in order to formulate problems and plan action. Psychiatric diagnoses have fitted Faber's description of the function of diagnoses as well as any in this respect. In practice, the equivalence of psychiatric diagnoses can be disputed—as when one group (such as schizophrenias) is said to represent true illness or disorder in comparison with another (such as personality disorders). These arguments are not pursued here, as such attempts tend to obscure the way in which psychiatric diagnoses enjoy membership of a common conceptual pool. Certainly, the impulse to try to impose ontological divisions can reflect a philosophical confusion that was identified by Kräupl-Taylor (1980) in a scholarly analysis of parallels between arguments in medieval scholasticism and nosology. Nosologists have been as guilty as those early theologians in assuming that a choice has to be made between a realism in which diagnostic concepts stand for entities with a life of their own and a nominalism by which a label has no standing beyond those cases in which it is used. As Kräupl-Taylor points out, the scholastics' solution to this dilemma, conceptualism (in which terms that denote universal properties are acknowledged to have a distinct status in our minds, if not in the world), represents the epistemological situation in nosography extremely well. Conceptualism allows diagnostic terms to exist in the minds of diagnosticians and to fulfill a useful purpose, without implying that they individually correspond to a distinct biological state.

This "conceptualism" tradition certainly meshes well with Toulmin's view of conceptual priority in science and technology, and it may even have an added twist in psychiatry once the character of its diagnostic concepts is analyzed a little further. Kendell (1986), in a discussion of the epistemological status of "disorder," acknowledges the sense of conceptualism. All the major disorders are things that psychiatrists have to talk about and deal with. Recognizing that the weight of epidemiological evidence supports none of the divisions between symptom groups to which our diagnostic concepts correspond, he has gone on to observe (Kendell, 1989, p.51): "The old aphorism that classification is 'the art of carving nature at the joints' loses its force if nature has no joints."

In other words, however important it may be to have a system of diagnostic concepts, no set of concepts can yet claim to be superior as a classificatory system through an appeal to raw clinical data. It might appear that, judged by the standards of an established "compact" science, diagnostic concepts in psychiatry would have a limited value when used to explain the problems it addressed. However, they clearly remain useful to psychiatrists, suggesting that their greatest value may be found in relation to other disciplinary aims, such as the pragmatic one of alleviating mental distress. We have already noted how Toulmin's philosophy does permit pragmatic aims to dictate how a discipline's conceptual content is selected. Insofar as psychiatry differs from other branches of medicine by owning diagnostic concepts serving pragmatic aims at the expense of explanatory power, it might, somewhat paradoxically, approximate rather better to Toulmin's ideal of the "single-value" discipline. The extent to which this is actually the case is considered in the final section.

Philosophically, important questions remain which are not pursued here. For instance, how far, for medicine in general and psychiatry in particular, does nosology represent a more fitting arena than many scientific fields for Toulmin's views on the place and function of concepts? The second key area of Toulmin's thinking, his account of conceptual selection, will now be examined in the context of psychiatry.

▪ ▪ Conceptual Change and Psychiatric Values

The patterns of conceptual change Toulmin charted in other disciplines can be applied to psychiatry rather easily. The types of changes that have occurred over time in the membership of the pool of diagnostic concepts, and in the scope of psychiatry as a discipline, seem to fit his model well. A simple illustration (figure 5.4) can be provided with what is prob-

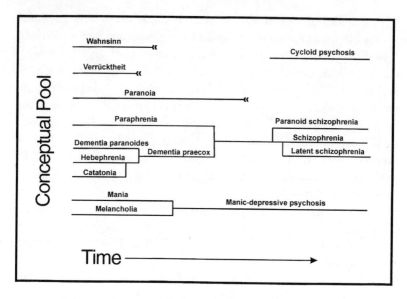

FIG. 5.4. Patterns of conceptual change in the nosology of psychotic illness

ably the most commonly taught piece of conceptual history within programs of clinical training in psychiatry, the nosology of psychotic disorders immediately before and after the introduction of "schizophrenia." (Data illustrated are based on accounts in Berrios and Porter, 1995.)

As will be evident from the direct correspondence with figure 5.1, nosological changes illustrate all the key processes of obsolescence (the fate of *Wahnsinn* and *Verrücktheit*), the formation of new concepts through hybridization (the genesis of dementia praecox and then schizophrenia), the differentiation of concepts once adopted (the variegation of schizophrenia into paranoid, latent, and other subtypes), and the mutation of new diagnoses such as cycloid psychosis to fill a residual need.

Beyond this concordance between the types of conceptual change found in psychiatric diagnosis and those described by Toulmin, Toulmin's detailed account of the mechanisms that prompt conceptual change in response to disciplinary values can help to explain critical developments in diagnostic history. To illustrate its utility, a critical example will be considered. The diagnosis of hysteria is frequently derided as one that has been not only useless but essentially prejudicial and harmful—that is, it represents a rationalization of extrinsic values that have little to do with the identification of disease (Showalter, 1985; Micale, 1995). This presumption of weakness is reflected in the way that Thomas Szasz, having the entire spectrum of psychiatry from which to choose, singled out hysteria as the primary target for his polemical attempts to discredit diagnosis in situations attributed to mental illness (Szasz, 1960). Yet Toulmin's account allows essential steps of hysteria's history as a diagnosis to be explained in terms of the internal needs of the conceptual systems in which it has been part, but without having to appeal to extrinsic values. The primary difficulty posed by hysteria is simply that, as a concept that has traversed disciplinary boundaries, its relationship to professional ideals has been unusually complex. As in the previous example, my concern here is to illustrate principles, not to provide a definitive historical account. I have detailed elsewhere the process by which conversion hysteria joined the class of "mental diseases" within official taxonomies early this century (Mace, 1992) and draw on this now. The emergence of the diagnosis of conversion hysteria was the resultant of three complementary developments in which the impact of changing professional ideals rather than extrinsic values was decisive.

These developments are summarized in figure 5.5, which highlights the rapidly changing interrelationships of the disciplines of neurology, psychiatry, and psychoanalysis around this critical time. A first development was a move within neurology to disown any "functional" disorders that

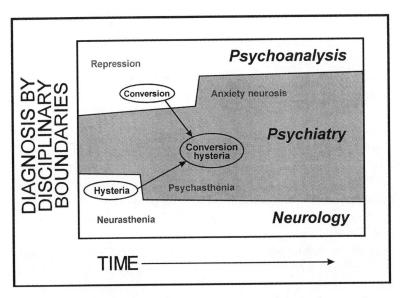

FIG. 5.5. Conceptual change and disciplinary boundaries in the mutation
of conversion hysteria

lacked an anatomical basis, represented (at the bottom of the figure) by the shift in its envelope away from the spreading terrain of psychiatry. This left the diagnostic concepts of hysteria and neurasthenia particularly vulnerable to exclusion from the neurological pool. A second change was the development of psychoanalysis (in the person of Freud) toward a systematic metapsychology that was transcending its origins in psychopathology. (This is represented by its complementary move off the top of the figure away from the medical disciplines.) As its conceptual pool had little further use for mechanisms identified exclusively with one narrow band of psychopathology, conversion was vulnerable to obsolescence within it. The third development was a new receptivity in psychiatry to neurotic illness as it extended beyond asylum-based "alienism." (This is represented by a considerable broadening of its envelope in the center of the figure.) A set of diagnostic niches was created for which there was a relative paucity of candidate concepts. Freud had been able to introduce anxiety neurosis as a diagnostic concept within this vacuum, and it proved a receptive environment in which the psychoanalytic neurological hybrid of conversion hysteria could be translocated as it became a psychiatric diagnosis.

Historically, convincing psychological explanations of the features of hysterical illness had been formulated several times before Freud came along, but these had not led to major diagnostic change (Mace, 1992). The acceptance of the concept of conversion as a diagnostic category where those previous concepts had failed cannot be accounted for without reference to contingent shifts in each discipline. This dynamic meant that the specific merits of Freud's psychodynamic theory were of marginal importance to the adequacy with which it met the needs of the moment. These were dictated by a process that would permit all three disciplines to consolidate, establish, and pursue clearly independent aims.

This example illustrates several central features of Toulmin's account of scientific development. First, a time-worn concept such as hysteria is transformed in its associations and modified in its terminology without being jettisoned. As is often the case in nosology, the familiar concept is qualified and subdivided, in this case into conversion and dissociative hysterias. And as with many scientific concepts, more precision attaches to these qualifiers than the core concept itself.

Second, the major conceptual changes that occurred reflected disciplinary activity. The scale of the changes in individual concepts was linked to realignment in the scope of the disciplines of neurology, psychoanalysis, and psychiatry.

Third, in understanding the character of the change, the relevance of the analogy with Darwinian selection is especially apparent. Toulmin's recognition of "genealogical" and "ecological" factors in speciation has already been cited. In the former, the new development is explained in terms of its continuity with previous variants, the novel design recommending itself through its novel integration of qualities that its predecessors only partially realized. An "ecological" account, conversely, emphasizes the "fittedness" of the new variant to environmental requirements irrespective of its relationship to previous concepts. The acceptance of conversion hysteria as a diagnostic concept was a situation in which ecological factors were paramount, the phenomena it embraced having come for the first time within the ambit of a discipline that suddenly found itself needing a container in which to place them.

It is especially important to remember this when considering subsequent developments in "conversion" within psychiatry. It maintained its place, minor modifications in terminology notwithstanding (e.g., the replacement of *hysteria* by *reaction, disorder,* etc.—cf. Mace, 1992, table 2) despite the progressive attrition of components (symbolization, secondary gain, etc.) central to its definition during earlier phases. This suggests it has survived on the basis of its pragmatic rather than its explanatory function, in the way I have been proposing is most typical of diagnostic concepts in psychiatry.

Finally, we should observe how far a development that has been controversial both within medicine (because of its ambiguity and resistance to reliable definition) and beyond (e.g., in accusations it is a rationalization of antifeminine prejudice) can be explained by reference to internal disciplinary aims.

If Toulmin's tools appear so effective in such a controversial instance, demonstrating the extent to which apparently indefensible diagnostic developments can be understood by reference to the apparently progressive aims of the disciplines concerned, what light can they shed on current psychiatric nosology as exemplified in the DSM-IV?

▪ ▪ The Current Situation

Diagnostic concepts have been considered up to this point without reference to the current treatment in diagnostic manuals. If diagnostic concepts in psychiatry are oriented around pragmatic rather than explanatory values, the idea of a manual that is both diagnostic and statistical could be contradictory if *statistical* implied a descriptive validity that is incompatible with other properties common to concepts that are *diagnostic*. The descriptions of diagnostic categories in manuals such as the DSM-IV seem antithetical on several counts to Toulmin's account of concepts in science and technology.

It may help to ground our discussion with a familiar example of a contemporary diagnosis. One that recommends itself here is somatization disorder, a descendant of some of the concepts discussed in the previous section. Although it had antecedents such as hysteria and Briquet syndrome, it was specifically devised for the DSM-III (American Psychiatric Association, 1980). Criteria for its diagnosis have subsequently been continually revised in specification, but not in kind. The current criteria are summarized in exhibit 5.1.

These criteria for diagnosis are remarkable in a number of interesting, if superficial, respects. For instance, no characteristic psychological features are identified in what is supposed to be a psychiatric syndrome. The many somatic complaints that qualify as symptoms of this syndrome can substitute for one another with extreme fluidity within each broad category. There is no apparent rationale for requiring more pain symptoms than reproductive symptoms, or more gastrointestinal symptoms than pseudoneurological ones. And so forth. However, these are only indicative of a basic weakness of the attitude to diagnosis represented here. This is a particularly clear example of how attention to replicability and minimization of diagnostic overlap occurs at the expense of any coherent theme to link the various components in the definition, so that associations between its components, and between these and its name, appear to be accidental rather than necessary. As a concept, somatization disorder emerges as an entity with an identifiable boundary but no core. Because the basis on which it is recognized is divorced from any reference to psychological dysfunction, clinicians may learn how to apply it, without learning to think with it.

At the same time, this conception of somatization disorder is one that, from a purely clinical standpoint, is at risk of being marginalized. Evidence for this might be found in a 1992 survey of 148 British psychiatrists on the use of somatization disorder (and its European equivalent) as a diagnosis (Stern, Murphy, and Bass, 1993). More than half of this sample had not used it, more than 40 percent did not believe it represented a distinct syndrome, and more than 20 percent of respondents provided additional comments explaining their reservations. The authors summarize these opinions in stating that "such a label implied a false sense of understanding, masked a heterogeneous group of conditions, and was atheoretical" (p. 465). The comments they quote also expressed impatience with any label the psychiatrists felt did not carry clear implications for treatment.

EXHIBIT 5.1. **Diagnostic Criteria for Somatization Disorder**
(adapted from APA, 1994)

A.   A HISTORY OF MANY PHYSICAL COMPLAINTS:

beginning before age thirty;

occur over several years;

lead to treatment seeking or functional impairment.

B.   EACH OF THE FOLLOWING TO HAVE OCCURRED DURING ITS COURSE:

Pain affecting four different sites or functions
(e.g., in head, abdomen, back, joints, extremities, chest, rectum; during menstruation, intercourse, or urination)

Two gastrointestinal symptoms (excluding pain)
(e.g., nausea, bloating, vomiting [excluding pregnancy], diarrhea, intolerance of different foods)

One sexual or reproductive symptom (excluding pain)
(e.g., sexual indifference, erectile or ejaculatory dysfunction, irregular menses, menorrhagia, vomiting in pregnancy)

One pseudoneurological symptom or deficit (not pain)
(e.g., impaired coordination or balance, paralysis, localized weakness, difficulty swallowing, lump in throat, aphonia, urinary retention, hallucinations, loss of touch or pain sensation, double vision, blindness, deafness, seizures, dissociative amnesia, loss of consciousness [excluding fainting])

C.   EITHER:

(1) Each symptom under B cannot be fully explained by a known medical condition or as the direct effect of a substance after appropriate investigation;

OR:

(2) When a related medical condition is present, the physical complaints or resulting impairment exceeds that expected from the history, examination, or lab findings.

D.   SYMPTOMS ARE NOT INTENTIONALLY PRODUCED OR FEIGNED.

Somatization disorder does not appear, therefore, to be a category without which psychiatrists "cannot live, cannot speak, cannot act" (p. 211; cf. Faber, 1923). This modern diagnosis is also very far from some philosophical conceptions of what a diagnosis is, as an ideal and in practice. The most quoted philosophical discussion of psychiatric diagnosis remains that by Carl Hempel. Believing that "the concepts determining the various classes or categories distinguished now are no longer defined just in terms of symptoms but rather in terms of the key concepts of theories which are intended to explain the observable behavior, including the symptoms in question" (Hempel, 1965, p. 326), he went on to cite with approval the typologies of Sheldon (somatic types), Kretschmer (character and physique), and Jung (personality) as indicative of this trend. The only actual diagnosis he cites in detail, conversion hysteria, has been regarded as an anomaly in subsequent DSM manuals because of its theoretical content, while the diagnostic principle quoted above seems irrelevant to the specification of somatization disorder.

If Hempel's philosophical images fail us when grappling with present-day diagnosis, Toulmin's analysis of the nature of shared concepts does not. His understanding of scientific concepts suggests that attempts to make diagnostic concepts absolutely explicit are inherently problematic. They ignore the superordinate status of many concepts necessary in diagnostic thinking and the implicit content, acknowledged by Toulmin's philosophy and traditional diagnostic practice, which each inevitably carries. Instead, the rigor that might reasonably belong to testing of theoretical propositions concerning the factors responsible for features attributed to mental disorders, as Hempel had supposed, appears to be applied to clinical labels, whether or not these represent theoretically coherent entities.

It is Toulmin's interest in conceptual change which indicates still deeper difficulty with recent diagnostic practice, however. Although manualized diagnoses are highly specified in their attempts to be definitive, they can be curiously blind to their own transience. Successive editions of the DSM and ICD will set out widespread revisions, sometimes involving considerable discontinuity between a concept's description in the new edition and its predecessor, while the basis for revision remains unclear, if not incomprehensible. Again, the career of somatization disorder is a clear case in point. Progressively fewer symptoms, of different kinds, have been required to qualify for the diagnosis through its three incarnations in the DSM within a brief fourteen-year career. The episode is very instructive because Toulmin can offer a diagnosis of the difficulty. Normally, concepts within a discipline are revised in the light of its guiding aims and the set of problems it encounters at any given moment. As a matter of recent medical history, the concept of somatization disorder had been introduced in response to a number of significant needs. Among these, the overriding practical need was to have a concept for diagnostic use which safely identified patients with somatic symptoms for whom further unnecessary medical investigations and treatment could legitimately be refused. Accordingly, the concept of hysteria was redefined as a chronic polysymptomatic disorder by Perley and Guze, symptoms being selected according to whether they improved its predictive validity. They summarize their project as follows: "When the diagnosis of hysteria was based on defined clinical criteria, there was a 90 percent probability that the clinical picture would remain unchanged over a number of years and that no other disorder that might explain the original symptoms would develop" (Perley and Guze, 1962, p. 426).

Their set of criteria were then successfully tested for their discriminatory potential in a population of women having multiple symptoms attributable to medical disorders (Woodruff, 1967). However, as the criteria for polysymptomatic hysteria have weakened through its metamorphoses as Briquet syndrome and somatization disorder, they have not been subjected to comparable tests of their predictive validity. There is no evidence a diagnosis of somatization disorder retains the practical implications of Perley and Guze's diagnosis, inviting understandable skepticism about its utility. One study finding that diagnoses of the DSM-III–defined somatization disorder are often retained at follow-up does not report how often other disorders supervene to account for symptoms with this weaker diagnostic requirement (cf. Cloninger et al., 1986).

In a short time, therefore, this diagnostic concept has come adrift from the problem it was meant to address. Criticisms quoted earlier of the atheoretical status of somatization disorder were not wholly fair because modern psychiatry has valued pragmatic over theoretical aims in a way that is widely reflected in its selection of diagnostic concepts. However, instead of revisions of this concept representing successive attempts to meet a specific pragmatic aim more adequately, we find that aim being abandoned with no clear alternative taking its place. This is not how rational disciplines are supposed to behave. If this erratic progress is typical of diagnostic change in the era of operationalized manuals, how should it be accounted for?

One major development likely to affect the role and form of modern diagnostic concepts has been their removal, in formalized manuals especially, from the exclusive preserve of psychiatry. Other interests are asserting themselves, ranging from those of medical scientists concerned primarily with diagnoses' operational reliability, to administrators seeking inclusiveness at any price (Carson, 1991). If the clinical needs of psychiatrists are having less influence on how the categories of psychiatric nosology are shaped, other influences seem to be growing. It is evident in specific instances how nonmedical values influence where lines are drawn; for instance, once "major depression" becomes a prerequisite for an admission to the hospital to be funded when a patient is dysphoric, then the criteria for "major depression" will represent a consensus of what the requirements are for hospital admission. The very wish to draw diagnostic boundaries in absolutely clear lines, not essential to traditional diagnosis, has become necessary through extraprofessional values. Explicit criteria are bureaucratically tidy, and they are demanded as summary statements of patients' problems and needs are increasingly communicated between administrative workers lacking clinical training or responsibility.

In one sense, the exploitation of psychiatric diagnosis for ends that remain pragmatic, even if they go beyond the normal limits of medical intervention, is a logical extension of aims that had previously informed it. However, it still contradicts a central element of Toulmin's account of progressive conceptual change. The link between host discipline and conceptual system has become attenuated and threatens to break altogether. Until recent times, this had not been of huge practical significance because, if official classifications were out of step with clinical thinking, they were by and large ignored. (The discussion of somatization disorder illustrated how clinicians will still do this when working in a culture in which a weak diagnosis remains outside the administrative system.) Currently, clinicians are under unprecedented pressure to adopt diagnostic systems that may be at odds with the way they have been trained to construct their professional experiences.

Toulmin's account of professional evolution, claiming to be descriptive rather than prescriptive, provides a yardstick against which it is easy to see that a change has occurred. It also implies that the current situation, in which the development of diagnostic concepts has lost its clear link with the disciplinary aims that had previously informed it, is unstable. If it carries no necessary message for what will or should follow, it tells us that something must give and why. I shall conclude by returning to Toulmin's analysis to indicate two of the possible directions change could take. These correspond to Toulmin's distinction between changes that are a response to a major change in environmental demands (the ecological account) and those that are a response to existing problems within the discipline which, in leading to major conceptual change, also change its scope (the genealogical account).

One scenario, in the absence of major conceptual innovation, would be for further disciplinary diversification to develop within the present sea of activity. As research, administrative, and clinical disciplines encompassing psychiatry and clinical psychology were reformed according to distinct aims and values, each would have its own morbid classification in which the form of diagnostic concepts as well as their delineation would be sensitive to their differing needs. There would be scope for many new concepts to fill gaps in these three independent classifications following partition. This would be rationally defensible in that classifications of mental disorder devised for clinical use by mental health specialists do not enjoy the same validity among other patient populations (Jenkins, Smeton, and Shepherd, 1988). However, the twin engines of managed care and evidence-based practice seem to militate toward imposition of classificatory systems on clinicians whether or not, at the nosographic level, the categories reflect the realities of the clinicians' daily practice.

Alternatively, if genealogical factors proved decisive in future change, the present impasse might be resolved by a radical disciplinary shift or reorganization that was secondary to a major conceptual change like those that, historically, followed the widespread recourse to morbid anatomy or discovery of the microbial basis of disease transmission. These events are, by definition, impossible to predict, but they involve a shift toward or away from other disciplines by virtue of the new discovery. The involvement of ever widening circles of people in discussion of diagnostic classification, in the absence of clear criteria or mechanisms for reform, means that its rationale is being appraised in principle as well as detail. Although there is growing confidence among those claiming that nosology can be placed on a sound biological footing, basic questions about the content validity of morbid categories right across psychiatric classification are being raised (Radden, 1994), and cogent proposals can also be made for reformed classifications that are grounded in the theory of social science (e.g., Sadler, 1994). Toulmin's analysis of conceptual change would suggest that any internally driven change would inevitably require professional realignments. Whether a future set of rational classificatory principles were phenomenological, etiological, pragmatic, statistical, or economic, neighboring disciplines would undergo considerable readjustment. At the same time, a new professional grouping could be expected to appear whose aims and values were relatively cohesive and were directly reflected in the system of clinical concepts which its members used and maintained.

Technical Reason in the DSM-IV:
An Unacknowledged Value

JAMES PHILLIPS, M.D.

THE OFFICIAL GOAL of the DSM-IV is apparent: it is to provide a scientifically grounded nosology that will be useful to both practitioners and researchers. In the DSM-IV the twin standards of construct validity and reliability are balanced to accomplish in correct proportion an accurate description of existing psychiatric disorders as well as reliable communication among users of the system, whether practitioners or researchers. In this chapter I wish to suggest another value that is implicit in the nosology—and not acknowledged as such—which I identify as the value of technical reason. My argument is that the manual is constructed so as to allow the maximal exercise of technical reason. This is, of course, not without consequences for all the user populations involved with the DSM-IV: patients, practitioners, researchers, insurance industry, public policy makers. That the technicist approach I describe is not inevitable will become clearer when it is contrasted with an alternative approach, that of practical reason.

In arguing that the DSM-IV allows maximal use of technical reason, I am not claiming that this represents the intention of the authors. There is every reason to think that their goal is a balance of the practical and the technical. My claim is rather that the DSM-IV lends itself readily to the strong technical bias in contemporary psychiatry. Technical reason is indeed an *acknowledged* value in contemporary psychiatry; its status as an *unacknowledged* value in the DSM-IV stems from the way in which it can be used to support the acknowledged technical bias in contemporary psychiatry.

The distinction between technical and practical reason as developed in this chapter follows the original differentiation articulated by Aristotle, and his early analysis and its legacy are described below. This effort to associate psychiatry with Aristotle's concept of practical knowledge, or phronesis, follows attempts by others to bring medicine in general under the rubric of Aristotelian phronesis. Typical of those attempts is Pellegrino and Thomasma's statement about medicine that "in the Aristotelian sense it is a habit of practical understanding refined and perfected by experience in dealing with patients" (1981, p. 59). (See also Beresford, 1996; Hunter, 1989; Widdershoven-Heerding, 1987.)

▪ ▪ Technical Reason

What do I mean by technical reason? The standpoint of technical rationality is that for any problem area there is a systematic body of generalized knowledge, with specific rules for application, which can define the handling of a particular case and thus minimize or eliminate the need for real judgment on the part of the individual practitioner. From this point of view knowledge is essentially instrumental, organized into means-ends structures; any problem can be analyzed in a way that allows for a means-ends formulation and a formulaic solution. A particular problem is always an instance of a general type, and knowledge of the type allows for application of the appropriate means to accomplish the respective end of that type of problem. The application of this kind of knowledge to the field of psychiatry—as well as to all of medicine—should be immediately clear. The schematic formula is not difficult to state: the patient's problem is an instance of condition A, which requires treatment B. Thus, if the patient has condition A, apply treatment B. The only requirement of the practitioner in this model is that he or she be able to recognize the particular case as an instance of the general disease (or disorder) type and be able to apply the relevant treatment. This technical approach to diagnosis and treatment is not that different from the technical attitude in other problem domains, in which the image of broken object and repair manual prevails. With the technicist strategy in psychiatry we are close to seeing the patient as something broken which can be fixed with a correct use of the psychiatric repair manual.

Two aspects of this technical approach to diagnosis and treatment in psychiatry need to be emphasized, the first relating to the patient, the second to the treater. The first is that the focus is on the general type of problem or disorder, not on the individual instantiation of the general type.

Thus the critical question becomes, What is the diagnosis and treatment of schizophrenia, of major depression, and so on, not, How do I think about and treat this individual? Stated in the instrumentalist formula, the end is the diagnosis and treatment of schizophrenia; the means is the treatment modality that works for this general disorder. Variations among individual schizophrenic patients are accorded importance only to the extent that they can be aggregated into subgroups, thus again into general subtypes.

A second aspect of the technical approach is that the reduction of the treatment to a generalizable structure tends to eliminate the individuality of the treater. The field abounds in examples of this tendency. When we are offered an algorithm for the treatment of depression or panic disorder, the clear implication is that any competent psychiatrist can apply the algorithm and carry out the treatment. We then have the generic psychiatrist doing generic treatment, just as any physician can prescribe the appropriate antibiotic for a sinus infection and accomplish the same treatment goal. We even have the example of the currently faddish dialectical behavioral therapy (Linehan, 1993), in which the specific claim is that practically anyone can be quickly trained to do the treatment, with no regard for prior training. Still a further example of this tendency to eliminate the individuality of the treater is the now fashionable "evidence-based treatment." Here again the practitioner refers to a database of controlled studies and allows his or her treatment to be dictated by those studies. As one writer describes it, "evidence-based medicine trains doctors to search medical journals and databases for tests and treatments that have helped large groups of patients. Then, they apply the information to their own patients, under the statistical assurance that what holds true for groups is likely to be valid for individuals" (Zuger, 1997). At its worst, this approach results in what we can call a robotic treatment, a treatment in which the practitioner assumes the qualities of an unthinking robot.

What is missing in this technicist model? The answer, of course, is the dimension of the practical experience of the seasoned practitioner. Or to use another language, what is left out is the *art* or *craft* of psychiatry, as opposed to the *science* of psychiatry. What the model of technical reason assumes is that the scientific basis of psychiatry can be made so strong that there will be virtually no need for individual experience and judgment. Psychiatry as craft will give way to psychiatry as science (for discussions of this debate, see Clouser, 1977; Forstrom, 1977; McWhinney, 1978; Munson, 1981; Toulmin, 1976). This is an illusion of technical mastery in which serious doubt and fallibility in the diagnosis and treatment are eliminated. The contrasting situation—which I argue is that faced by practitioners most of the time—is one of uncertainty and fallibility in the actual treatment (Gorovitz and MacIntyre, 1976; Greenblatt, 1980). The diagnosis may be unclear, the range of possible treatment approaches may be varied, and the patient may have his or her own ideas about how to proceed. The direction of treatment will ultimately depend on the clinical judgment of the individual practitioner, in conjunction with—and in dialogue with—the patient's expressed wishes. The scope of practical knowledge is developed further on in this chapter, but I want to mention now that a practical approach does not exclude the use of technical knowledge, any more than psychiatry as craft would exclude psychiatry as partial science. The experienced practitioner will use all the technical knowledge available in determining how to deal with the individual patient. What the practical approach *does* exclude is the illusion of technical mastery. What the experienced practitioner is *not* is a robot.

With this description of technical reason as background, it still remains to be clarified how the nosological approach of the DSM-IV (as well as the DSM-III and DSM-III-R) depends on or fosters technical reason. Since the manual says nothing about treatment and only formulates diagnoses, the answer to this question may not be immediately apparent. The answer is in the effort of precision that goes into the manual. The technical, instrumental formula, as described above, was: first define the problem (the end) precisely, then define the means for resolving it. The DSM-IV, in giving the impression of great precision in the first half of the instrumental formula, the problem to be solved—that is, the diagnosis—fosters the belief that the second half, the exact treatment, will follow. The manual thus fosters the technical attitude and its illusion of mastery in the various populations of users. If major depression can be precisely described, then a precise treatment will surely follow. It could certainly be argued that the statement of a precise definition does not guarantee or necessitate a precise treatment. For any precisely defined condition, it may, for instance, eventuate in the empirical world that there is not any treatment—or that there are several possible treatments. The issue here is more one of attitude. Does the diagnostic approach of the DSM-IV foster the kind of knowledge and treatment approach being described as that of technical reason? I am, of course, arguing that it does, but we need to examine the evidence to the contrary.

To begin with, it can be argued that diagnostic criteria sets, rather than fostering an illusion of technical mastery, and rather than eliminating the role of clinical judgment in psychiatric practice, merely provide guidelines for the practitioner in the assessment of a particular patient. In this sense they may be seen as quite practical rather than as overly technical. In this regard we should pay due attention to two statements from the DSM-IV introduction. In a section entitled "Issues in the Use of DSM-IV," and under the heading "Limitation of the Categorical Approach," we find:

> In DSM-IV, there is no assumption that each category of mental disorder is a completely discrete entity with absolute boundaries dividing it from other mental disorders or from no mental disorder. There is also no assumption that all individuals described as having the same mental disorder are alike in all important ways. The clinician using DSM-IV should therefore consider that individuals sharing a diagnosis are likely to be heterogenous even in regard to the defining features of the diagnosis and that boundary cases will be difficult to diagnose in any but a probabilistic fashion. This outlook allows greater flexibility in the use of the system, encourages more specific attention to boundary cases, and emphasizes the need to capture additional clinical information that goes beyond diagnosis. In recognition of the heterogeneity of clinical presentations, DSM-IV often includes polythetic criteria sets, in which the individual need only present with a subset of items from a longer list (e.g., the diagnosis of Borderline Personality Disorder requires only five out of nine items). (American Psychiatric Association, 1994, p. xxii)

And under another heading, "Use of Clinical Judgment," we find this statement:

> DSM-IV is a classification of mental disorders that was developed for use in clinical, educational, and research settings. The diagnostic categories, criteria, and textual descriptions are meant to be employed by individuals with appropriate clinical training and experience in diagnosis. It is important that DSM-IV not be applied mechanically by untrained individuals. The specific diagnostic criteria included in DSM-IV are meant to serve as guidelines to be informed by clinical judgment and are not meant to be used in a cookbook fashion. For example, the exercise of clinical judgment may justify giving a certain diagnosis to an individual even though the clinical presentation falls just short of meeting the full criteria for the diagnosis as long as the symptoms that are present are persistent and severe. On the other hand, lack of familiarity with DSM-IV or excessively flexible and idiosyncratic application of DSM-IV criteria or conventions substan-

tially reduces its utility as a common language for communication. (American Psychiatric Association, 1994, p. xxiii)

These are certainly both statements that *discourage* an overly technical use of the DSM-IV. If we can assume that the authors of the DSM-IV are not being disingenuous in their introduction, we must conclude that the technicalized use of the manual by managed care and other sectors of contemporary psychiatry does not represent the goal of the authors. On the other hand, their caution regarding the use of the manual in a cookbook fashion is an implicit acknowledgment that the manual does lend itself to that kind of use. As suggested in the introduction to this chapter, my argument is not about the intentions of the authors of the DSM-IV but rather about the technicalized use that the manual readily fosters.

▪ ▪ The Aristotelian Legacy

The discussion of different kinds of knowledge which is at the basis of this chapter has its origin in Aristotle, specifically in the distinction he draws between technical and practical knowledge. For that reason it will be useful to frame the discussion in the context of Aristotle's analysis and in the legacy of his thought.

Aristotle distinguishes between technical knowledge, *technē*, which is concerned with the process of making something, *poiēsis*, and practical knowledge, *phronēsis*, which is concerned with action and living well, *praxis*. The master of a technique has a firm idea of the thing to be made and is able to work from this clearly held idea to the production of the object. The idea of the completed object can be understood separately from the means, the techne, of producing it. Aristotle's model for techne and poiesis is the skilled craftsman, who possesses expertise in the principles governing his particular area of production, such as house building. This is an expertise that has a strong theoretical component—a knowledge of cause and effect in the particular area—and which can be taught to other potential craftsmen. Distinguishing the theoretical knowledge of the technical master from the more modest knowledge of the man of experience, Aristotle writes:

> We think that *knowledge* and *understanding* belong to techne rather than to experience . . . and this because the former know the cause, but the latter do not. For men of experience know that the thing is so, but do not know why, while the others know the "why" and the cause. Hence we think also that the master-workers in each craft are more honourable and know in a truer sense and are wiser than the

manual workers, because they know the causes of the things that are done . . . thus we view them as being wiser not in virtue of being able to act, but of having the theory for themselves and knowing the causes. And in general it is a sign of the man who knows and of the man who does not know, that the former can teach, and therefore we think techne more truly knowledge than experience is; for masters of technique can teach, and men of mere experience cannot. (1941a, 981a, p. 690)

Practical knowledge, or phronesis, is sharply contrasted with the theory-laden expertise of techne. Concerned with action and the question of how to live well, practical knowledge is bound to the particular situation and the unique challenges it poses. The particular situation is an area in which unvarying universal principles are not available which will dictate what is to be done. The general principle is there for guidance, but in each circumstance it will be applied—and indeed understood—somewhat differently. Practical knowledge cannot be simply taught—or learned from a manual; it is learned through experience, for which there is no substitute. Aristotle writes:

Practical wisdom on the other hand is concerned with things human and things about which it is possible to deliberate; for we say this is above all the work of the man of practical wisdom, to deliberate well, but no one deliberates about things invariable, nor about things which have not an end, and that a good that can be brought about by action. The man who is without qualification good at deliberating is the man who is capable of aiming in accordance with calculation at the best for man of things attainable by action. Nor is practical wisdom concerned with universals only—it must also recognize the particulars; for it is practical, and practice is concerned with particulars. This is why some who do not know, and especially those who have experience, are more practical than others who know. (1941b, 1141b, pp. 1028–29)

In developing these Aristotelian notions we must note certain modifications of them in Aristotle's own thought (see Dunne, 1993, pp. 237–356). To begin with, there is a certain blurring of what falls under the rubric of the technical and what under the rubric of the practical. Formally, techne involves the making of something and phronesis ethical action. But Aristotle includes a variety of *activities* under the category of techne. And regarding phronesis he broadens the concept to activities other than ethical action. A clear example of the blurring of techne and phronesis is medicine. Although often called a techne, it is action rather than production, and it shares all the uncertainty that is part of phronesis. In fact, when describing the conditions of practical knowledge, rather than calling on an instance of ethical behavior for an example, Aristotle often invokes the example of medicine.

> The whole account of matters of conduct must be given in outline and not precisely, as we said at the beginning that the accounts we demand must be in accordance with the subject matter; matters concerned with conduct and questions of what is good for us have no fixity, any more than matters of health. The general account being of this nature, the account of particular cases is yet more lacking in exactness; for they do not fall under any art or precept but the agents themselves must in each case consider what is appropriate to the occasion, as happens also in the art of medicine or of navigation. (1941b, 1104a, p. 953)

A further modification, related to the one just indicated, is that technical knowledge is formally quite theory laden but is in fact often described in the experiential terminology of practical knowledge. Medicine is again a ready example. The consequence is that activities such as medicine or navigation might be alternatively described by Aristotle either as technical expertises, but with all the experiential limitations of practical knowledge, or as practical activities.

Still another modification of Aristotle's thinking has to do with the respective values placed on the domains of technical and practical knowledge. Given his general privileging of theoretical knowledge and his statements—as the one above—concerning the superiority of techne *as theoretical,* one would expect a derogation of practical knowledge as inferior to more theoretical forms. In all his complexity, however, this is not the whole story with Aristotle. There are other occasions of his showing an appropriate respect for practical knowledge as a quite worthy contender with the more theoretical types. In this vein he writes:

> With a view to action, experience seems in no respect inferior to techne, and men of experience succeed even better than those who have theory without experience. (The reason is that experience is knowledge of individuals, techne of universals, and actions and productions are all concerned with the individual; for the physician does not cure *man,* except in an incidental way, but Callias or Socrates or

some other called by some such individual name, who happens to be a man. If, then, a man has the theory without the experience, and recognizes the universal but does not know the individual included in this, he will often fail to cure; for it is the individual that is to be cured. (1941a, 981, pp. 689–90)

Finally, we may summarize this discussion of Aristotle by saying that his distinction between techne and phronesis ultimately translates into the more modern distinction between theory and practice, or theory and experience. Aristotle's importance is indeed that he is at the origin of this modern distinction. As indicated above, techne stands in sharpest contrast to phronesis when its theoretical side is emphasized. And phronesis, once it is broadened beyond ethical activity to any human endeavor that engages one in the challenges of the particular situation, easily translates into practice and experience.

▪ ▪ The Modern Tradition

To complete this historical review it will be useful to trace the course of Aristotle's legacy into the contemporary era. The significant step into the modern era occurred with the transformation of knowledge and epistemology in the seventeenth century, a transformation we associate with the names Descartes and Galileo. With the assimilation of Aristotle's theoretical techne into modern rationalism, the role of practical knowledge or experience was brutally devalued into the unreliable categories of secondary qualities or subjectivity. In the rationalist view the world is viewed as a mechanistically understood nature from which the knower can take distance and form an objective picture, uncontaminated by human subjectivity and uncertainty. In Thomas Nagel's description, this is a "view from nowhere": the attempt is made to view the world not from a place within it, or from the vantage point of a special kind of life or awareness, but from nowhere in particular and no form of life in particular at all. The object is to discount for the features of our prereflective outlook which make things appear as they do and thereby to reach an understanding of things as they really are. We flee the subjective under the pressure of an assumption that everything must be something not to any point of view but in itself. To grasp this by detaching more and more from our own point of view is the unreachable ideal at which the pursuit of objectivity aims (Nagel, 1979, p. 208).

Charles Taylor analyzed modern rationalism as an effort to take a disengaged stance toward the world and then read the features of the rationalist, disengaged attitude into the very constitution of the mind. "The disengaged perspective, which might better have been conceived as a rare and regional achievement of a knowing agent whose normal stance was engaged, was read into the very nature of the mind" (1995, p. 66). He isolates three features of the disengaged mind: an atomism of input, a computational picture of mental function, and a view of the input as value-free "facts." These features, which derive from Cartesian and empiricist seventeenth-century epistemologies, are quite congruent with contemporary mechanistic, computer-based models of the mind and for that reason have continued to maintain their influence, despite their, for Taylor, blatant incoherence. Taylor's argument against the "disengaged stance," for which argument he finds support in Heidegger and Wittgenstein, is the failure of the rationalist position to take account of the context or background in which all knowing occurs. What this means is that I do not have a "view from nowhere" of the world. My contact with the world is always situated in a context. I am always in some fashion "engaged"; there is always a "background" for that on which I am focusing. "When we find a certain experience intelligible, what we are attending to, explicitly and expressly, is this experience. The context stands as the unexplicited horizon within which— or to vary the image, as the vantage point out of which—this experience can be understood. To use Michael Polanyi's language, it is subsidiary to the focal object of awareness; it is what we are 'attending from' as we attend to the experience" (Taylor, 1995, pp. 68–69). In contrast to the disengaged stance, Taylor argues that knowing is always finite and situated. There is always a background of implicit assumptions against which any act of focused knowing takes place. We make the effort to bring the background into focal awareness, but this is always an unfinished task.

While Taylor's argument is implicitly—and at times explicitly (1985, pp. 45–76)—hermeneutic, we may continue this excursus into the fate of theory and experience and at the same time circle around back to Aristotle, by focusing on the hermeneutic thought of Hans-Georg Gadamer and his reappropriation of Aristotle. The point was made above that in the modern era Aristotle's distinction between techne and phronesis was translated into that between theory and experience and that theory took on the features of disengaged, objective knowledge of a neutralized, mechanistic world. The development of hermeneutics in the nineteenth and twentieth centuries may be seen as a reaction to this notion of theory and as a rehabilitation of experience as a valid source of knowledge. In the hermeneutic tradition, especially as developed by Wilhelm Dilthey, the re-

habilitation of experience took the form of the assertion that the experi-
ence-based human studies, the *Geisteswissenschaften,* have a methodology
that is independent of and different from that of the natural sciences, the
Naturwissenschaften. It is hardly surprising that we find in Dilthey a focus
on the individual which is reminiscent of Aristotle's practical knowledge.

It is, however, in Gadamer's development of hermeneutic thought that
we see the full reappropriation of Aristotle. For Gadamer hermeneutic understanding in the human sciences always involves interpretation; the two
form a unified process. Gadamer insists, however, that a third component
accompanies understanding and interpretation, namely, application. For
him application is not an add-on that may or may not accompany understanding and interpretation; the three form an indissoluble unity. Hermeneutic understanding is thus in its essence practical. It is because of this
integration of application into the process of understanding and interpretation that Gadamer accords to legal and theological hermeneutics a priority over literary hermeneutics as models of understanding in the human
sciences.

This practical dimension of hermeneutic understanding is what brings
Gadamer to Aristotle's phronesis. It is in the dialectic of the universal and
the particular found by Aristotle at the very heart of practical knowledge
that Gadamer finds a critical link with the hermeneutic unity of interpretation and application which he investigates. "If the heart of the hermeneu-
tical problem is that the same tradition must always be understood in a different way, the problem, logically speaking, is that of the relationship
between the universal and the particular. Understanding is, then, a particular case of the application of something universal to a particular situation. This makes Aristotelian ethics of special importance for us" (Gadamer, 1975, p. 278). Just as the Aristotelian ethical man must sort out how to
apply a general moral principle to the concrete situation in which he finds
himself, so must the Gadamerian interpreter sort out how the historical
text or phenomenon engages him- or herself now in the present. And, of
course, so must the clinician sort out how to apply the general diagnostic
categories to the individual facing him or her.

Finally, we may complete this trajectory of theory and experience by
focusing on some of the contemporary discussion of theory and practice
in medicine. Although in spirit both Aristotelian and hermeneutic, such
discussion is not necessarily articulated in the language of either. Stephen
Toulmin, for instance, reasons from a philosophy of science perspective
about the multilayered structure of medical knowledge and the primacy of
focus on the individual patient.

The spectrum of medical knowledge runs all the way from a general extreme (e.g., the fundamental principles of biochemistry as applied to physiology) to a particular extreme (e.g., a practitioner's understanding of the cardiovascular distress of his immediate patient). It embraces both idealized, or Platonic, theoretical models, as in parts of neurophysiology, and more concrete, or Aristotelian, analyses, as in general pathology. Yet the generality characteristic of biomedical science has to achieve an effective union with the particularity of clinical treatment, most particularly with the individuality of the relationship between the patient and his personal physician. From this latter standpoint, the doctor's mission thus has more in common with the historian's or biographer's—not to mention the minister's—than it does with physics or zoology. A medical history is just what its name suggests: the chronicle of an individual human life considered and digested with selective attention to the episodes significant for current treatment. Though the physician's particular understanding of some individual patient may rely on general principles, whether physiological or psychological, the principles themselves will have medical significance only insofar as they can be related to a personal understanding of the particularities of clinical practice with actual patients, that is, individual human beings coming for professional advice. (1976, p. 40)

In an excellent review of the rise of technology in medicine, McWhinney shows how the "misuse" of technology has led to the devaluation of the craft dimension of medical practice.

As a generalization, it can be said that technology is harmful when its values override other human values without any substantial net benefit. . . . We will see that a constant theme is the tendency for medicine to be dominated by the mechanistic values of objectivity, precision, and standardization. The dominance of mechanistic over other values has not only affected our actions but also our concept of medical knowledge. Although the understanding of patients and their illnesses requires a blend of objective and subjective knowledge, medical education has become concerned overwhelmingly with objective knowledge. The *episteme* of technology has become the *episteme* of medicine. (1978, p. 299)

In another study Sadler and Hulgus (1994) reintroduced the nineteenth-century German philosopher Wilhelm Windelband's distinction between nomothetic (i.e., oriented toward general laws) and idiographic (i.e., oriented toward the unique event) science in an effort to critique the DSM-IV as tilting too much toward the nomothetic ideal. Their argument for a large idiographic component in psychiatry and psychiatric classification is clearly quite consistent with the argument being made in this chapter.

A final example of contemporary discussion is Richard Zaner's *Medicine and Dialogue* (1990), in which he reviews many aspects of medicine as a praxis oriented toward the suffering individual, including the therapeutic necessity and benefit of the unique doctor-patient relationship. Zaner emphasizes that medicine is in its essence a moral, rather than scientific, practice and that its proper focus is the patient's *illness* rather than the patient's *disease* (the latter is a biological concept, the former a broader concept that includes the patient's experience of his or her condition). Further, Zaner underscores the fact that the physician will come to an understanding of the patient's experience only through a dialogue with the latter.

▪ ▪ Theory and Practice in the DSM-IV

In an earlier section the argument was made that the DSM-IV fosters the aims of technical reason in psychiatry. With the immediately preceding section as background, the question of technical versus practical reason in the DSM-IV can now be discussed in more depth. Technical reason, it may be recalled, is the theory-laden generalized knowledge that has its origins in Aristotle's techne and its more recent incarnation in modern rationalism. Practical reason, in contrast, is knowledge oriented to an understanding of the individual in which the general principle is tailored to the individual situation and is thus viewed somewhat differently in each of its instantiations. In the case of technical knowledge the practitioner must be an expert in the general principles of the respective discipline; he or she must know the manual's details well. In the case of practical knowledge the practitioner must be an expert in the understanding of individuals; he or she must know how to subordinate the manual to the particularities of the individual. (Each kind of practice will, of course, require its own kind of experience. The expert DSM-IV diagnostician will be someone experienced in working with this manual. In this chapter, however, *experience* is used in a different sense—as a *contrast* to theory; it is used to describe the kind of practical knowledge which comes from a long experience of working with many individuals and which cannot be neatly formulated into general principles.)

It might be objected at this point that I am drawing too sharp a distinction between technical and practical knowledge in the DSM-IV. The DSM-IV diagnostician must, after all, diagnose the individual. Being an expert in the manual does not relieve one of the task of *applying* the manual to the individual in the consulting room. Where, then, is the difference between the so-called technical expert and the so-called practical expert? When all is said and done, each must find an appropriate diagnosis and treat the patient. Although there is indeed some validity to this objection and thus some overlap between the activity of the two experts, I argue that the distinction does hold—that the DSM-IV, even in its application, tends to privilege technical over practical knowledge. This will become clear with the use of an example. Let us take up the group of psychotic disorders.

The psychotic disorders are typical of DSM-IV disorders in that each condition is organized around an elaborate criteria set that attempts to delimit the respective disorder sufficiently to allow most clinicians to agree on a diagnosis. Schizophrenia is typical of the precise, obsessive DSM-IV style. The patient must manifest at least two of a list of symptoms for a substantial part of at least one month. The patient must have shown evidence of the condition for at least six continuous months (and during at least one month of which must have shown the psychotic symptoms from the first criterion). For much of the period of illness the disorder must have caused dysfunction in work, socialization, and so on. Finally, the diagnosis is made only in the absence of mood disorders and schizoaffective disorder, medical conditions and substance use that cause psychosis, and developmental disorders. Other psychotic disorders are analogously defined and can often be cross-related to one another. Thus schizophreniform disorder is used for patients who meet criteria for schizophrenia except for the six-month duration; schizoaffective disorder shows symptoms of schizophrenia but with the presence of prominent manic or depressive symptoms; and so forth.

The question we must pose is this: What kind of knowledge or expertise is required to make these DSM-IV diagnoses? To begin with, the clinician will have to know the manual pretty well, or at least be adept in referring to it and using it when confronted with a patient to be diagnosed. This will require not merely knowing the various definitions and criteria sets but also having an understanding of the terms used in the definitions and an ability to evaluate them in patients. Thus, for the psychoses one will have to understand symptoms such as delusions, hallucinations, thought disorder, and flat affect and be able to diagnose them in particular patients.

The critical question here is how this diagnostic application to the individual patient is made. It is in fact made, not through an appreciation of the individuality of the patient, but rather through a mechanical listing of symptoms and diagnostic criteria, in which process the patient appears only as an instance of a disorder. Far from discouraging an *atomistic* approach to the symptom and criteria clusters, the DSM-IV virtually invites such an approach. Each symptom or diagnostic criterion is treated as a piece of data which is aggregated with other pieces into the recognizable criteria sets. In the case of schizophrenia, for instance, one is asked to find and aggregate symptoms, not to relate them to one another to develop a coherent picture of the illness presentation. A duration of illness of five months, for instance, defines a different illness than a duration of seven months. All the cautions of the manual introduction notwithstanding, the diagnostic system does not encourage one to question whether it is indeed the same illness but only to make the distinction and place the individual into the correct diagnostic category (Miller, 1990). The tendency to aggregate and cluster symptoms and criteria into the respective diagnostic categories is dramatically formalized in the graphical, computational algorithms that are popular as a method to aid the diagnostician in navigating his or her way through the diagnostic quagmire of the DSM-IV.

This atomistic procedure is certainly reminiscent of the manner in which modern rationalism was described above by Charles Taylor: an atomism of input and a computational analysis of the input. It is thus possible to view the DSM-IV as an undertaking in the modern rationalist tradition. The world (i.e., psychiatric patients) is objectivized into a field of observable pieces of data. These data are then subjected to a computational analysis and aggregated into defined clusters. With such an approach it is hardly surprising that the DSM-IV fits neatly into computerized protocols and diagnostic algorithms. Nor is it surprising that the DSM-IV can be used rather robotically by minimally trained clinicians. Nor, finally, is it surprising that clinicians begin to view their patients, their patients' disorders, and the treatments of those disorders through the atomistic lens of the DSM-IV. In this we have a final confirmation of Taylor's analysis. His point, it may be recalled, was that "the disengaged perspective, which might better have been conceived as a rare and regional achievement of a knowing agent whose normal stance was engaged, was read into the very nature of the mind" (1995, p. 66).

We have something very analogous with the DSM-IV and the current state of psychiatry. The atomistic/computational method of the DSM-IV could be regarded as a limited but useful approach to diagnosis, chosen for its efficacy in achieving reliability across diagnosticians. The fine-tuned obsessiveness in symptom counting allows for a precision and reliability in diagnosis—whatever its validity—which is clearly useful for communication among researchers and clinicians. But it is quite another thing to mistake this heuristic achievement for an accurate picture of the reality in question. People—and psychiatric conditions—are not atomistic clusters of behavioral traits and symptoms. Yet that is how they have come to be seen in the era of DSM-IV–oriented psychiatry. Just as, according to Taylor, the atomistic, disengaged approach was read into the constitution of the mind, so has the atomistic approach to psychiatric disorders been read into the constitution of those conditions.

As was indicated in an earlier section, the apparent technical mastery of achieving diagnostic reliability in the DSM-IV fosters a similar illusion of objectivity and mastery in the area of treatment. Viewed as atomistically defined, objectivized conditions that can be *diagnosed* by following the rules of a technical diagnostic manual, the same conditions can now be *treated* by following the rules of a technical treatment manual. As discussed earlier, this approach to treatment reduces the expertise of the clinician to that of knowing what treatment fits a particular diagnostic entity. Within this technical paradigm we witness a spectrum of therapeutic experience and expertise. At one extreme there are the treatment modalities, such as dialectical behavioral therapy, which actually boast of being manual-driven therapies that can be done by anyone. At the other extreme are the experienced psychopharmacologists who develop an expertise in complicated pharmacologic combinations that are targeted at specific subgroupings of the various psychiatric disorders. These clinicians do indeed possess a kind of practical, experiential expertise in psychopharmacology. Between these two extremes of the technical therapeutic spectrum are the treatment manuals, organized to target the DSM-IV disorders; the treatment algorithms that mimic the DSM-IV decision trees; the manuals for various behavioral and short-term treatments; and finally the guides for primary care physicians to recognize and treat anxiety and depression with the latest selective serotonin reuptake inhibitor.

In light of this description of the DSM-IV as a product of technical reason and its modern presentation in scientifically oriented rationalism, how might we approach psychiatric diagnosis (and then treatment) from the standpoint of practical reason? Let us first recall Aristotle's words, speaking of conduct and invoking his familiar examples of medicine and navigation:

> The whole account of matters of conduct must be given in outline and not precisely, as we said at the beginning that the accounts we demand must be in accordance with the subject matter; matters con-

cerned with conduct and questions of what is good for us have no fixity, any more than matters of health. The general account being of this nature, the account of particular cases is yet more lacking in exactness; for they do not fall under any art or precept but the agents themselves must in each case consider what is appropriate to the occasion, as happens also in the art of medicine or of navigation. (1941b, 1104a, p. 953)

With these words Aristotle sets the tone for every formulation of practical knowledge into the present. He argues that there are areas of human activity which do not lend themselves to a knowledge that can be formulated in precise, general principles. The relationship of general to particular will thus be different from that of the so-named nomological sciences in which universal laws predominate and individual cases are only instances of the universal law. Practical knowledge, in contrast, is inexact and focused on the individual. Although general principles are certainly invoked, they are used and revised as fits the individual case. As Gadamer put it in speaking of history, "the same tradition must always be understood in a different way" (1975, p. 278). Finally, in practical knowledge the experience and judgment of the knower, interpreter, or practitioner assumes great importance. In tacking back and forth between the particular case and the relevant general principles, the practitioner draws on his or her hopefully large experience in the matter at hand. Needless to say, this practitioner will not be able to rely on a technical formula or a manual to relieve him or her of the burden of making a reasoned judgment.

Let us apply this structure of understanding to the example of the psychotic disorders. In doing so it makes most sense to focus on the difficult cases; it is these that raise the question of judgment and experience. For someone who is obviously schizophrenic, the difference between technical and practical knowledge will not stand out. All will be in agreement, and the actual application of DSM-IV criteria will be but a formality that will in reality decide nothing. With the difficult cases the matter is different. Clinicians are all familiar with the (not infrequent) cases in which the presentation of psychosis leaves one uncertain whether he or she is dealing with a schizophrenic process or a mood disorder with psychosis, whether the psychotic agitation represents a manic psychosis, an agitated depression, or schizophrenic excitement, or, finally, whether there is enough mood lability to shift the diagnosis from schizophrenia to schizoaffective disorder. We are also familiar with the ambiguities inherent in the longitudinal course of illness, in which, for example, we are evaluating a patient at any particular point on a course that has initially looked schizophrenic and ends up looking bipolar. Again, there is all the ambiguity inherent in schizophrenic-like presentations that involve a history of significant substance abuse.

Although these may be all cases in which the atomistic approach of the DSM-IV has technically failed—that is, cases in which the patient does not neatly and clearly fit any criteria set—the DSM-IV approach to these patients will still be to get them correctly categorized. This task may realistically require bending the criteria sets to match what the clinician intuitively thinks the diagnosis to be—and thus may turn the DSM-IV diagnostician into a "closet" practitioner of practical knowledge. The approach of practical knowledge, on the other hand, will be to leave the case in its ambiguous status and to draw on one's own experience in making a considered guess as to diagnosis. The experienced practitioner will in all probability *not* let the question of diagnosis in one of these ambiguous and uncertain situations be decided by which criteria set comes closest to matching the patient's symptom checklist. Further, the experienced practitioner will *not* adopt the atomistic approach of just adding up symptoms and other criteria. He or she will try to develop a coherent picture of the patient which will lead in one diagnostic direction or another. To take the rather gross example mentioned above, it would be absurd from the standpoint of practical knowledge to decide to call a patient schizophrenic or schizophreniform on the basis of on which side of the six-month threshold the patient falls. Finally, this rejection of diagnostic atomism will probably involve the inclusion of diagnostic features that are not included in the DSM-IV. Many practitioners, for instance, will feel quite comfortable including psychodynamic factors in their diagnostic evaluations.

One reason for the experienced practitioner's greater casualness about diagnosis is that he or she is oriented toward treatment and does not sharply separate the diagnostic phase of patient encounter from the treatment phase. Recall here Gadamer's dictum that there is no understanding without interpretation and no interpretation without application. If application/treatment is then paramount for the phronetically oriented practitioner, the diagnosis is useful only to the degree that it suggests a direction for treating the particular patient. Contemporary psychiatric practice indeed bears out the degree to which practical considerations concerning the particular patient override the directives of the technical model. In our example of the psychoses, the technical pharmacologic approach would, for instance, dictate neuroleptics for schizophrenics and mood stabilizers for bipolar conditions. Such a dichotomy follows the clean technical categories of diagnosis and treatment. In actual practice, however, what we see is a widespread use of both kinds of medications for both kinds of conditions. Clinicians, whatever their official allegiance to the technical model may be, seem to recognize that their patients require treatments that are individualized and which do not necessarily follow the neatly partitioned categories of the DSM-IV. One response to this looseness of actual practice might be that it represents the current limitations of scientific psychiatry and that, with further scientific advances, treatment will be more precise and differentiated. Only time will provide the answer to this question. The alternative response, the one more consistent with a sense of psychiatry as a kind of practical knowledge, is that psychiatric conditions will never allow the kind of precision in diagnosis and treatment required by the technical model and will thus always depend on the judgment of the experienced clinician.

▪ ▪ Another Approach to Nosology

The question with which we are left is, If the DSM-IV fosters the values of technical reason over those of practical reason, what kind of nosology would provide a better balance between the two? There has already been a good deal of discussion about alternatives to the technical rigidities of the DSM-IV and its DSM predecessors. The replacement of monothetic category sets by polythetic sets is already an acknowledgment within the DSM-IV of a failure of the technical ideal. Efforts to think of categories in terms of "fuzzy" sets (Agich, 1994), prototypes (Genero and Cantor, 1987), or family resemblances (Blashfield et al., 1989) all suggest abandoning the illusory precision of the DSM-IV in favor of more loosely defined categories that resemble the general principles of practical knowledge, that is, categories that can be applied judiciously by the clinician working with the individual patient. These are, however, all piecemeal suggestions aimed at fine-tuning and softening up the DSM-IV. A more thorough nosological alternative is that proposed by Schwartz and Wiggins (Schwartz and Wiggins, 1987; Schwartz, Wiggins, and Norko, 1989; Wiggins and Schwartz, 1994), who suggest a nosology based on ideal types. In recognition of the limited scientific basis of current psychiatric knowledge, ideal types are recognized to be nominalistic concepts that do not represent the real world as such but rather serve as heuristic notions for putting order into the psychiatric field and promoting further inquiry.

The ideal types endorsed by Weber and Jaspers embody a nominalist approach to classification. Ideal types, as developed by Weber, create a conceptual order that, when imposed on reality, merely permits inquiry to begin. Ideal types delineate in reality a certain pattern that may not actually exist in reality but which can at least orient and structure scientific inquiry into it. As the inquiry proceeds, however, the ideal type will likely require modification and redefinition to conform to the investigator's findings. (Wiggins and Schwartz, 1994, p. 95)

Ideal type categories—which, by the way, comfortably coexist with prototypical and dimensional concepts (see Wiggins and Schwartz, 1994, pp. 96–97)—represent an approach to nosology which is quite consistent with the standpoint of practical knowledge. With this kind of nosological system, the practitioner will not be counting off diagnostic criteria. He or she will be looking carefully at the individual patient to determine what ideal type diagnosis will best guide his or her approach to understanding and treating the patient.

The question about these alternatives is whether they lean so much in the direction of practical reason that they forfeit all the advantages of a more technical approach. Fuzzy categories are not of much use in carrying out statistically based research that depends on sharply defined concepts and categories. A fair conclusion to this analysis may be that the DSM-IV, with its tilt in the technical direction, favors psychiatric research, while the more practical nosological approaches just mentioned favor psychiatric practice. The authors of the DSM-IV certainly want a balance between the technical and the practical. Although they may want to argue that the DSM-IV *can* be put to practical uses, the argument of this chapter is that it too readily lends itself to an overly technicalized use. A reasonable goal for the authors of the next edition of the DSM is to balance the manual more evenly between the technical and the practical—not a small task!

7

Implications of a Pragmatic Theory of Disease for the DSMs

GEORGE J. AGICH, PH.D.

IN THIS CHAPTER I discuss the implications for the DSM project of a pragmatic theory of disease which has been described elsewhere (Agich, 1997). In speaking of the DSM project, I limit my comments to the DSM-III, DSM-III-R, and DSM-IV (American Psychiatric Association, 1980, 1987, 1994). I first discuss the relation of disease concepts and theories to nosology. Second, I outline the main commitments of a pragmatic theory of disease and argue that although elements of a pragmatic approach are evident in the DSM project, the central significance of this theory of disease has not been fully incorporated into it. Third, I argue that opposition to this incorporation will likely be based on a competing view of disease which tends to deny a value-charged view of disease and refers instead to the atheoreticism initiated in the DSM-III. And fourth, I argue that atheoreticism can be interpreted as a methodological commitment that was adopted as a pragmatic stratagem to bypass the complex conflicts associated with the theoretical and scientific commitments of American psychiatry.

▪ ▪ Disease and Nosology

In order to gain perspective on the question of the relation of nosology and disease, I begin with a brief and highly selective discussion of the some historical examples of nosologies which reveal several important points that are relevant for understanding the DSMs. Disease does not come from thin (or thick) air. Even though at one time miasma was believed to be a source of disease, such a view seems quaintly misguided today. Nor does disease come from disease entities, though such an ontological view sits more comfortably with commonsense and scientific views that tend to reify disease language. Such views of disease may seem contemporary, but the recognition and rejection of ontological theories of disease were features of nineteenth-century thought. For example, Rudolf Virchow argued persuasively that the idea of an infectious agent as the cause of disease involves a melding of the cause of illness and the disease. When the disease, tuberculosis, is identified with *Mycobacterium tuberculosis*, a hopeless, never-ending confusion results, because the ideas of the disease as entity (*ens morbi*) and causation of disease (*causa morbi*) are arbitrarily thrown together (Virchow, 1958), resulting in an oversimplified view.

When the bacterium is regarded as the disease, the pathological process in which it is involved is slighted. Virchow himself took the *causa morbi* as the central aspect of disease. Preferring the *causa morbi* to the *ens morbi* reflects a number of important preferences. For example, knowing the cause of disease may help to advance therapeutic effectiveness, and searching for the cause of disease undoubtedly promotes certain kinds of scientific research. Either preference can have profound effects on nosology. A nosology of causes, depending, of course, on one's understanding of cause, might stress infectious processes over other pathological processes or stress identification of infectious agents over the immune response. This commitment is more than an idiosyncratic preference for a certain branch of medical science over another; it reflects and is influenced by what is technically and scientifically feasible at any particular moment in history and so is, importantly, a product of social process.

From the beginning of the modern period, nosologies have featured preferences for certain kinds or features of disease concepts. For example, the anatomical approach developed by Jean Fernel correlated disease and bodily structure. His anatomically based classification divided diseases into general and special types. The latter were subdivided into those that involved anatomical parts above the diaphragm, those affecting parts below the diaphragm, and external diseases. He further subdivided special diseases into those that are confined to a part of a single organ, those that affect the entire organ, and complex types that affect several organs and their interrelationship (Veith, 1957, p. 387). So regarded, diseases were to be identified and understood based on their anatomical location, not in terms of the pathological process. One consequence of this kind of approach is the way that specific organs are highlighted and seen as the substrate of disease.

Seventeenth-century nosological efforts introduced classification based on symptomatology, not anatomy. Driving the effort of Felix Plater, for example, was the goal of constructing a nosology composed of irreducible and constant units. Observation, it was hoped, would reveal these units to represent different diseases. If diseases could be specified in this way, one might better understand their similarities and differences. In this conception of nosology, however, disease was seen as a static condition built of constant and easily recognizable entities. As a consequence, disease was conceived in a way that was removed from the clinical experience of the patient or from a dynamic clinical manifestation of the disease (Sherrington, 1946). This nosological ideal held forth the promise of a rational nosology, one whose principles were unsullied by unwieldy clinical details and messy manifestations of pathology.

Such a view of disease as something having a relatively independent nature, unrelated to the patient, was challenged by Thomas Sydenham, who "proclaimed the need for a sharp separation between those symptoms that are always present in certain diseases and those that occur only infrequently" (Veith, 1957, p. 387). Drawing such a distinction would allow one to develop a scientific nosology, namely, a classification of disease which displayed its true rational structure. Stressing commonalities led Sydenham to insist that disease is "uniform and consistent; so much so, that for the same disease in different persons the symptoms are for the most part the same" (1848, p. 85). Sydenham thus focused on disease as manifested in patients. His goal was to develop a view of disease as a specific kind of entity that would be amenable to specific and, it was hoped, effective therapy applicable across patients. By correlating the recurring symptoms with the history of the individual patient and recognizing the similarity of the manifestation of these symptoms, Sydenham established a basic correlation between clinical states that otherwise appeared to be different from one another. This marked an important advance in the history of medicine, because it gave a clinical and empirical focus to the idea of disease. The seventeenth-century faith in the primacy of observation was remarkably congruent with the era's basic conception of science: a guided inspection of the world to reveal the basic rational structure of nature.

The implications of this conception of disease for nosology, however, were most evident in the work of the eighteenth-century nosologist François Boissier de Sauvages, who grouped diseases into classes, orders, and genera in the same way that the contemporary natural scientists arranged systems of plants and animals (Veith, 1957, p. 388). What resulted was a complex and richly articulated catalogue of diseases which was meant to display clinically constant patterns and relationships among diseases. Despite the empirical observational commitment, the inevitable tendency of his approach was to treat each symptom presentation as a distinctive type of disease, thereby proliferating disease entities. Sauvages was, in modern slang, a "splitter" whose nosology yielded more than twenty-four hundred different diseases grouped under ten classes, forty orders, and seventy-eight genera (Veith, 1957, p. 388). In effect, symptoms and symptom clusters came to be identified as diseases; a remorseless logic of difference led him away from the original insight of Sydenham to discern recurrent patterns in the constantly changing clinical manifestations of illness.

These historical reflections provide a cursory illustration of the profound implications that disease concepts have on nosology and the reciprocal influence that nosological ideals can have on concepts of disease. Because nosologies always contain normative features that direct the proper employment of disease language, a nosology provides at least minimal guidance for the clinical identification of disease. Nosologies thus influence clinical perception, but the operative clinical concepts of disease also influence the kind of nosology which is conceptually feasible. The exact effect or influence of nosology on clinical diagnosis and treatment, however, is much harder to identify, because clinical judgment and experience play an important role as well. However, it is safe to say that current ideas about the nature of science and beliefs about the rational character of disease shape the nosology. This shaping, of course, is limited by the practical, clinical bearing of modern medicine, though such a bearing seems remote indeed in the case of the seventeenth century's idealization of scientific rationality, warning us that nosology can promote or make irrelevant clinical experience.

As a whole, a nosology presumes to establish the range of legitimate diagnoses; whether a nosology actually directs diagnosis in any significant way, of course, depends on the particular nosology and its degree of acceptance by practitioners. In the modern period, however, there is a marked tendency to view disease and nosology as scientific; in this view, the term *science* reflects the reigning orthodoxy regarding scientific method. The principles or criteria by which illness states are included or excluded from the nosology may reflect the clinical evidence, accepted scientific theories, experimental or research findings, or any of a large set of other considerations. These conditions vary over time. Specific criteria for membership in a class of disease are included or excluded on the basis of a complex set of judgments regarding how the clinical and other scientific evidence "fits" the underlying nosological purposes or interests, interests that are unsurprisingly shaped by the intellectual climate of the time. The epistemological, logical, and methodological character as well as the descriptive and explanatory ideals of nosologies are a historical product. For convenience we can say that these features are the logical consequence of choices and commitments that were made in the course of constructing the system of classification, but this certainly oversimplifies matters. There are always background assumptions and beliefs not only about the nature of disease but about science and scientific methods that play a role as well. These beliefs include normative standards for evidence, the relevance of theory and clinical phenomenology of illness, and the background purposes or goals that guide the nosological effort.

The history of psychiatric nosology clearly shows that nosology is strongly shaped by underlying conceptions of disease (Wallace, 1994; Berrios, 1996). If this is true, then disease concepts cannot be purely descriptive or evaluatively neutral, as some would have us believe (Boorse, 1975, 1982; Wakefield, 1992a, 1992b, 1993). Disease concepts incorporate a wide range of historically determined theoretical and practical preferences. As Engelhardt has argued, these commitments are ultimately "to medical intervention, the assignment of the sick role, and the enlistment in action of health professionals" (1975, p. 137). These value-laden purposes influence and shape not only the clinical use of disease language but also its organization and integration into a system or classification.

▪ ▪ The Classification of Disease

Understanding the intellectual influences on nosology is obviously important, but it may overcomplicate our understanding of the nosological process. After all, a nosology could be regarded as nothing more than a taxonomy or classification of disease concepts. On this reading, a nosology might be claimed to be less a product of historical circumstance and more the outcome of a purely conceptual or intellectual enterprise (Hempel, 1965). The clarity and simplicity in defining nosology as a classification of disease, however, yield not only an austere portrayal of nosology but a murky and complex array of questions once we focus on a specific type of disease concept such as psychiatric disorder and on a historically specific yet evolving nosological project such as the American Psychiatric Association's DSMs. But perhaps these contingencies are a distraction that can (and perhaps should) be set aside in the interest of achieving better insight into the DSMs.

From this Hempelian point of view, a nosology is first of all a classification or taxonomy of disease *concepts*. So it would be natural to assume that the influence comes from the patterns of description and explanation which define the disease concepts. Like any set of complex objects, psychiatric disorders can be grouped and ordered in terms of any number of features, but some stand out or exhibit a salience that nosologists find compelling. The question that naturally arises is what gives rise to this salience? This is less a genetic question asking "From where do the nosological commitments come?" than it is a logical question asking "Should nosology reflect the conceptual commitments and features of disease language?" Asking the question in this way attempts to remove the historical contingencies to yield the logical features. The focus now becomes: If nosology is the classification of (the concepts of) disease, a nosology should be based on and reveal the logical features or aspects of disease. This point, of course, assumes that classification is guided primarily by the nature of the things classified. This admittedly attractive way of looking at nosology presumes that diseases are the sorts of things which are amenable to classification by dint of some logical or conceptual operation. If this is true, then the classificatory choices made by nosologists have to be seen as a rather esoteric kind of choice.

This way of looking at matters, however, does not get us very far, once we realize that even simple objects or concepts can be ordered in various ways and that complex concepts or objects are even more malleable from the point of view of classification. There is no guarantee that the things will simply fall into place as a matter of logic without a good deal of tinkering. Once we *have* the classification, it might *seem* to be logical, but it would be a mistake to read the "obviousness" back into the nosological process.

This evidently simplified view of classification has one attractive feature, namely, it claims an objectivity that derives from the implied neutrality of the logical features of disease. Such a view is supported by the belief that diseases are the sorts of concepts which are amenable to being known or characterized in a descriptive language that neutrally displays the essential features of disease. Unfortunately, this view not only minimizes the considerable and creative contribution of the nosologist but ignores the preexistent meanings and uses of disease language in clinical practice. These uses and meaning are hardly evaluatively neutral. Classification of disease may be able to capture only the salient features of the concepts of disease which are already present in everyday clinical experience and perception (Schwartz and Wiggins, 1987; Schwartz, Wiggins, and Norko, 1989). If so, then nosology might be far more dependent on clinical practice and its evaluative commitments than it first appears.

To be sure, efforts can and indeed have been undertaken to strip away these confounding evaluative features. The controversial atheoretical approach of the DSM-III and DSM-III-R, for example, represents a conscious and sustained nosological decision to pursue a kind of descriptive neutrality (American Psychiatric Association, 1980, 1987). It would be otiose to claim that this commitment was motivated by the aforementioned simplistic view of nosological construction. Rather, this commitment is understandable only when it is seen in terms of the DSMs' two guiding purposes, namely, the medicalization of psychiatry and the promotion of effective communication among clinicians and researchers (Wiggins and Schwartz, 1994, p. 91). These practical goods shaped the atheoreticism and limited its scope. Given the broad acceptance of the DSM nosologies, the purposes of medicalization and communication were evidently important for contemporary psychiatric practice and research, but their deep relation to nosology and disease concepts is hardly clear. No matter how reformist the nosological effort might be, it starts with the contemporary understanding and perception of clinical phenomena. The failure or success of a nosology ultimately depends on its contribution to the care of the sick. If the DSM seems to have gotten matters "right," it is because of the adequacy of the nosological work for its intended purposes and not simply because the nosology captures the distinctive descriptive features of psychiatric disorders. These general points can be best illustrated by considering a classification of a common type of everyday object, namely, books.

■ ■ The Pragmatic Vector of Classification: An Everyday Example

Books are common everyday objects, at least for this audience, so it might seem that they would be amenable to a straightforward logical ordering based simply on some obvious and observable features of the books themselves. Besides physical properties such as size or color, books could, and indeed should, be viewed in terms of features that are arguably essential to their being of a certain kind of cultural object—they have a distinctive author, year of publication, or subject matter. The question that naturally arises is whether one classification is better or truer based on one or another of these properties or on one or another system of these features. Unfortunately, this is a question that cannot be adequately answered without specifying some purpose or use for the classificatory scheme. Each scheme has advantages and disadvantages, though we might be inclined to think that the range of possibilities is actually quite small and familiar, because of our own experience with libraries. However, that would be a mistake. Any one scheme might be better in the sense of being more suited to a particular purpose than another, but in no significant sense can one scheme be truer than another.

An obvious objection to this line of analysis is that it applies only to classifications in which subjective purposes or interests outweigh or predominate over objective features of the objects themselves. So, although it might be argued that classification by an "objective" property such as size would provide a descriptively based and objective system whereas a categorization of books predicated on use or interest would be value infected and thus relative or arbitrary, this apparently obvious point is misleading. It misleads because it presumes that size, which I stipulate to be an objective property, is more relevant than authorship or the subject matter of a book. Even if this were so, would we really want it to affect the way common things such as books are classified?

Imagine entering a major bookstore, a Barnes and Noble or Borders, for example, to be greeted by a smiling and enthusiastic young clerk inviting you to shop to your heart's content, "The large books are on the left and the smaller ones on the right!" A categorization of objects based on such a measurable "objective" property such as size (or weight) derives its usefulness not because it neutrally classifies things but because it serves an accepted purpose or use. Only a cultural Philistine would consider (and use) books solely based on size. We might, however, not be surprised to find that a shipping department arranged its shipments of books by size and weight. Goal, purpose, and use are utterly central to any classification. To suggest that the order or priority of the categorical scheme comes from the objects considerably minimizes the often creative contribution of the ones who classify the objects and the purposes the classification serves.

It is certainly true that a categorization of books based on use would be relative, but it is not true that such a categorization would be arbitrary in the sense that it would lack a rational ground or justification. Consider categorizing books by author. Such a classification scheme might be so eminently useful that it would appear to be objective, but this would be so only because it coheres with our typical expectations or routine uses. Similarly, a classification of books based on subject matter might appear to capture the objectively important features of books, but only on the condition that the subject matter closely correlated with the way the books were used. The classification appears transparent or "objective" only to the extent that there is an intersubjective agreement, tacit or explicit, about the relative importance of various features of the objects classified. Thus, it is not the objectivity of the objects which supports classification but the shared or common purposes that link the classificatory effort with the use of the concepts. Intersubjective agreement regarding use is a fundamental epistemological court of appeal for any classification.

I suspect that many academics group their own books—of course, without bothering to develop a formal classification system—based on their usefulness for a certain project. Thus, a set of books for the project of this chapter might include not only the DSMs and related books on psychiatric nosology but also books on the philosophy of science, history of medicine, and so. Of course, each of these books has common themes or common features, but they do not "hang together" without specifying the particular interest or set of interests which guides the project. What thus makes a classification appear to be "rational" is the ease with which we see through the reasons so that in using the classification the categories appear transparent.

A classification of books based on the order in which they were read by a certain individual might be accepted as rational, but not in any important sense. However, if the reader was a major thinker, such a classification might well be compelling for a scholar trying to understand the literary influences on the thinker in question. The important point is not the variety and relativity of use, which many devout defenders of the DSM might wish to highlight in opposition to these points, but simply that purposes provide a necessary and regulative function for classification. Without a set of purposes or uses and without intersubjective agreement about the purposes and uses, no classification—much less a psychiatric nosology—could find any significant degree of acceptance.

Talking about a necessary agreement regarding purposes and uses does not imply that a "complete" agreement, whatever that might mean, is needed, but only that there needs to be a broad enough acceptance of the central guiding purposes and rationale to establish and sustain the classification's "relevance." In the case of psychiatric nosology, the acceptance cannot simply be conceptual but must also be practical enough to enjoy a sufficiently broad adoption and use in clinical and research settings if it is not to be consigned to momentary mention in the history of psychiatry. Sometimes, as in the case of the periodic table of elements, a classification provides predictive power and, over time, seems to be confirmed by scientific evidence to such an extent that it seems to mirror the world (Polanyi, 1962). While this might be a hope for a classification, it is not a logical requirement and certainly cannot be an epistemological standard. When a classification does appear to capture the objective sense of things, we rightly marvel at the remarkable coincidence. For most classifications, and for the DSMs in particular, such a state of affairs is unlikely and, in any event, unnecessary.

▪ ▪ The Relevance of Context for Nosology

A pragmatic theory of disease highlights the ways that disease language reflects specific kinds of practical concerns related to human suffering and disability (Agich, 1997). So said, it is important to characterize what gives rise to disease language from the base phenomena of human suffering and experiences of disability or incapacity. A defensible view is that there is a loose but nonetheless important relationship between the language of illness, sickness, and disease, a relationship in which explanatory control and interest are greater at the level of disease language than at the level of illness, and that concern for the amelioration of human suffering moves from isolated, individual responses to the plight of ill or suffering individuals to the social organization of ways to respond effectively. The modern development of effective responses to illness features the use of disease language within a practice of medicine which is characterized by a commitment to scientific methods. This possibility of scientific explanation legitimates treatment of illness within the sick role and is sustained by, rather than sustains, the practice of caring for individuals with psychiatric illness. For present purposes, I simply note that a pragmatic account of disease concepts can accept scientific interest as one—perhaps, even as the paramount—interest among others that shape disease language and its systemization in a nosology. But this interest is related in complex ways to at least two other kinds of regulative ideas: first, the standards internal to the social practice of medicine which give primacy to clinical utility and efficiency over scientific proof, and second, standards contained in both the implicit and explicit practical goals of each DSM. What is too often overlooked and too easily forgotten is that a fully adequate theory of nosology needs to account for its practical functions in addition to its scientific or explanatory status. This need is even more apparent in the case of the DSMs, a project conceived as a collective task yielding not a definitive ideal taxonomy of psychiatric disorders but an evolving set of nosologies with anticipated future revisions.

The DSMs, at least from the DSM-III forward, is an archetypal pragmatic nosology in the sense that it is constructed to achieve a range of practical results. As C. S. Peirce argued: "In order to ascertain the meaning of an intellectual conception one should consider what practical consequences might result by necessity from the truth of that conception; and the sum of these consequences will constitute the entire meaning of the conception" (Peirce, 1965, vol. 5, p. 9). Disease is part of a broad historical and socially determined therapeutic response to sick persons. The construction of disease concepts can be expected to reflect a broad spectrum of human interests that interplay in shaping the historical and social forms of response. Disease concepts sometimes follow the experience of illness and sometimes shape it. Regardless of the direction of influence, the influence is essential to the nature of disease and nosology. One need not go so far as did Charcot, who claimed that "there are no diseases; there are only sick people (Feinstein, 1977, p. 192), but diseases are constructions, and classifications of disease are constructed to satisfy a range of interests and needs. Importantly, disease language arises from a response to the everyday experience of illness, namely, the individual experience of feeling bad or of not being able to perform some normal action (Fulford, 1989). Although its explanatory power derives from appeal to pathophysiological functions, diseases concepts link empirical scientific explanation with the specific failures of action which define illness.

Disease language is best regarded as a particular kind of response to human illness which is organized with a commitment to scientific methods. It is important to remember that magic, incantation, religious ritual, and alternative healing practices are also responses to the phenomena of human illness and suffering. What first distinguishes the specifically medical approach to illness is the implicit claim to the possession of a distinctive expertise for treating sickness which is based on scientific knowledge. It is worth pointing out, however, that belief in the scientific basis of medical practice was accepted by society long before any reasonable empirical basis for this belief was evident. The social belief in the scientific basis of medical practice thus precedes its actuality, and this point helps us to see that expectation of results is central to the use of disease language in medicine. The scientific nature of disease language is founded on deep cultural and social beliefs that themselves involve primarily pragmatic as opposed to epistemological commitments. Because of the generality and practical foundation of these beliefs, they cannot be validated as cognitive claims. To understand fully the basis of these beliefs, we would need to analyze medicine's role in the emergence of scientific thought in the modern period. Moreover, we would need to relate this development to the assimilation of ideals of health into the modern view of the good life and the ideas of control (over nature) and progress. Although such an exploration is beyond the scope of this chapter, it is important to stress that although scientific explanation is an important goal of medicine and psychiatry, other pragmatic interests underlie disease language and hence shape the DSM nosological effort.

Two points follow from these observations. First, disease language is essentially evaluative. It is bound up with the evaluative concepts of illness, and it incorporates these into an explanatory framework that itself introduces additional explanatory judgments into the underlying experiential notions of harm. Second, disease language serves important clinical functions, namely, to provide a scientific foundation for caring for sick individuals including making possible the treatment and cure of the disease states, controlling factors contributing to the disease so as to prevent and modify its course, and promoting effective communication for clinical, research, and administrative purposes (Agich, 1997). For these reasons, disease language always involves what has been called a normativist stance.

Disease language essentially includes evaluative (or normative) as well as descriptive components. However, unlike better-known strong normativist views, which insist on a *separation* of the descriptive and evaluative elements and which seek to restrict disease language to the explanatory function, a pragmatic theory accepts the complementarity of description and evaluation as ineliminable aspects of disease concepts. The implication of this approach for interpreting the DSMs is obvious: explanatory interests, though important, are not primary. Other interests and purposes are also important. A pragmatic understanding of the DSMs simply requires an openness to the nonscientific motives influencing a DSM.

A pragmatic approach to the DSMs offers two distinct advantages over other approaches. First, it encourages a historically and socially situated analysis of the construction and use of disease concepts. For example, a pragmatic approach to the DSM-III-R offers a way of understanding the apparent contrary, if not conflicting, tendencies implicit in its overall conceptual framework as well as in the treatment of specific disorders such as antisocial personality disorder or substance abuse disorders (Agich, 1994; Goodman, 1994). Such an approach to the DSMs encourages an analysis that accepts from the start the practical interests guiding the development, use, and justification of the taxonomy. Indeed, such an approach requires that philosophical approaches to the DSMs are conversant with not only the conceptual issues in the DSMs and their development but also its application and function in the clinical practice of psychiatry (Sadler, Wiggins, and Schwartz, 1994b).

▪ ▪ The DSMs and Pragmatic Purposes

In the case of the DSM-III and following, there is no compelling evidence of an unbridled faith that the classification scheme would, over time, achieve the ideal of descriptive purity or value neutrality that some of its defenders imply. Value neutrality is not an epistemological or logical feature of the nosology for two important sets of reasons: first, the system is explicitly designed to serve a *variety* of purposes including diagnosis, research, and reimbursement (not to mention coherence with the ICD), and, second, the classification is designed to allow for *change* over time. The latter commitment, if not the former, indicates that the DSMs are not founded on any faith in the objectivity of the disorders themselves or of the criteria by which they are specified; rather, the disorders and their criteria are provisional in an important yet nonetheless scientifically sound sense.

The ideals of scientific objectivity and universality are interwoven with the goals of record keeping, diagnostic consistency and efficiency, and coherence with current knowledge and research programs on diagnosis and treatment of mental disorders. Allen Frances and coauthors have noted in this regard that they did not fully resolve or expect to resolve these issues. Instead they attempted to find balanced, if imperfect, solutions that reflected the best available knowledge and would stimulate research that would allow for more incisive solutions in the DSM-V (Frances et al., 1991, "Toward a More Empirical Diagnostic System"). As the authors of the DSM-IV expressed it, there are various sets of purposes and goals for the manual. The "highest priority has been to provide a useful guide to clinical practice. . . . An additional goal was to facilitate research and improve communication among clinicians and researchers" (American Psychiatric Association, 1994, p. xv). Although it might seem controversial and certainly contentious to say that all knowledge is structured by human interest (Habermas, 1968), it is clear that medicine is so guided. Thus, the pragmatic thrust of the DSM should not surprise anyone, but its effect on the manuals has not been adequately appreciated. The function of disease language in contributing to medicine's commitment to care, cure, control, and communication about the illness of individuals is not a passing fashion but is a historically influenced feature of medicine as a practice (Agich, 1997).

If we insist that the taxonomy have a certain logical structure, then we might believe that disease language will itself be shaped by our nosological interests. This is plausible only if the nosology has a special practical normative power over psychiatric research and practice. Another way of expressing this point is to say that although the concepts of disease with which one works influence the kind of classification which can be developed, it is also true that the kind of classification which one is developing will influence what one regards as a disease. The possibility of such reciprocal shaping is just that—a possibility, not a necessity—and the exact relation might be expected to vary from disorder to disorder, making generalization risky. Furthermore, one need not look too far afield to find this influence. As Margolis (1994, p. 109) argued, because operational definitions cannot be relied on to be constant in actual use, the very definition of the categories in question requires a strong consensual agreement on the exemplars of the categories. This fact undoubtedly yields a degree of relativity which is a problem only for those who insist that descriptive or diagnostic categories require a constancy of use which ideally would occur if psychiatric nosology did conform to a set of logical empiricist covering laws or if it actually described natural kinds that fell under covering laws. Although there is evidence of the influence of such a Hempelian model on the DSM-III (Hempel, 1965), this model cannot explain other features of the nosology (Margolis, 1994).

A pragmatic understanding of the DSMs does look to the other goals guiding the DSMs beyond the specifically cognitive or taxonomic commitments. These other goals, such as completion deadlines, consistency with the ICD, and the need to make nosologic decisions based on less than full information or evidence, interplay with the basic organization and administration of the DSMs and cannot but affect the end result. These process aspects (for want of a better term) of the DSMs need to be understood independent of a critical assessment of them, though it should be noted that much of the literature in which the process aspects are discussed has a decidedly partisan tone. It is clear, however, that the practical commitment to consensus both in the development of the nosology and in the process of clinical application inevitably predisposes the definition of disorders in a particular direction, namely, toward an inclusivity that supports wide clinical adoption and application and away from the kind of specificity of criteria which requires a theoretical grounding.

Try as it may, a nosology cannot completely control for variation in practice, though mitigation of variation can be accomplished to some degree. Why the goal of reliability was preferred over, for example, validity is, of course, a different question. Whether for uniformity in coding treatments for reimbursement, consistency with the ICD, or record keeping for clinical and research purposes, the DSM's choice of reliability over validity is guided by a pragmatic choice (Mirowski and Ross, 1989). For present purposes I ignore the controversy that has surrounded the question of reliability and instead note that certain background commitments played a central role in deciding this question. Once the goal or purpose of producing a nosology that is reliable and suitable for a relatively wide variety of uses is adopted, a number of significant effects predictably result. These effects are supported by the regulative idea guiding the nosology, namely, that the nosology achieve adoption in clinical practice and research. Of course, this goal is related to an unstated set of background beliefs about how psychiatry should comport itself in order to participate legitimately in the biomedical clinical and research enterprise as an equal partner along with the other specialty areas of medicine.

One set of common responses to these points, however, is not helpful and actually detracts from this analytic task. For example, shrouding these background choices in the language of science and claiming that they rest on empirical evidence or that these concerns are already dealt with in the DSM's analysis and reanalysis of data and research results significantly misunderstands the status of these commitments. This tendency is evident in both defenders and critics of various aspects of the DSMs. For many critics the tendency to complain about—or for defenders the tendency to insist on—the project as a whole may relate to a central misunderstanding of the necessary function that regulative ideas play in science and, by extension, in a science-based nosologic project. Arguing for this point would take me too far afield, but thinkers from Immanuel Kant (1933, 1987) to Mary Hesse (1980) have shown that regulative ideas are necessary for science (or, in the case of Kant, for reason itself) yet cannot be validated empirically.

The importance of regulative ideas is critical for properly understanding a central tenet of a pragmatic theory of disease applied to psychiatric nosology, namely, that nosologies are ultimately a component of a historically based practice. What guides the DSM nosological process is an idea of relevance which is not captured by any one of the many contending theoretical orientations at work in contemporary psychiatry. Indeed, the lack of a dominant and validated scientific orientation in psychiatry (McHugh and Slavney, 1983) assures that scientific or theoretical consensus is, at best, an ideal and, at worst, a fantasy. Fortunately, regulative ideas in research and practice are not subject to the same kinds of disagreement or to the same types of proof or disproof which plague theories.

Regulative ideas cannot be established by empirical data but themselves provide norms or standards whereby experience is transformed into data or into evidence for scientific reasoning. Regulative ideas not only structure the general process of scientific work but also allow the analysis and interpretation of data to proceed in a methodical fashion, and they are essential for establishing causal connections and constructing laws to explain observations. The regulative ideas that guide the DSM project are much more than cognitive preferences. Regulative ideas exhibit features of the imagination as much as or more than of understanding, theoretical, or practical reason. The DSMs have successfully tapped into the powerful ideas that structure the process of scientific investigation and clinical diagnosis and treatment at the end of the twentieth century; understanding the function of these ideas in the nosology is essential for future DSMs.

Many have criticized the atheoreticism of the DSM-III and following and called for an abandonment of such atheoreticism without fully appreciating its methodological function. The ideal of scientific objectivity and universality is motivated by the need to bypass somehow the complex conflict and disagreement that characterized psychiatry in the 1970s. It is bypassed by the remarkable claim that a classification of psychiatric disorders *could* be theory neutral. Although there is no need to suspect that the authors of the DSM-III were disingenuous, there is nonetheless a covert commitment to a behavioral theory (Mishara, 1994, p. 130) as opposed to the not yet dead psychoanalytic orthodoxy. This has had the undesirable outcome of turning away from phenomenological approaches as well. These historical facts, however, often distract commentators from the main purposes of the DSM. Implicit is the purpose of moving psychiatry toward an empirically grounded and evidence-based research paradigm and away from the clinically oriented commitment of the DSM-II. Atheoreticism was simply a ploy to achieve this purpose. That much seems clear, but is the commitment to atheoreticism a continuing value for the DSMs? This is a more difficult question. To answer it we need to understand better the implications that atheoreticism has had for the DSM project.

A pragmatic interpretation of the DSMs would require that the purposes guiding the atheoreticism be fully understood before it is criticized. Recommendations for a theoretical pluralism or agnosticism as alternatives to atheoreticism should be regarded with some skepticism, because atheoreticism *only partly* serves and incompletely expresses the epistemological commitments central to scientific explanation. Certainly, these commitments were at work in the DSM-III through DSM-IV, and these commitments do seem to reflect an unanalyzed and relatively uncritical acceptance of what is now a much criticized theory of science. Nevertheless, it would be mistaken to conclude that the DSMs are decisively attacked by targeting its atheoreticism or its implicit commitment to a Hempelian view of scientific taxonomy. Beneath the text of the strictly scientific (explanatory) project of the DSMs, there is a more diffuse set of pragmatic purposes which needs to be better understood.

Theories of disease which highlight the scientific and theoretical aspects of disease language often do so in a way that idealizes the scientific process. As a result, they can fail to account for the actual historical and social processes that influence scientific investigation. In Hanson's terms, they focus on the logic of justification rather than logic of discovery (Hanson, 1958). Excessive attention to the demands and structure of scientific explanation and the kind of disease concepts that are imagined to meet these demands, however, has not really advanced the conceptual analysis of psychiatric disorders, because they have left pragmatic values and concerns stranded on the side of the road.

▪ ▪ A Look Ahead

A pragmatic theory of disease helps to explain the treatment of certain specific disorders and some of the contradictions, paradoxes, or tensions within the DSM-III, DSM-III-R, and DSM-IV schemes (Agich, 1994). A pragmatic approach to the DSMs places emphasis on the implicit and taken-for-granted practical goals and purposes that actually shape the nosological enterprise, rather than on the dominant debates. The explicit purposes of record keeping, diagnostic consistency and efficiency, and coherence with current knowledge and research programs on the diagnosis and treatment of mental disorders are supplemented, even guided, by commitment to the scientific ideal of objectivity in science on the one hand and the practical need for consensus and agreement in a world that exists somewhere short of this ideal on the other hand. Keeping the concerns of science and clinical practice apart does not serve this end (Wiggins and Schwartz, 1994).

The animating spirit of the DSM project since the DSM-III incorporates a process of revisions and is committed to critical review and self-examination. Indeed, the DSM-III Task Force openly states that its members have been guided by the "best judgment" made by themselves and other experts. In the DSM-III, the aim of the classification is threefold: to facilitate communication among clinicians and researchers, to provide a classification system that may be of help in planning treatment programs, and to increase the possibility of comparing the efficacy of various treatment modalities. Similarly, Frances, Widiger, and Pincus pointed out (1989, p. 374) that nothing in the DSM-III-R is sacred but that revision should not just be based on opinion but substantiated by explicit statements of rationale and a systematic review of the evidence. They wrote that "consideration should be given to clinical utility, user friendliness, and the impact on other diagnoses or criteria within the DSM. It is very important to achieve greater compatibility with ICD-10, but this should not be at the cost of sacrificing important clinical concepts or distinctions." This marked a change from the process of the DSM-III and the DSM-III-R, which largely relied on expert group consensus subject to the limitations of group process. The DSM-IV, in contrast, was designed to "provide the first well documented psychiatric nosology" (Frances, Widiger, and Pincus, 1989). In this regard, a pragmatic theory of disease highlights this reflective and critical aspect of the enterprise of constructing a psychiatric nosology not for all time but precisely for present purposes and uses with a clear commitment that those uses are openly identified and open to further discussion and analysis in the future.

8

Rethinking Normativism in Psychiatric Classification

ALLYSON SKENE, PH.D.

One of the commonest complaints about psychiatric classification is that its categories lack both reliability and validity because of the value content in the categories. Both the DSM and the ICD have responded by aiming toward an increasingly descriptive taxonomy that provides what is often termed "operational" criteria for diagnosis. Despite these modifications, however, the validity and reliability of psychiatric diagnostic classification are still challenged on the grounds that values are presupposed at almost every level of analysis. At the most general level, terms that describe the domain of psychopathology, such as *disorder, dysfunction,* and *impairment,* connote specific values. A more specific example would be *personality disorder,* which is defined as an "enduring pattern of inner experience and behavior that deviates markedly from the expectations of the individual's culture" (American Psychiatric Association, 1994, p. 629), thus making the relation between individual and social norms the common feature of this type of disorder. Finally, the repeated use of adjectives such as *unusual, bizarre,* or *inappropriate* to describe perceptions, thoughts, or feelings reveals that both diagnosis and classification require a multitude of value judgments.

There are, generally speaking, two opposing solutions to the problem of value in psychiatric classification, which, following Agich, I refer to as "realism" and "strong normativism." The "realist" position is exemplified by Hempel's early essay (1965) in which he argues that psychiatric classification must aim toward increased reliability by introducing operationalized criteria for diagnosis and removing evaluative components. Hempel points out that the predominance of value terms within psychiatric taxonomy decreases reliability because their application must be somewhat subjective and inferential. Psychological tests such as the Rorschach are available but require a high degree of interpretation and consequently do not offer a method of developing unequivocal diagnoses. Operational criteria, as clear, precise, and public tests that can determine application of concepts, will increase the objectivity of diagnostic classification, which will in turn allow for the formulation of theoretical concepts to explain, predict, and control. Hempel admits, however, that it is "unreasonable and self-defeating" to expect too high a level of precision in the beginning and suggests that the concept of "operational criteria" must be understood in its widest sense (such that observations will count as operational criteria) and may only provide a partial definition of the theoretical concepts in psychiatry.[1]

"Strong normativism," in contrast, is exemplified by antipsychiatrists such as Szasz and Laing and labeling theorists such as Scheff and Goffman, who argue that mental illnesses are merely labels applied to social deviance. Psychiatry, they agree, is the only branch of medicine which will treat a "disease" in the absence of biological abnormality and without a patient's consent.[2] This, combined with the fact that the primary target of psychiatric intervention is behavior and psychological states, leads to the conclusion that psychiatry is a form of social control which represses socially undesirable behaviors.

Both Agich and Fulford reject the dichotomy between these two positions and attempt to account for both the evaluative and the descriptive aspects of psychiatric nosology. I argue that although they offer much in the way of a critique of a value-neutral psychiatry, neither "weak normativism" nor a "value-based view" is sufficient to counter the critics who maintain that diagnostic categories are no more than labels applied to forms of social deviance. Agich does not distinguish clearly between theory ladenness and value ladenness and thus does not address the implications of a largely value-based classification. Fulford attempts to circumvent these problems by posing a "reverse view" in which value is primary in both physical and mental illness, but I argue that it is precisely because values in the domain of psychopathology are highly contentious that the implications of value for psychiatric classification are so far-reaching. I then introduce Foucault's claim that knowledge, treatment, and practices of the mental health industry are necessarily situated within a historical context. This differs from Agich's position in that it considers explicitly the problem of cultural or historical relativity. It differs from Fulford's in that it questions the source of any intersubjective agreement and emphasizes the importance of value in psychiatric classification. Once values are accepted as a fundamental component of psychiatric taxonomy, the empirical sciences are revealed as inadequate to the task of explaining or defining mental disorder.

▪ ▪ The Weak Normativism View

In developing the position he terms "weak normativism," Agich is rejecting the dichotomy between "realism" and "strong normativism" and attempting to develop a middle ground that will account for both aspects. Agich is critical of the DSM claim to be atheoretical and purely descriptive on the grounds that it presupposes a naive view of science which imagines that observations or classifications can be independent of theory. Citing Kuhn, he argues that a modern philosophy of science recognizes that observations, descriptions, and classifications are necessarily theory dependent as well as influenced by social values and norms.[3] Further, as psychiatry is a practical discipline as well as scientific one, it is necessary to use some interpretive judgment in the application of concepts. "All diagnoses are fictions: they are interpretations of findings which have an empirical basis in the clinical and experiential reality of the patient" (1994, p. 242). Agich prescribes a "weak normativism" that allows for a more sophisticated view of the fact-value interplay. He requests that values be made explicit, not with the intention of eliminating taxonomic conflicts, but with the aim of allowing discussion as to what values ought to be expressed and how they ought to influence psychiatric diagnosis and research.

Whether Agich is correct that all science is both theory laden and evaluational is debatable, but what I want to focus on here is that he does not make the distinction between these two claims clear. On the one hand, he claims that "psychiatric diagnostic categories are not only evaluative but also theory laden" (p. 234), suggesting that he does distinguish between the two concepts. On the other, he conflates them when he states that "the issue of theory ladenness of diagnostic categories is really an aspect of the larger issue of the relation of descriptive and evaluative elements" (p. 235). Certainly, one of the reasons that Agich is concerned that values must be made more explicit and open to discussion is his view that value is a fundamental component of psychiatric classification because all theories will presuppose social and cultural preferences.

It is, however, possible to distinguish theory dependence from value ladenness more clearly. Theory dependence need not preclude objectivity, testability, and value neutrality. Hempel, for example, predicts that psychiatric classification will increasingly incorporate theoretical considerations without suggesting that we merely accept purely evaluational definitions. (In this regard, see Gottesman, Chap. 19 in this volume.) Increased operationalization of defining criteria will allow for a gradual reduction of the subjective and interpretive elements with a concomitant increase in objectivity. This does not entail an elimination of theory, for it is theory that gives a framework for explaining observed phenomena, allowing predictions, and, ideally, discovering etiology. Theory must imply assertions that can be tested to be true or false, which in turn will provide confirming or disconfirming evidence. Value, on the other hand, is that which is based on preference, whether individual or social. Thus, to claim that psychiatric classification is theory laden is not the same as to argue that it is value laden. Theories are intended to be both explanatory and predictive, while values judge phenomena in relation to norms or ideals. Further, theories—at least scientific ones—are developed with the objective of determining truth or falsity. Values are justifiable in terms of ethical or practical implications but are not, strictly speaking, true or false. How would we test for the validity of social norms?

It might be objected here that there is no neat distinction between theory and value because theories necessarily presuppose values. Even if this claim is granted, however, I think that there is still good reason to distinguish between the two concepts. Values in theories do not necessarily presuppose moral evaluations of the object of study but reflect judgments of what is accepted as a "good" theory. Thus, the values presupposed by a theory might include simplicity, explanatory force, or comprehensiveness (Sadler, 1996a). While these values may lead to the acceptance of a theory that is false, or, conversely, the rejection of a theory that is true, the truth or falsity is determined on the basis of how well the theory explains the phenomena in question. Further, reasons for maintaining value commitments serve to justify choice of value but do not further explicate the object of study. Values, then, are not proved false by further investigations into the object of study but are accepted or rejected according to quite different criteria.

Because values are not the kind of thing which can be tested for truth or falsity, their prevalence in psychiatric diagnostic classification must detract from the overall validity of the categories. This Agich does not deny, but he argues that it is practical reasons that legitimate the continued use of the categories. He says that "the alleged presence of contradictions, paradoxes, or tensions in the DSM III-R classificatory scheme can be regarded as an expected outcome of its pragmatic approach to nosology" (1994, p. 236). Because psychiatric diagnostic classification serves practical as well as scientific aims, the validity of the categories will not be absolute but "workable" or "generally agreed to." For Agich, the problem is not that there are values in psychiatric nosology but that they are implicit and hidden rather than explicit and openly discussed.

The appeal to a practical justification, however, does not circumvent the accusation that psychiatric diagnostic categories are labels applied to social deviance. If it is value that leads to the identification, description, and explanation of madness, and if validity is only a matter of expert consensus, and if there is no way to disentangle fact from value, then Agich must concede that all facts are relative to the values that form them. Agich does not deny this, but it is for this reason that it is difficult to distinguish his version of "weak normativism" from the conclusions reached by the "strong normativists." The reasons he uses to justify "weak normativism" (i.e., the inseparability of value and fact), combined with his justification of current nosology (i.e., practicality and intersubjective agreement), are the same reasons that antipsychiatrists use to argue that the major function of psychiatry is to exclude and repress socially undesirable behavior. If Agich maintained a "realist" position that only asserted theory dependence, he would have grounds to assert that validity as well as the truth or falsity of description could be established through testing. In maintaining that it is evaluation that is central to psychiatric classification, he is making a claim virtually indistinguishable from Szasz's assertion that "psychiatric diagnoses are stigmatizing labels, phrased to resemble medical diagnoses and applied to persons whose behavior annoys or offends others" (1974, p. 267).

Agich, however, rejects the conclusions of the "strong normativists." Although he admits that current classification contains a large evaluative element and this component detracts from the validity of current categories, he argues that this is not sufficient reason to reject them or accept the thesis that mental illness is a myth. On the contrary, he believes that even though what is funded, what is controversial, and what is important will in part determine what is studied, the values that shape nosology do not override the fact that there is a situation, condition, or behavior that can be described, known, and treated. Consider, for example, Agich's admission that he regards psychiatric diagnosis as a matter of practical ethics (Agich, 1994) but also his wish to preserve the descriptive aspects because "all disease concepts inevitably involve both descriptive and evaluative components"

(Agich, 1994, p. 243). If Agich allowed for a clear distinction between fact and value, this claim would be largely unproblematic. Because these so-called descriptive aspects, however, are also admitted to be both theory and value laden, there is no way to isolate the "facts" of the conditions from the values that judge them. This implies that the "facts" are, at least in part, determined by social factors such as economics, politics, and public opinion, which would make them relative to the cultural and historical context in which they are situated. This Agich does not deny, but it makes distinguishing "weak" from "strong" normativism even more problematic.

If Agich agrees that there are no essential aspects of disease, then he needs some justification of why categorization of conditions that are defined in terms of social norms is "descriptive" rather than purely normative. What is, for example, the state of affairs independent of social norms for antisocial personality disorder (APD)? He offers two possible ways of answering this question. The first is to pay closer attention to context, and the second is to refer to the pragmatic goals of psychiatric classification. Although attention to context will serve to narrow the scope of the category, it is not clear that it will remove the evaluative components at the level of description and classification. "Running away from home," for example, is one early sign of APD. According to Agich, this behavior is too general and does not account for the fact that people "run away from home" for a variety of different reasons. If the home is a bad one, it would seem that running away from it is a reasonable response. Thus, by including context, Agich is attempting to isolate those behaviors that are a sign of a "dysfunction" in the person.

Agich admits that his solutions are insufficient to remove the problem of value altogether, but he claims that it will be confined to the level of application. Expanding contextual understanding ensures that diagnosis is not made arbitrarily in the sense that it will exclude certain conditions from the labeling. Narrowing the scope, however, does not circumvent the problem that it is not self-evident that running away from any home, even if it is a good one, is anything more than deviation from expected norms. Because there is no biological evidence for such a disorder and because it is still defined and described in evaluational terms, Agich's solutions are not sufficient to counter the arguments of "strong normativists" that psychiatry is exercising social control—for it is precisely the continued use of labels that identifysocial deviance without reference to underlying pathology which leads them to their critique of psychiatry.

I agree with Agich's assessment that what is required is critical discussion of what values are presupposed and the degree to which value ought to play a role in psychiatric classification. It is not clear, however, that "weak normativism" provides the solution to the problem. Because he fails to distinguish clearly between theory ladenness and value ladenness, he does not establish the theoretical elements as testable or as true or false but makes them the equivalent of judgments of preference. Thus, he offers no ground to support his assertion that psychiatric categories are as much descriptive as they are evaluative. Further, his analysis of APD indicates that he is willing to admit that subjective judgments and social norms are acceptable criteria for classification. Once these are admitted to be inescapable components of psychiatric diagnostic classification, there are no grounds to counter the conclusions of the "strong normativists."

▪ ▪ The Value-Based View

Fulford takes a different tack and argues that antipsychiatrists make the same mistake as advocates of medical models: assuming that "disease" is conceptually prior to "illness" (Fulford, 1989, 1994). That is, in the debate as to whether mental illnesses are "real," both antipsychiatrists and advocates of a medical model presuppose that the criteria of "disease" ought to be applied to these disorders. Antipsychiatrists emphasize the lack of biological evidence for the disorder, whereas advocates of the medical model emphasize similarities, but both sides presume that, in determining the reality of mental illness, criteria associated with medical disease must be met.

Fulford rejects this "conventional" view and argues for a "reverse" view that posits that "illness" is conceptually prior to "disease." That is, "illness," construed as a harmful syndrome, cluster of symptoms, or complaint, is prior to disease concepts, which entail knowledge of pathogenesis or etiology. According to Fulford, "illness," whether medical or mental, is an evaluational concept. Using kidney dysfunction as an example, he argues not only that the term *dysfunction* is evaluative in that it implies harm but also that value terms are imported into the concept of a functioning kidney because it functions to eliminate waste. Fulford recognizes that this example may be somewhat artificial, as there are no obvious evaluative terms in other bodily functions such as circulating blood, but he maintains, nonetheless, that when a physical organ is said to be dysfunctioning, an evaluative component is imported. As such, the fact that categories and criteria for mental illness are value laden does not necessarily detract from legitimately identifying them as "illnesses." Fulford concedes that mental illnesses are more problematic than medical illnesses, but the antipsychiatric conclusion that they are not legitimately so called is mistaken. The crucial defining feature of all illness is "failure of ordinary doing," which, according to Fulford, is evidenced in both medical and mental illness.

The first difficulty with his view is his comparison of medical and mental functions. What identifies a kidney dysfunction is not only the purpose of the organ but its mechanisms as well. Further, the purpose is identified within a nomological network of well-established theories about the nature and processes of the physical organism. Claims of dysfunction in mental processes, however, refer only to the failure to meet a particular end state without reference to mechanism or to well-substantiated theories about why that end state is crucial to the proper functioning of the human being. If blood is not cleansed, toxins will accumulate, resulting in a number of possible diseases and eventually death. There is no equivalent theory or body of evidence for mental functioning. A failure to be happy, at peace, sober, or rational may be unpleasant, but it is not clear that the individual has failed in either purpose or mechanism.

Fulford recognizes that it is difficult to analyze mental functioning because of problems in sorting out the intentions and desires of ordinary doing, but it is not clear that his solution is sufficient to counter arguments from the antipsychiatrists. Of primary importance is the question, Who decides when there has been a "failure of ordinary doing"? A condition that is "undesirable" for the patient may be significantly different from one judged to be "undesirable" by a third party. Consider, for example, the criteria for diagnosing a manic episode in which there is "an abnormally and persistently elevated, expansive or irritable mood" (American Psychiatric Association, 1994, p. 328).[4] (Not surprisingly, manic patients tend to be committed by a third party rather than volunteering to get help.) Feminists have argued against the inclusion of "gendered" categories such as self-defeating personality disorder and late luteal phase dysphoric disorder on the grounds that they presuppose certain unacceptable values.[5] In the case of self-defeating personality disorder, there is outright conflict: psychiatrists argue that there is an impairment of function, and feminists argue that categorizing this behavior as pathology negates the fact that an oppressive society has conditioned women to behave this way. Pathologizing it removes the blame and responsibility from the oppressive social conditions and places it on the shoulders of individual women who are said to be "disordered" because they are living under certain expectations of their role. The category of homosexuality was finally eliminated from psychiatric classification because it could not be established with any empirical evidence or intersubjective agreement that homosexuality is a harmful way to live one's life.[6]

Even if those seeking help concur that symptoms do interfere with important areas of functioning; however, this only justifies the practical needs for service but does not answer the epistemological or ontological questions raised by the prevalence of value terms. It is not just that psychiatric problems are negatively evaluated or that an individual may desire help. It is that the conditions themselves are described in terms of social norms and expectations. For example, describing hallucinations as (culturally unusual) mistaken perceptions is not sufficient reason to make schizophrenia a distinct diagnostic category, especially since the symptoms overlap with bipolar disorders.[7] Thus, when Fulford hints that categories such as obsessive-compulsive disorder or anxiety seem to fit with his conception of illness as a "failure of ordinary doing," he does not address the problem that while it may be true that the person cannot stop washing his or her hands or cannot erase feelings of anxiety, this does not necessarily imply underlying pathology, categorical distinction, or another disorder.

Fulford concedes that mental illness concepts are largely evaluative, that there are difficulties in distinguishing moral fault from mental illness, and that sorting out intentions and desires related to these questions are problematic, but he claims that his "reverse" or "value-based" view shows that mental illness is legitimately so called. I have argued that because he does not address differences between medical and mental illness in terms of theory of functions and because he does not address the ontological and epistemological questions of how these "failures" come to be "illness," let alone distinct diagnostic categories, it is not clear that a reverse or value-based view of illness is sufficient to overcome the objections of the antipsychiatrists.

If Agich and Fulford are correct, what holds psychiatric classification together is the intersubjective judgment that certain kinds of failure to meet social expectations are distinct from others and warrant the label "illness." This, however, is exactly the problem Szasz refers to in his famous work *The Myth of Mental Illness*. Psychiatrists, he asserts, are all too willing to support efforts that will increase their power and professional status; thus, appeals to intersubjective agreement may only point to the desire of psychiatrists to extend their field. "Practical applications" are no doubt intended to allow for service to be provided where there is an obvious demand, but it is not clear that drugs, electroshock, and even talk therapy are not simply forcing people into a mode of behavior considered "appropriate" for their role. Fulford intends to counter this problem by making the patient's subjectivity primary, but he does not address what is to be done in situations in which treatment is involuntary, that is, when it is clear that another decides what is desirable, appropriate, or necessary. It seems, then, that efforts to render explicit the values in psychiatric classification lead to serious problems in maintaining a scientific or objective classification. Once it is admitted that value terms predominate, the artificiality of the categories combined with difficulties in practical application makes a strong case for the argument that mental illness is a myth and psychiatry exercises no more than the imposition of social norms.

▪ ▪ Strong Normativism Revisited

The key reason that leads both Agich and Fulford to reject "strong normativism" is their insistence that psychiatric diagnostic classification offers more than a categorization of social norms and a practice of imposing social control. There is a state of affairs that can be described, studied, and known. More important, there is also a patient who requires care—and giving this care is more than arbitrarily imposing a set of norms and expectations on an individual. My concern here is to argue that "strong normativism," at least insofar as this term applies to the work of Foucault, need not deny either of these claims.

Philosophers and psychiatrists have been quick to categorize Foucault among the antipsychiatrists and dismiss his "strong normativism." Richer (1992), for example, interprets Foucault's analysis of power and knowledge as leading to the conclusion that all of psychology is a form of the police.[8] Foucault is, no doubt, critical of psychiatry, but his analysis extends far beyond the rejection of mental illness as myth and the assertion that psychiatry is a form of social control. According to Foucault, the negative status we attribute to madness actually has little to do with our knowledge of it. It matters not whether we revere or despise; what is relevant is the how the forms of behavior are described, understood, and treated. "In fact, a society expresses itself positively in the mental illnesses manifested by its members; and this is so whatever status it gives to these morbid forms: whether it places them at the center of its religious life, as is often the case among primitive peoples; or whether it seeks to expatriate them by placing them outside social life, as does our own culture" (Foucault, 1987, p. 63).

Foucault's point is not that society judges a behavior or an act as undesirable and attempts to restrain it but that social practices, institutions, and knowledge serve to construct the phenomena of madness. "Loosening of associations," for example, is one of Bleuler's four "A's" crucial to the diagnosis of schizophrenia. Under the social control model, in the attempt to cure this disorder—or alleviate the symptom—psychiatrists are merely imposing a certain concept of rationality in which thinking is linear, coherent, and organized according to specific rules. The easy analysis, the one that asserts social control, is that the positive value of rational, logical, and linear thinking would lead to a negative evaluation of its opposite. This is not necessarily true, however, as "loose" associations can also be connected to creativity, dreaming, or even psychoanalysis, none of which are necessarily negatively evaluated.

But it is not simply the observation that we negatively evaluate certain behaviors which interests Foucault. His claim, rather, is that social values constitute these symptoms—not just as symptoms but as possible phenomena. One of Foucault's examples is regression (1987, p. 80).[9] In order for regression to be a pathological phenomenon, it is necessary that we have a concept of the individual in which time progresses linearly and the past is distinct from the present and not recoverable. Further, childhood must be construed as an escape from problems—where such an escape is expected of the child but refused to the adult. By extension, it could be argued that "loosening of associations" presupposes a certain concept of rationality which is linear as well as rules as to what types of thoughts properly go together but also recognizes the limitations of this same concept of rationality. It is, for example, possible that it is the positive components to "loose" associations which lead many a schizophrenic to refuse treatment.

To say that madness is constructed as mental illness, then, is not to say that the phenomena do not exist but that they are dependent on a host of conditions that make their existence possible. How does this happen? For Foucault the answer lies in how practices, institutions, knowledge, and power create possibilities. The study of individuals and the study of society intersect at a crucial point such that "at any given instant, the structure proper to individual experience finds a certain number of possible choices (and of excluded possibilities) in the systems of society; inversely, at each of their points of choice the social structures encounter a certain number of possible individuals" (Foucault, 1970, p. 380). These possibilities are not merely hypothetical. Rather, the idea that social factors construct individuals suggests, as Hacking observes, that "what it is to be a person is in part determined by the possible categories which you and others may use to describe you" (1986, p. 63). Unlike the classification of things, the classification of human beings makes a difference in how we view ourselves, our sense of self-worth, and even how we remember our own past (Hacking, 1995). Because classifications influence both others' perceptions of us and our own perceptions of ourselves, classifications are not merely practical/theoretical but organize who we are.

Further, although Foucault asserts that power and knowledge constitute the individual, the conclusion that it is the expert with the power who gets to decide what people are (or ought to be) is based on a misinterpretation of Foucault's conception of power. For Foucault, the claim that power represses the individual assumes the stance that power is essentially negative, prohibitive, censorial, and uniform.[10] A repressive conception of power allows only two mutually exclusive conclusions. Either liberation is possible, or we are forever trapped. Foucault contrasts this with a conception of power which recognizes its positive, productive, and heterogeneous aspects. Power is neither held nor imposed solely from the top down. Rather, it is exercised in all directions through local and specific struggles. Although power constitutes the individual, it does not necessarily determine what each and every individual will be like as an individual, because it determines in multiple, heterogeneous, and often conflicting ways. "Relations of power-knowledge are not static forms of distribution, they are 'matrices of transformations'" (Foucault, 1990, p. 99). Power is everywhere, not in the sense that it is imposed on everything but in that it is exercised from all points and in all directions. Thus, individuals are not merely subjected by hegemonic power but create this power through daily practices. Because the relation between power and knowledge is constitutive of madness and not merely its oppressor, it can be argued that there is a "real" state of affairs to be described. Thus, to say that madness is constructed is not to say that mental illness is myth or that psychiatry is merely the exercise of social control. It is to suggest that the phenomena of madness are constructed by a complex relation between a variety of conditions.

How, then, does Foucault's conclusion differ from Agich and Fulford? First, it agrees with the "strong normativist" position that insofar as the phenomena of madness are relative to history, culture, and social values, psychiatric taxonomy will fail to identify objective disorders and "operational" criteria will be subjective and inferential to some degree. If Foucault is right, once we begin peeling back the layers of theory and value which go into the development of psychiatric nosology, we begin to see that there may in fact be no disorder independent of our historical and cultural milieu.

> To sum up, it might be said that the psychological dimensions of mental illness cannot, without recourse to sophistry, be regarded as autonomous. To be sure, mental illness may be situated in relation to human genesis, in relation to individual, psychological history, in relation to the forms of existence. But, if one is to avoid resorting to such mythical explanations as the evolution of psychological structures, the the-

ory of instincts, or an existential anthropology, one must not regard these various aspects of mental illness as ontological forms. In fact, it is only in history that one can discover the sole concrete a priori from which mental illness draws, with the empty opening up of its possibility, the necessary figures. (Foucault, 1987, pp. 84–85)

None of this is to dismiss a priori the need for research or intervention, nor is it to abandon our practical goals of developing knowledge of, and solutions to, the problems of psychopathology. It is to suggest that these things in isolation do not account for the degree to which our theories, values, institutions, and practices actually produce the phenomena of madness. Further, if Foucault is right that madness is constituted by social and historical factors, the empirical sciences, whether natural or social, are not sufficient to develop an understanding of psychopathology. This does not mean that we must reject science or the study of madness, as research into individual biology, psychology, and history has much to teach about mental health or illness. It does, however, imply that the empirical sciences must be complemented with critical analyses that attend to the ways in which social conditions create possibilities as well as cross-cultural and cross-historical differences.

Two implications for psychiatric nosology can be drawn from these points. First, the extent to which value constitutes madness is also the extent to which psychiatric nosology will be relative to culture, history, and social situation. Thus, in their efforts to preserve the current concepts of mental illness, Agich and Fulford are overlooking the possibility that what is being described is not a "dysfunction" but a set of social norms in relation to expected roles and behaviors. This means that the categories are, to some degree, artificial and subject to change. Second, insofar as mental illness is historical rather than ontological, the development of a psychiatric nosology requires looking beyond the empirical sciences to an analysis of the conditions that constitute the phenomena. Agich and Fulford recognize that it is essential to be attentive to how values shape facts, but this must be complemented with a recognition that once the problem of value is brought to the fore, deep questions arise as to the ontological status of mental disorder as well as the epistemological foundations of psychiatric classification.

Notes

1. It is, perhaps, in this widest sense that DSM categories can claim to offer "operational" criteria, but even still they allow for too much latitude in interpretation to count as clear and unambiguous public tests (Hempel, 1965, p. 323).

2. This is technically not true, as medicine has provided and still will provide painkillers or other therapies without knowledge of organic pathology and will in some instances treat a person against her or his will. Still the point that psychiatry treats behavior of unknown etiology in the absence of biological pathology—and frequently involuntarily—is for the most part true.

3. Here Agich is referring to Kuhn, 1970. Note that Kuhn's view of the relation between theory, value, and fact differs from that of other philosophers of science who do not presuppose a "naive realism." I discuss this in more detail below.

4. To be fair, three additional symptoms must also be present for the diagnosis of a manic episode. Note, however, that the list includes increased involvement in goal-directed activities, excessive involvement in pleasurable activities with a high potential for painful consequences, inflated self-esteem or grandiosity, and decreased need for sleep.

5. The result of these arguments is that self-defeating personality disorder was not included in the DSM-IV and late luteal phase dysphoric disorder (now called premenstrual dysphoric disorder) has been relegated to the section on "criteria sets and axes provided for further study." See American Psychiatric Association, 1994, pp. 715–18, and American Psychiatric Association, 1987, pp. 371–74.

6. There is no diagnosis in the DSM relating to sexual orientation. In the ICD-10, no disorder can be diagnosed on the basis of sexual orientation alone, but there is a diagnosis for egodystonic sexual orientation (which includes homosexual, heterosexual, and bisexual orientations). See World Health Organization, 1992a, p. 368.

7. It has been suggested that the features said to distinguish schizophrenia from bipolar disorder are largely arbitrary and to some degree a matter of decision. See Berner, Katschnig, and Lenz, 1986, pp. 70–91.

8. Richer is not the only one to make this claim; I refer to him only because he makes it so boldly and unambiguously.

9. It must be noted that this is a very theory specific example and does not apply to current diagnostic categories. Other examples he refers to include mania, melancholia, and hysteria, which may be argued to be outdated. All the same, the point that certain conditions are required for a phenomenon to exist can be extended to include other examples. See also Foucault, 1965.

10. The section in which Foucault is most explicit about the positive and productive aspects of power can be found in Foucault, 1990, pp. 83–100. See also Foucault, 1980.

Part Three

Diagnostic Categories and Values

9

. . . .

Evaluation and Devaluation in Personality Assessment

LEE ANNA CLARK, PH.D.

SYSTEMATIC DESCRIPTIONS of individual differences in human behavior have ancient origins in natural language and the Greek theory of bodily humors and temperament. Focusing on the domain of personality disorder, I examine the conceptual basis for judging whether a behavioral pattern is "excessive"and the link between behavioral extremes and disorder. I analyze the DSM definition and diagnosis of personality regarding how evaluative judgments are inherent in the language and process of diagnosis; discuss inconsistencies in the DSM treatment of judgments of extremity, motivation, and relations between behavior and personality traits; and consider how culturally relevant standards of comparison are determined and applied in personality disorder diagnosis. Finally, I propose an alternative approach to defining personality disorder grounded in understanding deviations from normal personality structure and processes. Personality diagnosis using this approach requires elucidation of the functions of personality and the ways in which these functions are not fulfilled in personality disorder.

As far back as there are adequate written records, human languages are found to be rich in words used to describe variation in individuals' behavior. Individual differences in physical abilities (*fast, weak*), cognitive abilities (*verbal, dull*) and style (*deliberative, intuitive*), emotional reactivity (*hot-headed, calm*) and expressiveness (*enthusiastic, gloomy*), and myriad aspects of interpersonal behavior (*friendly, hostile, considerate, manipulative*) are all encoded in languages around the globe. Cross-cultural studies of these lay terminologies, which developed gradually over millennia to describe common human behaviors, have revealed both striking commonalities as well as notable differences in how this broad domain is parsed across the range of languages. What is important to note in this context is that human behavior is sufficiently systematic so as to be noticed and labeled in the course of ordinary discourse (however unconsciously that process may have occurred).

Further, long before even the earliest versions of the DSM, astute observers of human behavior consciously discerned broader patterns in this variation than are typically encoded in common words. Consequently, attempts were made to describe certain of these patterns that appeared to occur with regularity and, moreover, to provide causal explanations for these behavioral patterns. For example, focusing on the domain of behavior which has come to be called "temperament," "character," or "personality" (and sidestepping for the moment the problem of defining this domain), the ancient Greek physician Hippocrates described four primary temperaments, each defined in terms of a characteristic emotional style: sanguine, or cheerful and optimistic; melancholic, or sad and gloomy; choleric, or angry and irritable; and phlegmatic, or calm and passive. Moreover, he proposed that these personality types each were associated with one of four "humors," such that the person's temperament reflected the internal balance of the humors, and excesses of humors led to extremes of personality. Thus, an extremely sanguine or active, hypomanic personality stemmed from an excess of blood; a morbidly melancholic or depressive personality reflected an excess of black bile; excessively choleric or angry, violent types had an overabundance of yellow bile; and a phlegmatic or apathetic, unresponsive personality was caused by too much phlegm.

Several aspects of this ancient Greek formulation are important for the purposes of this chapter. First is the idea that human behavior is not random but is regular enough that it can be described systematically not only at a level useful for ordinary human discourse, as noted with regard to natural language, but also at a greater level of abstraction. A second and related point is that this systematic variation in human behavior has natural causes, which be sought through scientific inquiry. That Hippocrates posited biological factors as the causal explanation for observable personality characteristics is tangential to this point—a hypothesis of environmental causes would have served as well. That Hippocrates' system maps remarkably well onto modern descriptions of personality (see Eysenck and Rachman, 1957) is fascinating—and humbling—but also tangential.

A third aspect of the Greek formulation launches this chapter, the idea that excesses or imbalances in the underlying causal factors lead to extremes of temperament. With the introduction of such notions as "excess," "imbalance," and "extreme," we are no longer simply describing variations in internal processes or observable behavior but are additionally *judging* both the physiology and the behavior. In doing so, we are positing that— or at least posing the question of whether—something has gone wrong with these processes and behaviors. That is, we are raising the suggestion of disorder.

It is important to note that the question of whether an extreme condition represents "disorder" is not intrinsic to extremity. As a counterexample, consider weather phenomena. Wind speed is a continuum from still air at 0 mph to hurricanes with wind speeds in excess of 300 mph. Meteorologists could provide a frequency distribution of wind speeds, which likely would be highly skewed, with most values falling below 20 mph and fewer and fewer values at higher and higher wind speeds. No doubt, the rate of precipitation in a twenty-four-hour period could be similarly plotted. Based on these distributions, one could say that winds of 300 mph or 12 inches of rain in a day is excessive. Yet, when a hurricane whips through Florida, a torrential rain falls on Indonesia, or Texas has a six-week period of 100-plus degree scorchers, we do not conclude that the weather is disordered. We might make analogies to disease or dysfunction ("this weather is really crazy"; "it just isn't *right* for it to stay this hot *this* long"), and we might wish that we could "fix" or "cure" the bad weather, but it is only in science fiction or fantasy that people speak seriously of "unnatural weather," caused by some demonic force.

One might object that the difference is that weather is not a living organism and that we link extremity to disorder only in organic systems. This may be true if we restrict ourselves specifically to the term *disorder,* but if we more broadly consider the phenomenon of "something gone wrong," then counterexamples are easily available. For example, mechanical devices of all sorts may behave in extreme ways that we consider "disordered." If a computer crashes too frequently, if a car uses an excessive amount of gas or oil, or if a television picture is too fuzzy to make out, we take these as signs that something has gone wrong with the device, that it is disordered.

In the human domain also, extremity and disorder may be correlated but are not isomorphic. For example, being extremely tall or intelligent does not automatically raise the question of disorder. Certainly, people who are unusually tall, short, or unintelligent *may* have a disorder that leads to the condition (although I know of no dysfunction that leads to unusually high intelligence), but clearly excesses, extremes, and unusual phenomena in natural processes are not inevitably considered "disordered" in the sense that something has "gone wrong." Rather, extreme phenomena may be considered undesirable without anything being "wrong" (e.g., unattractive, uncoordinated), or they even may represent desirable conditions, as in the case of an extremely tall basketball player or an extremely bright individual.

Thus, the link between extremity and disorder is, to a certain extent, a domain-specific concern, as extremity in natural systems is not necessarily considered disordered and extremity in nonliving systems *may* be a sign of disorder (i.e., something gone wrong). Therefore, the emergent question in this chapter's focal domain of personality (and the psychiatric domain to which we may wish to generalize) is, What *is* the conceptual basis for determining, first, whether a specific behavior or general behavioral pattern is excessive or extreme, and second, whether such excesses and extremes represent "disorder" in the sense that something has "gone wrong" and "needs to be fixed." I do not intend to answer these questions but only to raise a range of issues that arise in their consideration. In this discussion I do not tackle the difficult task of defining *disorder,* which most recently has been debated vigorously by Wakefield (1992a, 1999, 2000) and Lilienfeld and Marino (1995, 1999). Rather, I take as a basis for my considerations those elements of disorder which are consensual in this debate, namely, that disorder involves something that has gone wrong and that causes harm.

▪ ▪ Personality Disorder Criteria: Description and Evaluation

Overview of the Criterial Structure

GENERAL CRITERIA

Beginning with the third edition, the DSM (American Psychiatric Association, 1980) set forth descriptions of a set of disorders, collectively known as the personality disorders. The DSM definition of this set of disorders begins by defining personality traits as "enduring patterns of perceiving, relating to, and thinking about the environment and oneself that are exhibited in a wide range of social and personal contexts" (American Psychiatric Association, 1994, p. 630). Though not identical, this definition is quite compatible with those offered in the psychological literature on normal-range personality. For example, synthesizing from the more than fifty definitions of personality which have been offered over the years, Watson, Clark, and Harkness (1994) presented a composite view of personality as internal, organized, and characteristic of an individual over time and situations, adding that, typically, personality traits are viewed as motivational or as having adaptive significance. Trait theorists thus distinguish enduring traits from more transient states (although it is important to recognize that states may be manifestations of associated traits) and distinguish internally organized behavior patterns that are more generally characteristic of an individual from more situationally based behaviors, which are driven by the demands (including clear reinforcements and consequences) of particular circumstances.

The DSM then proceeds to specify further certain qualities that personality traits must have to constitute a personality disorder. First, the behavioral pattern must *deviate markedly* from the *expectations* of the individual's culture and be manifested in two or more of the following areas: cognition, affectivity, interpersonal functioning, and impulse control. A number of relevant affective parameters—range, intensity, lability, and *appropriateness* of emotional response—are specifically mentioned. Consistent with the definitions of traits given earlier, other general criteria emphasize that the defining traits must show evidence of early onset, be longitudinally stable, and be "pervasive across a broad range of personal and social situations" (American Psychiatric Association, 1994, p. 633). Finally, to be considered disordered, the traits also must be "inflexible" and maladaptive, causing either "clinically significant distress or impairment in social, occupational, or other important areas of functioning" (p. 633).

Although readers may be familiar with these definitions, it is instructive to reflect on how many of these general criteria require evaluative judgment. It is also important to note that these evaluative judgments are distinct from the subjective decision making that is frequently involved in diagnosis and treatment of any sort, for example, a physician's judgment that an infection requires antibiotics or a mechanic's judgment that a starter should be replaced. These latter types of judgments involve expert prediction of probabilities and are based on very widely shared assumptions—or values. In these examples, the shared assumption or value is that no infection is better than infection, that a car starting is better than it not starting. These value judgments, of course, may be debated from certain perspectives or special circumstances. For example, the affected bacteria may not agree that no infection is better, since it represents their livelihood. Similarly, a person who believes that every living organism has equal status might not accept the judgment that infections should be treated with antibiotics. Or suppose that you missed a plane because your car wouldn't start. You likely would be quite upset, at least until you heard that the plane had crashed on takeoff, killing everyone on board. Now the car not starting seems like a blessing, even though the car is still "disordered." Raising these issues underscores that value judgments are pervasive, even when they are not obvious, because they are based on widely shared, typically unspoken assumptions.

In contrast to expert judgments that are grounded in widely shared values, in the case of personality disorder the diagnostician is asked to evaluate such qualities as the deviance of behaviors relative to cultural expectations, to judge the adaptability versus inflexibility of behaviors, and to consider the clinical significance of social, occupational, or other impairments. Each of these types of judgments invokes a process that is fundamentally, qualitatively different from deciding that a certain immune system will—or will not—be able to fight an infection without antibiotics or that a starter likely can be used six more months before it will fail to work.

Was Dennis Rodman's hairstyle markedly deviant? What standard should be used in making this judgment—the culture of sports and entertainment or that of Normal, Illinois? A thirty-six-year-old never-married client is socially anxious and maladroit. Does his behavior cause social impairment? If so, is it clinically significant? What standard should be used to make this judgment? Is it enough that he is unmarried at the age of thirty-six? Surely there are many unmarried thirty-six-year-olds who would not be judged socially impaired. I used the term *maladroit* to describe his behavior; an evaluative judgment is intrinsic to the very word. On what basis did I make the decision to use that term? Clearly, judgments of this type involve evaluation of behavioral patterns in relation to standards that are far from objective, absolute, or unchanging. I explore these judgments more fully in a later section, but first I describe briefly the structure of criteria for the diagnosis of specific personality disorders.

SPECIFIC CRITERIA

Each of the ten currently specified personality disorders (and the two appended categories) is introduced with a general statement of its primary defining characteristics, followed by seven to nine more specific criteria, a subset of which must be manifested as exemplars of the defining characteristics to merit the diagnosis. Two examples may be used to illustrate various subsequent points. Antisocial personality disorder is defined as "a pervasive pattern of disregard for and violation of the rights of others" (American Psychiatric Association, 1994, p. 649), which must be fulfilled by manifesting three or more of the following specific criteria: repeated illegal acts, deceitfulness, impulsivity, irritability and aggressiveness, reckless disregard for safety, consistent irresponsibility, and lack of remorse. Dependent personality disorder, by contrast, is defined as "a pervasive and excessive need to be taken care of that leads to submissive and clinging behavior and fears of separation" (p. 664), which must be manifested by five or more of the following specific criteria: has difficulty making daily decisions without excessive advice and reassurance, assuming responsibility for major life areas, expressing disagreement, initiating projects, doing things independently, and not being in a close relationship; goes to extremes to obtain nurturance and support; feels helpless when alone; and is preoccupied with fears of being left to take care of oneself.

It is important to emphasize that the diagnostic task posed by the DSM criteria is not only to determine whether the specific criteria are present but, just as important, whether the specific behavioral criteria reflect the primary pattern that defines the category. Take, for example, the antisocial criterion, "failure to conform to social norms with respect to lawful behaviors as indicated by repeatedly performing acts that are grounds for arrest" (American Psychiatric Association, 1994, p. 649). One can readily think of behaviors that meet this specific criterion but which may not reflect pervasive disregard for and violation of the rights of others—prostitution, civil disobedience, homosexual activities, and marijuana consumption all are possibilities. Upon initial consideration, it seems that this situation could be quite problematic if, for example, a person met multiple criteria for a disorder—in the sense that the described behavioral criteria were manifest—but in each case the manifest behavior did not reflect the primary target characteristic.

Such a possibility raises additional questions. First, to what extent are clinicians who make diagnoses aware that the overarching task set by the DSM is to determine whether the primary pervasive pattern is or is not present rather than the simpler, "lower order" task of determining whether the person manifests four or five or more of seven to nine specific criteria? And second, given the construction of the DSM Axis II diagnoses, does it matter whether they are aware of this overarching task? The first question is an empirical one, and I know of no data to answer it. However, rating the criteria rather than the pervasive pattern appears to be the task set forth by structured interviews used to diagnose personality disorder. For example, in one widely used structured interview, a single set of questions is provided to rate both the "inappropriate intense anger" criterion in borderline personality disorder and the "irritability and aggressiveness" criterion in antisocial personality disorder. And yet the primary target construct for these two diagnoses seems quite different: that for borderline personality disorder is "a pervasive pattern of instability of interpersonal relationships, self-image, and affects, and marked impulsivity" (American Psychiatric Association, 1994, p. 654), which contrasts with that for antisocial personality disorder, "pervasive disregard for and violation of the rights of others" (p. 649).

Certainly it is possible that clinicians could use a person's responses to a single set of questions about his or her anger and aggression to determine that the person met the borderline criterion but not the antisocial or vice versa, or that he or she met both criteria in the behavioral sense but only one of them in the sense that the behavior reflected the target construct. However, structured interviews typically do not even provide the target construct for the ten personality disorders to be rated; only the general and the disorder-specific criteria are listed. Thus, the clinician would either have to memorize the target construct for each diagnosis or have to consult the DSM when rating each interview. Extensive experience with these interviews suggests to me that this level of knowledge and differentiated judgment would be quite unusual for research or clinical use of structured interviews. It is interesting to speculate whether some of the poor convergence in diagnosis which has been documented between structured interviews and clinical diagnoses (e.g., Perry and Vailliant, 1989) may stem from the former's focus on criteria, with less regard for the general behavioral pattern, whereas the latter focuses on the general pattern of behavior which characterizes the diagnoses as a whole with less regard for specific manifestations. The poor convergence between clinical diagnoses, on the other hand, may stem from the fact that without the guidance of specific criteria, judgments about the presence or absence of a general behavioral pattern are very difficult to make.

These considerations lead to an examination of the second question: What difference does it make if clinicians rate the criteria alone rather than criteria as manifestations of the general pattern? Although not explicitly stated, the measurement model adopted by the DSM has many parallels to that used by most psychological tests (see Blashfield and Livesley, 1991, for an extended analysis). That is, the individual criteria were selected specifically because they were thought likely to reflect the primary characteristics of each diagnosis, just as test items are selected specifically as reflections of the underlying latent trait that a scale is intended to measure. In the case of psychological tests, psychometric indexes of internal consistency are used to assess the degree to which each item fulfills this function. Items that do not reflect the latent trait adequately are eliminated from the scale in the course of its development. The result is a set of intercorrelated items whose common variance reflects the target construct.

Similar analyses were performed in the latest revision of the DSM Axis II diagnoses, though with less rigor and less data than for most psychological tests. Results indicated that, for the most part, the criteria are moderately coherent and thus in the aggregate presumably reflect the target trait moderately well, though there is marked variation across diagnoses. The critical point is that in a well- constructed psychological test and, analogously, in a well-constructed diagnosis (at least those on Axis II), the items or criteria each reflect the target construct to some degree.

The phrase "to some degree" is critical in this statement, because no single item can perfectly reflect one and only one construct, nor can a construct of any meaningful breadth be captured by a single item. Assessment of a construct, therefore, requires aggregation across a set of imperfect indicators, each of which contributes to the overall measurement (Clark and Watson, 1996). The essence of classic reliability theory is that if enough such indicators are aggregated, the construct will be measured with good reliability. Thus, the hypothesis of classic reliability theory for personality disorder diagnosis would be: *If* each of the personality disorder criteria does in fact reflect the target construct to some degree, *and* a person exhibits a sufficient number of criteria, then the likelihood is high that the person's behavior reflects the target construct. From this viewpoint, a clinician's consideration (or lack of consideration) regarding whether a person's behaviors reflected a target construct when rating a criterion is irrelevant. What is important is the construction of the diagnosis itself. Again, however, it is an empirical question whether this hypothesis is true for each of the specific personality disorders set forth in the DSM.

This whole discussion may seem to be somewhat removed from the consideration of values in personality disorder assessment, but it is necessary in order to clarify how the Axis II diagnoses are constructed. That is, in some cases objective, descriptive judgments of the presence or absence of specific behaviors are separated from the more subjective judgments of the relevance of those specific behaviors to more abstract behavioral patterns. Thus, the clinician can determine whether a client is "suggestible and easily influenced by others or circumstances" independently of the judgment of whether this behavior reflects excessive emotionality and attention seeking. On the other hand, for many specific criteria, these two judgments are intertwined, with the primary characteristic literally or implicitly restated in the criteria themselves. Take, for example, the dependent personality disorder criterion "urgently seeks another relationship as a source of care and support when a close relationship ends." It would be difficult to find an example of this behavior which did *not* reflect a strong need to be taken care of, because "as a source of care and support" is part of the criterion.

This structural inconsistency in the DSM is manifested also with regard to the issue of extreme behaviors. In some cases, the decision of whether the behavior "markedly deviates" from cultural expectations is separated from the judgment of whether the behavior is present or absent (e.g., the antisocial personality disorder criterion "impulsivity or failure to plan ahead"). In many other cases, however, the specific criteria themselves require judgments of extremity or excessiveness (e.g., the dependent personality disorder criterion "feels uncomfortable or helpless when alone because of *exaggerated* fears of being unable to care for himself or herself"; emphasis added). In these latter cases, the specific behavior must be judged extreme or excessive for the criteria to be met, whereas in the former cases, the judgment of extremity is not made at the criterion level but at the level of the overall pattern of behavior; in still other cases, it may be unclear where this judgment is to be applied.

Clearly, in examining the various ways in which evaluative judgments come into play in personality disorder diagnosis, we must keep in mind that in the current DSM formulation evaluative judgments are involved inconsistently at different descriptive levels and that evaluation and description may or may not be intertwined for any given criterion.

▪ ▪ Judgment and Evaluation in the General Personality Disorder Criteria

The first of the general criteria for diagnosing personality disorder is "marked deviation from the expectations of the individual's culture." Rather than discuss each of the general criteria in turn, I focus on this criterion as an illustration of how evaluation pervades personality disorder diagnosis. Each of the two main parts of this criterion bears scrutiny. How deviant a behavioral pattern must be to be considered "marked" is left undefined in the DSM. At this stage of our knowledge and understanding of human behavior, this was a wise, indeed the only, reasonable choice. Clearly, if a behavioral pattern is "unremarkable," we have no reason to consider it further as a candidate for professional attention. On the other hand, research in human judgment and decision making indicates that consensus is more readily attained if the object of judgment is clearly defined (Shanteau, 1992), and, presumably, "markedly deviant" behavior is generally more clearly defined than behavior falling in the range between marked and un-remarkable, a range whose width will vary as a function of the object of judgment. For some behaviors, perhaps hallucinations being a good example, there is a steep gradient between "unremarkable" and "marked deviation," whereas for many others—likely the majority of behaviors relevant to personality disorder—the range is wide and the gradient smooth and gradual. Examples of such criteria include "self-dramatization, theatricality, and strong emotional expression," "miserly spending style," and "reluctant to take personal risks or engage in new activities."

In certain domains of behavior, such as cognitive abilities, the distribution of behaviors has been studied extensively, and we know a great deal about the meaning of different levels of behavior. In principle, similar investigations could be carried out for the range of behaviors relevant to personality and its disorder. Indeed, this is the aim of psychometric investigations of personality traits, both to define and to measure the relevant constructs so that questions of deviation may be framed in terms of a more complete and precise understanding of the full range of associated behaviors. If, for example, we had a reliable means of assessing emotional expressiveness ranging from extreme self-dramatization and theatricality to extreme lack of emotional expression, we could study the correlates of different levels of expressiveness. This might permit judgments about the need for treatment of self-dramatization to become more like the physician's judgment that an infection requires antibiotics. In essence, the basis for the judgment of whether a behavioral pattern is "markedly deviant" need not—and, by extension, if diagnosis is to be scientifically based, *should* not—remain forever undefined as it is currently.

The second phrase in this criterion—"expectations of the individual's culture"—is more problematic in terms of distinguishing objective description from subjective evaluation. It is necessary that some such phrase be included, because the question of whether a given behavior "deviates markedly" must be considered relevant to some standard, and cultural standards are diverse. Yet, like "deviates markedly," what constitutes "the individual's culture" is also undefined, again with good reason. Nevertheless, the decision of the standard against which the person's behavior is to be compared may be an important one in many cases. I say "may be" rather than "is" because it is possible that "markedly deviant" behaviors do not, for the most part, differ widely across cultures, however different cultural expectations may be. Whether there are certain extremes of behavior which are universally seen as "markedly deviant" or whether a strong relativist position more accurately reflects reality is an interesting and important empirical question that is widely studied by anthropologists. Delving further into this question would again take us away from our topic. Nevertheless, I note it as another example of a question that may not remain forever a point of subjective speculation but which potentially may be answered by future empirical research.

On the other hand, I say "may be important in many cases" and "for the most part" because there are clear cases in which the cultural standard of comparison is critical. For example, Americans typically are horrified by reports from India of fifteen-year-old girls who are shamed and outcast because they ran away from husbands who had handed them over to other men to have sexual intercourse with them; yet the tribunals that sit in judgment of the husbands find the men's behavior above reproach. Certainly, the decisions that diagnosticians will need to make regarding the appropriate cultural standard against which to judge a potentially deviant behavior will, in most cases, be less striking than this example; nevertheless, the relevance of the cultural standard of comparison cannot be dismissed lightly.

The situation is complicated by the fact that human judgment is highly influenced by prior information, including stereotypes and judges' expectations about individuals' behaviors. Clinical diagnosis of personality disorder, particularly when based on traditional unstructured interviews, is susceptible to gender, cultural, and ethnic biases (Widiger and Axelrod, 1995). There is very little empirical work to illuminate how clinicians take cultural background into account in judging behaviors, and it is far from clear how one would determine "accuracy" in this endeavor. To suggest that clinicians overcorrect, undercorrect, or are accurate in judging the effect of culture on behavior implies a known standard against which to compare clinical judgment. Although it is not inconceivable that we may someday be able to parse cultural influence from individual differences, the knowledge needed for such a task is well beyond our current understanding. For the foreseeable future, we will be relying on subjective judgments.

I have been focusing on the last word in this phrase—"culture"—but the modifier, "the individual's" also presents interesting problems. One reason that is it unclear what constitutes "the individual's culture" is that the notion of "the individual's culture" is itself subject to cultural variation. That is, in certain sociopolitical climates, what I term "microcultures" are held in high esteem, and the number of the "individual's cultures" is great; in other times and places, broad cultural conformity is prized, and fewer cultural distinctions are accepted. Currently, with the change to the new millennium, for example, multiculturalism is strong. The zeitgeist seems to be that the worldview of each self-defined subgroup—perhaps down even to ns of 1—should be respected and valued. The strength of this value system is such that it is difficult even to discuss the issue, because any specific example may be interpreted as disrespectful by one of the many possible microcultures. Suppose I wanted to consider the question of how one would determine whether a certain behavior—hostility at perceived discrimination, for example—was deviant if it occurred in an individual in subculture X. If I were to select an actually existing subgroup as an example, I might be questioned as to why I singled out that group; on the other hand, if, in an attempt to avoid offending members of any particular existing subculture, I were to make up a subculture—left-handers who have had encounters with aliens, for example—in order to consider the question of whether hostility at perceived discrimination is deviant from the viewpoint of that culture, I might be seen as disrespectful by making fun of all microcultures or of the idea of multiculturalism. Thus, in an era that values extreme microculturalism, "the individual's culture" is potentially infinitely variable, every individual's behavior must be judged by its own standards, and there may be social costs for violating this expectation. The cultural value of microculturalism thus sets one boundary for the task of judging whether a behavior is markedly deviant relative to the expectations of the individual's culture.

In contrast, microculturalism is a pendulum swing away from the value held in other times and places, whereby all individuals are expected to conform to broad cultural standards. This latter value comes in several varieties, exemplified by the "melting pot," the "moral majority," or the Chinese Cultural Revolution. It may be easier to judge marked deviance against a rigid cultural standard, but this also has its problematic aspects. Over the course of human history, people have judged and treated as deviant many behaviors that most of us today probably would agree should not be so judged. But clearly this reflects a revised evaluation of these behaviors, not a change in the nature of psychological disorder per se. Evolutionary psychologists Cosmides and Tooby have argued that we must separate the question of dysfunction—which they define in evolutionary terms—from that of conditions judged in need of treatment (Cosmides and Tooby, 1999). They cite the example of homosexuality as a condition that may represent a dysfunction from the viewpoint of evolutionary design but which, at least currently in the professional world of the United States, is nevertheless not considered a condition in need of treatment. Certain members of the deaf community similarly argue that deafness is not a condition in need of treatment (Lane, 1992). These considerations begin to take us afield of our topic. To return, the critical point is that for the range of behaviors relevant to personality disorder, evaluation relative to cultural standards is unavoidable and that there is relativism within relativism in this domain.

Many of the same considerations already discussed apply to the remaining general personality disorder criteria: appropriateness of emotional response, inflexibility, clinically significant distress, and impairment in social, occupational, or other functioning. In each case, questions arise regarding the standard against which "appropriateness," "inflexibility," "clinical significance," and "impairment" are to be judged. As noted earlier, the DSM is inconsistent as to whether these judgments are interwoven with the criteria. For example, "inappropriateness" is intrinsic to the "excessive social anxiety" criteria of schizotypal personality disorder. However, it is not at all clear that the schizoid personality disorder criteria of "appears indifferent to the praise or criticism of others" is intrinsically problematic. One can imagine that Maslow might have described ideal, "self-actualized" persons as so self-contained and self-confident that they are "indifferent to the praise or criticism of others." Thus, for this behavior, separate judgments must be made regarding whether the behavior betokens self-confidence or aloof detachment, regarding the appropriateness and flexibility of the behavior, and whether the behavior causes distress or impairment.

In this context, it is worth mentioning yet another way in which evaluation is intertwined with description in the DSM, and that is through the evaluative nature of the descriptive words themselves. Williams (1985) refers to concepts in which description and evaluation are combined as "thick" value concepts and contrasts these with "thin" value concepts, which are transparently evaluative, such as *beautiful* or *malicious*. I alluded to this issue earlier when I described a client as *socially maladroit*, a term in which evaluation is inherent in the common meaning of the word. There are many such instances in the DSM Axis II criteria: behavior that is odd, eccentric, or peculiar (schizoid personality disorder); identity disturbance (borderline personality disorder); shows arrogant, haughty behaviors or attitudes (narcissistic personality disorder); consistent irresponsibility (antisocial personality disorder); or shows rigidity and stubbornness (obsessive-compulsive personality disorder). It certainly may be possible to find specific circumstances in which at least some of these behaviors would be positively evaluated. For example, there are teen subcultures that appear to celebrate the odd, eccentric, or peculiar, but this is only relative to mainstream culture; if they themselves deemed a person odd or peculiar, the label again most likely would take on a negative evaluative tone.

Or, one can think of specific circumstances in which rigidity and stubbornness are called for and adaptive; traffic safety rules for small children must be rigidly enforced, for example. However, it is difficult to imagine cultural settings in which these various traits would be valued if they were longstanding and pervasive across a wide range of situations. More typically, these behaviors are prejudged by the very meaning of the words themselves as socially undesirable, if not frankly non-normal, deviant, or causing impairment.

Interestingly, however, there is nothing in the general personality disorder criteria which requires social undesirability for the behaviors constituting the pattern that is judged markedly deviant, inflexible, distressing, and so forth. I noted earlier that these judgments had to be made separately for some personality disorder criteria, and, indeed, some criteria describe behaviors that in less extreme forms are quite normal and may even be highly desirable. For example, perfectionism can be a virtue, if it is not so extreme as to interfere with task completion. There's certainly nothing inherently wrong with being self-dramatizing and emotionally expressive; people who are this way can be very entertaining, and I would imagine that actor Jim Carrey, even outside his roles, is not typically a subdued, restrained individual. Somewhere between antisocial personality disorder's "lack of remorse" and depressive personality disorder's "prone to feeling guilty or remorseful" there would seem to be a normal, appropriate, and desirable level of remorse. Similarly, it seems there should be a normal range of behavior between narcissistic personality disorder's "requires excessive admiration" and schizoid personality disorder's "indifference to praise and criticism." Nevertheless, a perusal of the criterion set reveals that most of them represent intrinsically undesirable behaviors in the sense of "thick" values or else they include either a term of extremity—such as exaggerated, preoccupied with X, excessive, or does Y to the point of Z, where Z contains a thickly evaluative term—or a motivational descriptor that makes the described behavior undesirable as a whole, again using thickly evaluative phrases, such as "because of feelings of inadequacy." In many cases, more than one of these evaluative types is used, for example, "*preoccupied* with details, rules, lists, order, organization, or schedules, *to the extent that the major point of the activity is lost.*"

▪ ▪ Personality: Adaptive versus Maladaptive

I have been considering the myriad ways that values are involved in the diagnosis of personality disorder. The involvement of values in this process is inevitable because the types of behaviors relevant to this domain are highly influenced by human culture, and human culture will always be sufficiently varied as to reflect a wide range of values that all fall within an adaptive range. However, the inevitable subjectivity involved in the diagnosis of personality disorder could be reduced considerably if time and effort were devoted to mapping out more precisely and comprehensively the structure—and eventually the underlying processes—of personality-relevant human behavior. In antiquity, the Greeks took the initial steps in this direction; in the past century, further great strides have been made in our understanding of this domain.

In this last section, therefore, I discuss briefly how we might use this information to develop a process for personality pathology diagnosis which would be more rational, consistent, and otherwise sensible than the system currently in place in the DSM. To do this, I return to the DSM definition of *personality*. As noted earlier, this definition has much in common with those put forth in the psychological literature on normal-range personality, yet the framers of Axis II chose to develop the diagnoses of personality disorders from within the medical, historical tradition and virtually to ignore the extensive existing work on normal-range personality. Given that personality disorders are essentially defined as personality trait patterns that have "gone wrong" in one or more ways, it seems more sensible either to start with normal trait patterns and study the ways in which these "go wrong" to the point that they are manifested clinically, or to start with clinical cases and study how their problems link back to normal personality traits.

As an illustration, I elaborate on the first of these research programs. Initially, one would consider the ways in which disordered forms of normal-range personality traits appear. Following the DSM for the purposes of this discussion, personality traits can be manifested in cognition, affect, interpersonal functioning, and impulse control, so if something has "gone wrong" with the personality, one would be expect that more than one of these areas would be affected. Similarly, one would expect that a range of life situations would be affected (e.g., work, social behavior, close relations). Moreover, problematic aspects of traits are likely to be either (a) extreme (i.e., markedly deviant from normal levels), (b) unstable (i.e., lacking the consistency normally observed in personality-related behavior), or (c) context insensitive or inappropriate (cf. rigid and inflexible). Finally, it is reasonable to use the criteria of distress or impairment as indicators that something has gone wrong. So far, this all is quite similar to the DSM; however, I propose one major change: that the starting point for describing, evaluating, and understanding personality-gone-wrong in all of these different ways be the knowledge we have about normal personality structure and processes and their relation to behavior, instead of the clinical tradition surrounding a small set of abnormal personality configurations.

Livesley and colleagues (Livesley et al., 1994) have elaborated this view, noting that the assessment of personality and the diagnosis of personality disorder are confounded in the DSM and suggesting that they be separated. They proposed that the notion of dysfunction, which currently is more easily applied to disorders on Axis I than Axis II, be extended to Axis II. To accomplish this, we would need to define the functions of personality which can go wrong. As a starting point, Livesley and colleagues suggested using analyses of universal life tasks or problems to be solved in personality development (e.g., Cantor, 1990). For example, Plutchik (1980) proposed four universal tasks that are basic to adaptation and survival: establishing and maintaining (a) group membership, including territoriality; (b) social structure (e.g., hierarchical relationships; complementary interactions such as dominance or control and submission) (Benjamin, 1993); (c) self-identity; and (d) intimate relationships, including dealing with loss and separation. Livesley and colleagues then offered a working definition of *personality disorder* as extreme personality variation associated with the failure to attain these universal tasks. The assessment of personality per se is thus separated conceptually from the diagnosis of personality disorder. With this separation, many of the problems with inconsistency noted earlier with regard to the DSM would disappear or at least be made more tractable.

Livesley and colleagues further note that our knowledge of personality structure far outstrips our understanding of personality processes, which involve the active and purposeful organization, integration, and regulation of behavior. If we are ever to understand personality disorder, we will need to go beyond understanding how behavior is structured and organized. We will need to understand the processes that maintain that structure and, conversely, how behavior becomes disorganized (i.e., disordered), how dysfunctional motivational states develop and are maintained, and the processes by which individuals come to develop maladaptive goals, that is, ones that will not serve them well in solving life's adaptive tasks. The challenges ahead remain formidable.

10

Values and the Validity of Diagnostic Criteria: Disvalued versus Disordered Conditions of Childhood and Adolescence

JEROME C. WAKEFIELD, D.S.W.

ACCORDING TO THE harmful dysfunction analysis of the concept of disorder (Wakefield, 1992a, 1992b), attribution of disorder requires not only a scientific judgment that a condition is due to an internal dysfunction but also a value judgment that the condition in question is harmful to the individual or to society. Thus, value judgments, although often implicit, are an integral part of the diagnosis of mental disorder. However, this involvement of values opens the door to a common fallacy, in which implicit value judgments are mistaken for a scientific judgment that a condition is due to a dysfunction. The invalid diagnostic criteria that can result from this confusion of values and facts are illustrated in this chapter using criterion sets for childhood and adolescent disorders. Specifically, I am concerned here with the role of values in the validity of child and adolescent diagnostic criteria of the kind that appear in the DSM-III, DSM-III-R, and DSM-IV (American Psychiatric Association, 1980, 1987, 1994). These DSM criteria are very widely used in mental health practice and research.

▪ ▪ The Harmful Dysfunction Analysis of "Disorder"

The form of validity with which I am concerned is what I have elsewhere labeled "conceptual validity" (Wakefield, 1992a, 1992b, 1993). A set of criteria for a mental disorder is supposed to pick out all and only disorders of a certain kind rather than nondisordered problematic conditions often labeled "problems in living" or categorized by the DSM as "conditions that may be a focus of clinical attention" but in which the individual has no mental disorder (1994, p. 675). Conceptual validity is simply validity with respect to picking out all and only disorders.

I work here within the framework of my "harmful dysfunction" analysis of the concept of disorder (Wakefield, 1992a, 1992b, 1993, 1997b, 1999), according to which "disorder" is a concept rooted in *both* (a) scientific notions of failed internal mechanisms of biologically designed functions and (b) everyday normative notions of harm. Only those failures of biologically designed functioning, or "dysfunctions," which actually cause harm to the individual are considered disorders, where "harm" refers to any negative outcome as judged by social values. Mental disorders are harmful dysfunctions of mechanisms involved in mental functions such as perception, language, thought, emotion, motivation, social relating, and so on. The harmful dysfunction analysis asserts that both factual judgments about dysfunction and value judgments about harm are necessary components of every attribution of mental disorder.

▪ ▪ The Normativist Fallacy

If the harmful dysfunction analysis is roughly correct, then there are two main fallacies about the concept of disorder. The first might be called the "normativist" fallacy. This is the belief that judgments of disorder are only just value judgments in the end. Generally speaking, disorders are bad things. Thus, antipsychiatrists, labeling theorists, and social constructivists of various stripes have argued that the concept of mental disorder is scientifically incoherent and is a value term used mainly as a tool of social control, to justify the application of medical power to socially disvalued conditions that are not really disorders in any factual sense.

However, disorders do seem discriminable on factual grounds from other negative mental conditions. There are many negative mental conditions that are not considered disorders, such as the pain of tragic loss, a lack of talent for activities that one ardently wants to pursue, and, within limits, a great variety of negative mental traits such as stupidity, selfishness, insensitivity, and so on. These conditions are believed to fall within the designed range of normal variation rather than to result from dysfunctions. Male aggressiveness is considered negative but, within limits, is not generally considered a disorder because it is seen as the result of the naturally selected design of the male sex. Many of these nondisordered conditions, such as lack of talent, may be due to internal states, so one cannot say that mental disorders are simply internally caused negative conditions. An additional factual requirement must be met, namely, the requirement that some mechanism within the organism is not performing a function it was designed to perform.

The factual component of disorder attributions is particularly clear in cases in which the very same negative state can be either a symptom of disorder or a normal reaction. For example, being moderately overweight is strongly disvalued in our society, yet few regard this condition as a disorder; it is rather viewed as a result of food preferences operating in our calorie-rich environment. However, when it was recently announced that researchers had found that some moderately overweight people may be suffering from a virus that causes a dysfunction in weight-regulating processes, it was immediately apparent that this condition would be considered a disorder. The negative nature of the manifest symptom is the same—being overweight is strongly disvalued in our culture, whatever its cause—and in both cases the cause was at least partly internal, in one case a virus and in the other a food preference. However, in one case, being overweight is caused by a virus-induced dysfunction, and in the other case overweight is due to voluntary food choices. The dysfunction-caused symptoms are considered disorders, but the others are not.

Similarly, vandalism is listed by the DSM as a symptom of conduct disorder, and it may sometimes result in part from dysfunctions of various mechanisms concerned with impulse control, empathy, and so on. Clearly, however, most vandals are not disordered, and if the facts suggest that a child is simply letting off steam or is being pressured by peers to engage in such behavior, we tend to dismiss the hypothesis that the youth is disordered. So, a mental disorder attribution is more than a value judgment. It is in part a factual *hypothesis* that a manifest disvalued condition is caused by an internal dysfunction of some mental mechanism. What makes the distinction here between dysfunction and nondysfunction a *factual* one is its basis in the evolutionary history of mental mechanisms (Wakefield, 1995).

The normativist fallacy, in which the factual component of "disorder" is ignored, leads to the mistaken view that disorder is entirely culturally relative and that cultures can "construct" genuine disorders at will simply by disapproving of a form of behavior or by labeling a condition as a disorder. In fact, cultures can be wrong about whether a condition is a disorder because they may wrongly believe it is caused by a dysfunction. The Victorian notions that female clitoral orgasm and masturbation are disorders, and the antebellum southern belief that runaway slaves suffered from a disorder, did fit the values of the cultures that labeled the respective behaviors as disorders, but these cultures were nonetheless incorrect to label the conditions disorders because, contrary to the cultures' beliefs, the conditions do not indicate mental dysfunctions. Similarly, we rejected the Soviet Union's classification of political dissidents as mentally disordered even though, by Soviet standards, the dissidents were violating social values, because we did not believe that the dissidents were suffering from dysfunctions but rather were expressing quite natural human motives.

What about the constructivist objection that judgments about the dissidents being dysfunctional changed just because the social/power relations that construct the notion of dysfunction changed in Russian society? From this perspective, the Victorian and antebellum southern judgments seem wrong to us merely because our power relations are different from theirs. But surely such judgments are objectively incorrect, based on false beliefs about human nature. Certainly, power relations can influence judgments of dysfunction and disorder, and power implications do go along with judgments of disorder. Such power issues are part of the overall social analysis of "disorder." But the conceptual question addressed here is, What is the structure of the concept "disorder"? To understand *which* judgments are influenced by power and carry power implications and *how* such uses of the concept of disorder work, we need to analyze "dysfunction" independent of power associations. Surely there is such a concept, for judgments of dysfunction are not in any simple criterial sense dependent on or defined by power considerations.

However, it does remain true that there is a degree of cultural relativity in disorder attributions. If a culture does not disvalue the effects of a dysfunction and the dysfunction causes no *harm* within that cultural context, then there is no disorder. For example, in a preliterate culture, a dysfunction of the corpus callosum which has as its only effect an impairment in the ability to learn to read would not be a disorder, whereas it is clearly a disorder in our own culture.

The Essentialist Fallacy

Opposite to the normativist fallacy is the essentialist fallacy (Wakefield, 1997c), the belief that, given the scientific underpinnings of mental health research, values are not a necessary part of the concept of disorder at all. To those engaged in the scientific study of disorders, it may seem an inconvenient distraction that disorder attributions involve value judgments, and it may be tempting to define mental disorder sheerly in terms of a factual description of an individual's internal state. In some cases, this can, in effect, be done, because a specifiable internal dysfunction may virtually imply harm as well. However, more often, the specified internal states are only correlated with harm and can exist without causing any symptoms and thus are not in themselves disorders. Defining disorder in terms of such internal states thus often runs into serious conceptual validity problems. Hans Eysenck's (1986, 1994) proposal to define disorders as extreme points on certain personality dimensions suffers from this problem, because those extremes are not necessarily associated with symptomatic harmful conditions (Wakefield, 1997c). For example, some of those who . score high on Eysenck's dimension of "psychoticism" show no psychotic symptoms and may show unusual creativity. One must add symptomatic criteria to get valid diagnoses. (Of course, even if not conceptually valid as a definition of *disorder,* Eysenck's "psychoticism" dimension may be high in construct validity.)

It is clear from the domain of physical disorders that a condition that involves no significant harm is not a disorder. Most people have what physicians call "benign anomalies," that is, minor malformations that are the result of genetic or developmental dysfunctions but which cause no significant problems, and such anomalies are not considered disorders. For example, it was recently discovered that, as a result of a genetic mutation, some people's cells are missing a certain immune system receptor; however, because the immune system is designed to be highly redundant, it turned out that the lack of these receptors caused no discernible harm, and consequently the affected individuals are not considered disordered. (This benign anomaly turned out to be important because the HIV virus apparently often latches on to these receptors at one stage of its life cycle, so the lack of these receptors appears to offer some protection against the development of AIDS in HIV-infected individuals.) Even when infectious agents invade cells and multiply in the body, one is not considered ill unless harmful symptoms result. For example, as many as 90 percent of people exposed to a cold virus become infected, but less than half of those infected actually become sick (Ramirez, 1996).

The requirement that valid criteria for mental disorder must imply harm was violated by the DSM-III's (American Psychiatric Association, 1980) definition of the childhood disorder of atypical stereotyped movement disorder, which read as follows:

> This category is for conditions such as head-banging, rocking, repetitive hand movements . . . , or repetitive voluntary movements that typically involve fingers or arms. These disorders are distinguishable

from tics in that they consist of voluntary movements and are not spasmodic. Moreover, unlike individuals with a Tic Disorder, those with these conditions are not distressed by the symptoms and may even appear to derive enjoyment from the repetitive activities. . . . These conditions are found almost exclusively in children. They are especially prevalent among individuals with Mental Retardation or Pervasive Developmental Disorders and among children suffering from grossly inadequate social stimulation, but they may also occur in the absence of a concurrent mental disorder. (p. 77)

Because stereotyped movement is often associated with serious developmental disorder, one may plausibly infer that such movement is caused by some unknown dysfunction, even when it occurs entirely alone, without any developmental disability. Nevertheless, the DSM-III's criteria were invalid as indicators of disorder because they did not require that the child or anyone else must be harmed by the movements. Indeed, the movements are described as voluntary—which distinguishes them from tics—as well as sometimes enjoyable. For example, some children who are otherwise normal engage in repetitive rocking motions at night before going to sleep, and they do so with seeming pleasure and with no interference with other functioning. Moreover, these behaviors can be expected to cease as the child gets older. In these cases, there would seem to be no grounds for considering the child disordered, despite the inferred dysfunction. The DSM eventually recognized this problem and in the revised third edition changed the diagnostic criteria to include the requirement that "the disturbance either causes physical injury to the child or markedly interferes with normal activities, e.g., injury to head from head-banging; inability to fall asleep because of constant rocking" (American Psychiatric Association, 1987, p. 95). This addition increased conceptual validity by insisting on harm. Note that the lack of a harm component in diagnostic criteria is a rare problem for DSM criteria because most categories are defined in terms of symptoms that are clearly harmful in and of themselves.

The harm requirement for valid diagnostic criteria obviously raises many questions that cannot be seriously addressed here, but a few such issues might be worth mentioning. First, must the harm be a direct result of the dysfunction, or can it consist merely of the fact that other people do not like the condition? To take the example of stereotyped behavior, if the dysfunction-caused behavior is entirely benign except that parents simply do not like their children rocking before bedtime, is that enough to validly classify the child's condition as a disorder? Neither answer seems immediately obvious or satisfactory. Second, must the condition be harmful on balance, when all the effects are taken into account, or can it consist of one harmful aspect even if other benefits outweigh the harm? Here, the answer seems to be that direct harm from a dysfunction is enough for disorder even if the harm is outweighed by good long-term effects. To take a well-known example, cowpox is generally a mild disorder in humans and protects against smallpox, so in certain environments or in certain periods of history it may be or may have been a good thing overall to contract cowpox, but cowpox is still a disorder because it does harm the individual. Finally, is harm judged from the patient's perspective, or is it judged by social values? This a complex question, but judging from our actual disorder attributions, it would seem that the concept of disorder tends to depend on a rather abstract notion of social values for the evaluation of harm. For example, a young man who is infertile is judged to have a disorder even if he himself does not want children and does not feel his condition is harmful. The fact that the concept of disorder seems to be based on a notion of social values raises interesting and difficult issues for the application of the concept in a pluralistic society like ours where the values of subcommunities may greatly differ. All these questions pose serious challenges for those interested in the role of values in valid diagnosis.

▪ ▪ Why It Is Easy to Mistake Disvalued Conditions for Disordered Conditions

So far, I have considered two fallacies about the concept of disorder. The DSM's definition of *disorder* commits neither of these fallacies. Its definition requires that a disorder be caused by a "dysfunction in the individual" and that the dysfunction cause impairment, distress, or some other kind of harm to the individual (1994, p. xxi; Spitzer and Endicott, 1978).

However, the DSM's diagnostic criteria for specific mental disorders often do not satisfy its own definition of disorder (Wakefield, 1996). The problem is due to a fallacy that involves not a misunderstanding of the concept of disorder itself but rather a misapplication of the concept to specific conditions. This fallacy, which I will call the "value projection" fallacy, occurs when one inadvertently projects one's values onto the world so that one mistakes what one values for what is naturally designed to happen and thus mistakes what is disvalued for a failure of designed functioning and, consequently, for a disorder.

It seems clear that values often influence diagnosticians to perceive dysfunction or disorder where there is none; the above-mentioned Victorian views of female orgasm and masturbation and the view that runaway slaves are disordered are examples of such value projections. It is no doubt much easier to see such errors when they are distant in time and space and when we do not share the values that led to the biased judgment of disorder. But, this mistake being so common, we must suspect that we are not immune to it ourselves. To take one example, when we use DSM criteria to diagnose children as "conduct disordered" partly on the basis of the fact that they have run away from home, are we being just as potentially oppressive to some children as were those who labeled runaway slaves as having a disorder? We owe it to ourselves and to our patients to take such questions seriously and to examine whether our values may not be mistaken for scientific facts about human nature and therefore yield invalid and over-inclusive criteria for disorder.

Disvalued conditions may seem disordered when they are not for several reasons. First, symptoms do double duty in attributions of disorder in a way that can be confusing. Symptoms must represent harms, but because we cannot look directly inside the individual and see whether there is a dysfunction, and because we do not really understand how most mental mechanisms work anyway, symptoms also have a second role; they are used as the basis for inferring that something has gone wrong inside the individual. It is easy to forget that symptoms are being used in diagnosis in these two entirely different ways and that different standards of evidence apply to each of these uses. It is thus easy to conclude from harmful symptoms that there is a disorder even when the evidential threshold for inferring dysfunction is in fact not met. For example, the painful symptoms of depression may be taken as a sufficient condition for disorder when in fact those same symptoms may exist when an individual is reacting normally to a serious loss. So, the inference of dysfunction would require more support than the mere existence of the typical depressive symptoms.

Second, socially valued conditions may be more statistically normal in a culture and thus may seem more functionally normal; although statistical normality is certainly not equivalent to functional normality, it is often a good indicator. Thus, it may spuriously seem as if some special dysfunction is required to cause deviation from the norm. For example, in a society in which disciplined behavior in school is the norm, a child who does not stay in his or her seat, who is not sufficiently quiet during class, and who is not responsive to the teacher's requests may be seen as suffering from an internal dysfunction and thus a disorder, though in fact the child's behavior may be a normal-range response to the constraining conditions of school, and it may be due only to a massive constriction of normal modes of childhood activity that children behave quietly in class in the first place.

Third, socially valued states are usually rationalized by the culture at large, so that their advantages are more manifest. Being so advantageous, they may seem like designed functions of inner mechanisms. For example, in our culture, the advantages of a child's doing well in school are obvious and constantly brought to the attention of parents and educators, and this may make it easier to get the impression that a child who is not keeping up must have a disorder, when in fact there are many reasons other than disorder for such below-average schoolwork.

Many such rationalizations of social values take the form of developmental theories that are claimed to capture what is natural and therefore define what is dysfunctional, but these theories themselves often capture instead the sequences that lead to the culture's preferred outcomes rather than any naturally developmentally privileged pathway. Thus, for example, one must be careful to examine the theory of attachment and separation, and accounts of the disorders of these processes, for value assumptions local to our culture, which prizes the ability of children to be autonomous and to separate early and often from parents. Or, consider the American belief that it is "natural" for babies to cry a lot, which was thrown into question by cross-cultural work showing that babies in cultures in which they are kept close to the mother simply do not cry at anywhere near the rate of American babies.

Fourth, socialization works in part by inducing in the individual's body and mind certain habitual feelings of "rightness" which can easily be confused with—indeed, are perhaps intended to be confused with—feelings of naturalness. That is, the feeling of naturalness which results from socialization can easily be confused with genuine naturalness. For example, each society defines a distance at which it feels natural for people of specific statuses to stand when they are talking together, and when talking to people from other cultures, one may get the uncomfortable feeling that they are violating one's space or otherwise acting in a bizarre manner when in fact they are merely standing at a distance that feels "natural" for them.

There are also obviously many self-interested motivational reasons—from reimbursement to turf maintenance—that professionals in particular would be prone to the value-projective fallacy. However, this fallacy is not limited to professionals and is common in the population at large. Seeing valued conditions as natural states maintains power relationships not just for the medical profession but for various social groups in general. For these and no doubt for many other reasons, it is often easy to confuse socially disvalued conditions with disorders.

▪ ▪ Invalid DSM-IV Criteria Sets Due to Value Projections

I now turn to the presentation of some examples of DSM-IV criteria sets that manifest this fallacy of confusing disvalued conditions with disordered conditions. I focus on disorders of childhood and adolescence because I think that the kind of diagnostic error I am considering, although widespread in the DSM, is particularly common and potentially most harmful when the diagnostic labels are applied to children and adolescents. Children are relatively powerless and least able to object to or correct a misdiagnosis, and yet they are also among those for whom such labeling can have the greatest impact on their subsequent lives.

It should be emphasized that the fact that DSM-IV diagnostic criteria for a category of disorder are overly inclusive does not mean that the category itself is spurious. Nothing said here about the invalidity of specific criteria sets should be taken to imply that the category does not refer to a genuine disorder. For example, there really are depressive disorders even if DSM criteria are overinclusive and classify some nondisorders as depressive disorders; the category is (potentially) valid even if the criteria are not. The problem is that diagnostic criteria may also encompass many disvalued nondisordered conditions as well as truly disordered conditions.

Learning Disorders

Educational failure is highly disvalued and potentially harmful in our society. It is clear that some cases of lack of educational attainment are due to internal dysfunctions in the brain mechanisms that are necessary for learning processes to take place. However, there are many other causes of failure to learn, from lack of opportunity to lack of interest. DSM-IV criteria for learning disorders require only that the child's achievement level, whether in reading, mathematics, or written expression, be substantially below average. For example, the criterion for a reading disorder is: "Reading achievement, as measured by individually administered standardized tests of reading accuracy or comprehension, is substantially below that expected given the person's chronological age, measured intelligence, and age-appropriate education" (p. 50). Below-average performance may be undesirable, but it is far from enough to infer an underlying dysfunction. As Kirk and Kutchins (1994) argue, bad penmanship should not qualify as a disorder of written expression, but DSM criteria do not allow for such a distinction.

Separation Anxiety Disorder

In a society where one or both parents often work in a location distant from the child, where children are expected to sleep apart from their parents and to go to day care or school without their parents quite early in life, and, in general, where the demands of the economic system and the pursuit of quality-of-life goals by the parents are generally agreed to take precedence over the desires of children for sustained contact with parents, it is not surprising that separation responses on the part of children which interfere with this system are disvalued and even seen as disordered.

Separation anxiety disorder is diagnosed in children on the basis of symptoms indicating age-inappropriate, excessive anxiety concerning separation from those to whom the individual is attached, as evidenced in at least three symptoms out of a list of eight symptoms, lasting at least four weeks. The symptoms include, for example, excessive distress when separation occurs, worry that some event will lead to separation, worry that harm will come to attachment figures, refusal to go to school because of fear of separation, and reluctance to be alone or to be without a major attachment figure. These are just the sorts of symptoms children experience when they have a normal, intense separation anxiety response. So, the validity of the criteria in distinguishing disordered responses from normal ones depends entirely on the interpretation of the notions of the age-inappropriateness or excessiveness of the child's anxiety, for which no guidelines are offered; the symptoms themselves are supposed to be the manifestations of the excessiveness. The problem here is that cultural demands placed on children or stressors, such as serious disruption of familial bonds, may arouse what could be construed as an excessive response in normal, nondisordered children. Such contextual factors are not taken into account in DSM criteria.

For example, a study of the mental health of children of military personnel at three bases (Bickman et al., 1995) happened to take place at the time of Desert Storm, when many parents of the children—including in some cases the mothers—were leaving for the Middle East, where children knew that parents could be killed or injured. The level of separation anxiety was high enough among many of the children that they could clearly qualify as having separation anxiety disorder according to DSM-IV criteria; relative to typical separation responses common at their ages, their reactions were "excessive" and "developmentally inappropriate." But in fact they could be considered to be responding with proportional, normal-range separation responses to a highly unusual environment in which an extraordinary kind of separation was taking place and in which they had realistic concerns that the parent would never come back. In these studies, to avoid wholesale pathologizing of these children, DSM criteria had to be modified (A. M. Brannan, personal communication). There is no question that there are real disorders of the separation anxiety response, but DSM's criteria for separation anxiety disorder seem inadvertently overinclusive and reflect our values as much as they do genuine dysfunction in the child's anxiety mechanisms.

Substance Abuse

The negative effects of teenage substance abuse, especially alcohol and marijuana abuse, have been much in the news lately. For example, binge drinking of alcohol by adolescents can lead to a great number of possible negative outcomes, from automobile accidents and vulnerability to unwanted pregnancy to the extreme effect of death from the direct physiological effects of rapid excessive alcohol intake. In addition to the real hazards of alcohol and drug intake, substance abuse in general is a target of our society's war on drugs, and such behaviors, especially in teenagers, are seen as challenging the social order to an almost hysterical extent in some quarters. These intensely held values about drug and alcohol abuse have been translated into grossly invalid diagnostic criteria for the DSM-IV disorder of substance abuse.

DSM-IV diagnosis of substance abuse requires that any one of the following four criteria be met: poor role performance at work or at home due to recurrent substance use; recurrent substance use in hazardous circumstances, such as driving under the influence of alcohol; recurrent substance-related legal problems; or social or interpersonal conflicts due to substance use, such as arguments with family members about it. For example, if an adolescent regularly drives home from parties under the influence of alcohol, that is sufficient for being diagnosed with substance abuse. Certainly we do not want our adolescents driving under the influence, but given how common alcohol is at adolescent parties and the frequent immaturity of adolescent judgment in this area, this criterion potentially inappropriately pathologizes a large segment of our adolescent population. It is clear that nondisordered adolescents and people in general are willing to risk driving under the influence of alcohol for all kinds of foolish reasons and that one need not have a mental disorder to do so. Or, if an adolescent repeatedly argues with his or her parents about alcohol or drug use, that is sufficient by itself for diagnosis. Given that parents are likely to argue with their children or adolescents about even minor experiments with alcohol or drugs, this criterion, too, is dangerously overinclusive with respect to adolescents. Being arrested more than once for driving while under the influence of alcohol or for possession of marijuana is also sufficient for diagnosis, making one's diagnostic status dependent on the diligence of the local police force, the vagaries of local drug laws, and sheer luck or evasive skill. Note that the use of social-individual conflicts, such as arrests for illegal activity or arguments with one's family, as criteria sufficient for diagnosis is inconsistent with DSM-IV's own definition of mental disorder, which asserts that conflicts between individual and society are not sufficient for inferring a mental disorder unless there is also an inferable dysfunction underlying the problem (1994, p. xxii).

Major Depressive Disorder

Depression is one of the most common diagnoses both in adults and in children and adolescents. Certainly, sadness is a painful and socially debilitating emotion. However, sadness, like other negative emotions, is a natural part of our biologically designed emotional repertoire and not in itself a disorder. Unfortunately, the DSM-IV's symptomatic criteria for diagnosing depression do not adequately distinguish extended periods of sadness, which, however painful, can be normal reactions to serious disruptions or losses in one's life, from disorders of sadness-generating mechanisms. Drug companies appear to be exploiting this failure by encouraging detection of DSM-defined depression in the population at large, for example, through education of physicians to detect formerly undetected depression, and the treatment of such detected depression with psychotropic medication. Thus, a wide range of disvalued conditions are being brought under the umbrella of medical treatment, not all of which may be disorders. Part of this trend is a recent move to give broader FDA approval to the use of psychotropic medication with adolescents for depression and other disorders, which raises serious ethical issues if indeed the DSM criteria tend to encompass normal youth.

Selective Mutism

Despite the traditional sentiment that children should be seen and not heard, sometimes our children refuse to speak when we very much want them to do so, as in school. Such a child can be diagnosed with the DSM-IV disorder of selective mutism, which in the DSM-III-R was called elective mutism. The changes in criteria for this disorder from the DSM-III-R to the DSM-IV illustrate how revisions of the DSM are rather unsystematic and are often a matter of trying to identify dysfunctional conditions better when initially the criteria overshoot the mark and encompass an overinclusive range of undesirable conditions. DSM-III-R criteria for elective mutism were simple enough: "(A) Persistent refusal to talk in one or more social situations (including at school); (B) Ability to comprehend spoken language and to speak" (American Psychiatric Association, 1987, p. 89). The voluntary refusal is critical here in distinguishing this disorder from the inability to speak: "In severe or profound mental retardation, pervasive developmental disorder, and developmental expressive language disorder, there may be inability to speak, but not a refusal to do so" (p. 89).

The problem with these DSM-III-R criteria is that they assume that refusal to speak is sufficient to indicate disorder, even when good reasons may exist for the refusal. For example, a note indicates that even when the language is a new one in which the child may feel uncomfortable, diagnosis is still warranted: "Children in families who have emigrated to a country of a different language may refuse to speak the new language. When comprehension of the new language is adequate but the refusal to speak persists, Elective Mutism should be diagnosed" (p. 89). But surely such children need not be disordered.

In the DSM-IV, the criteria for selective mutism were revised in an attempt to eliminate some of the most obvious false positives by the addition of a series of rather ad hoc exclusion clauses, each dealing with a particular type of situation. The disorder's criteria now require that the silence cannot occur only during the first month of school, that the failure to speak is not due to lack of knowledge of or comfort with the spoken language required in the social situation, and that the failure to speak is not better explained by some communication disorder such as stuttering. The last three requirements deal with obvious false positives. During the first month of school, many students are nervous and hesitant to talk; recent immigrants may feel embarrassed by their level of command of English and thus refrain from speaking; and those with speech impediments may feel anxious about speaking and thus may remain silent, but none of these conditions need be a disorder. The problem is that the DSM-IV does not take the next step and systematically analyze the source of the false positives so as to avoid further such mistakes. The criteria thus remain invalid. For example, a girl who refuses to talk because a bully has accused her of being teacher's pet and has threatened to beat her up if she opens her mouth in class can still be diagnosed as disordered under these criteria. Much more work obviously needs to be done to figure out how validly to distinguish selective mutism as a disorder from undesirable voluntary silence that is nondisordered.

Oppositional-Defiant Disorder

Obviously, the obedience of children would be high on everyone's list of desirable and socially approved conditions. However, child development by its very nature requires some independence and therefore some failure of obedience; moreover, many children and adolescents are under the control of adults who do not warrant obedience. Unfortunately, the DSM-IV overpathologizes difficult and disobedient children in the criteria for oppositional-defiant disorder. This disorder is defined by a pattern of negativistic, hostile, and defiant behavior lasting at least six months, during which four or more of the following "symptoms" are present: (1) often loses temper; (2) often argues with adults; (3) often actively defies or refuses to comply with adults' requests or rules; (4) often deliberately annoys people; (5) often blames others for his or her mistakes or misbehavior; (6) is often touchy or easily annoyed by others; (7) is often angry and resentful; (8) is often spiteful or vindictive. Of course, it is clear that these unpleasant behaviors are ones that many nondisordered children and adolescents engage in for periods of six months or more during their development. To deal with this problem, the DSM-IV adds that symptoms are to be counted only if the behavior occurs more frequently than is typically observed in individuals of the same age and developmental level. But this allows the upper half of the nondisordered population to be diagnosed, and in any event the nature of the child's situation rather than an internal dysfunction in the child might account for higher than average generation of such behaviors.

Conduct Disorder

Clearly, antisocial behavior by children and adolescents is highly disvalued. However, not all such behavior is the result of disorder. DSM-IV diagnostic criteria for conduct disorder inappropriately allow the diagnosis of adolescents as disordered who are responding with antisocial behavior to peer pressure, to the dangers of a deprived or threatening environment, or to abuses at home, even though such adolescents need not be suffering from a disorder. Rebellious children or children who fall in with the wrong crowd and who skip school and do a bit of shoplifting and vandalism also can qualify for diagnosis, despite the very high incidence of such behaviors among normal adolescents. Even Huckleberry Finn and Tom Sawyer seem to qualify (Richters and Cicchetti, 1993).

In the case of conduct disorder—but not in the cases of any of the other examples presented earlier—the DSM-IV acknowledges that the criteria are not conceptually valid as they stand and addresses how to correct the problem: "Concerns have been raised that the Conduct Disorder diagnosis may at times be misapplied to individuals in settings where patterns of undesirable behavior are sometimes viewed as protective (e.g., threatening, impoverished, high-crime). Consistent with the DSM-IV definition of mental disorder, the Conduct Disorder diagnosis should be applied only when the behavior in question is symptomatic of an underlying dysfunction within the individual and not simply a reaction to the immediate social context" (p. 88).

These comments do address the source of the invalid diagnoses described above. However, the DSM-IV did not attempt to incorporate such considerations into the criteria, so there is no guidance as to how to evaluate such possibilities. Yet it is the criteria, not textual comments, which are almost always used by researchers and clinicians. Moreover, as we have seen, the same kinds of problems afflict many other categories but are unrecognized even in the DSM-IV's text. The DSM-IV's textual comments thus provide not a solution but the opening for an agenda to improve the criteria for this and other categories.

▪ ▪ Conclusion

I have pointed to some obvious conceptual validity problems with DSM criteria for child and adolescent disorders, but I have not suggested substantive solutions, which would require a category-by-category detailed analysis. Clearly, considerations such as those in the DSM's text for conduct disorder must be directly incorporated into diagnostic criteria, and this must be done not just for conduct disorder but for a great number of DSM categories, including many of those applying to children and adolescents. At the heart of such changes to the criteria is the challenge of operationalizing the contextual factors that indicate whether a problem is a dysfunction or a normal response to the environment. Until this is done, the antipsychiatrists' accusation that psychiatric diagnosis is just a tool for the social control of undesirable conditions rather than truly the identification of disorders will not have been completely answered.

Last, I want to address a commonly heard objection to the kind of analysis I have provided. The objection is simply that it doesn't matter whether a condition is a disorder or not; all that matters is whether the practitioner can help the client with the client's problems. In one sense, this is absolutely right; what ultimately matters is helping people, not categorization of conditions as disorders or nondisorders. However, mental health professionals, in order to obtain considerable advantages and benefits including reimbursement by health insurance, do claim to the public to be treating mental disorders—indeed, a central theme of pronouncements to the public is that mental problems of the type treated by mental health practitioners are real disorders, just like physical disorders. In addition, most practitioners, to get reimbursement, label their clients as disordered. Moreover, clients themselves really care about the answer to the question, "Is there something wrong with me?" So, refusing to take seriously the distinction between disorder and nondisorder may be unethical and may have negative repercussions for clients. It's fine not to care about the distinction as long as one does not pretend that nondisordered conditions are disordered conditions or that what one is doing when one helps nondisordered clients is conceptually part of medicine just like any other medical treatment. Of course, there are also many medical rationales for treating nondisordered conditions, such as prevention, so nondisordered status does not mean no reimbursement—but those rationales depend on a prior distinction between the disordered and the nondisordered. In the end, the analysis of the concept of disorder must indeed matter to the ethical professional.

11

Implications of an Embrace: The DSMs, Happiness, and Capability

JENNIFER H. RADDEN, D.PHIL.

THAT VALUES ARE inescapable in psychiatric classification is accepted today. Not only are values inescapable, but they are also recognized to be important, as the criteria or warrant for disorder status. Happiness and capability are goods, the absence of which indicates mental disorder characterized by subjective distress or pain, and incapability or dysfunction.

Although they are explicit and agreed on and play a very central role in warranting the disorder status of numerous conditions, these values are only casually acknowledged in the DSM. The DSM would better serve its goal of providing a warrant or explanation of disorder status by eliminating ambiguities in its introductory discussion and noting that it may be on a different symptom model that emotional pain serves as a criterion for mental disorder. It would also be helpful if the DSM acknowledged the differing models of incapability on which its diagnostic descriptions rest and the theoretical and etiological implications they convey.

▪ ▪ Mental Health Norms Requiring Clarification

Rejections of earlier attempts to provide a value-free diagnostic classification (see, for example, Fulford, 1989; Sadler, Wiggins, and Schwartz, 1994a; Wakefield, 1992a, 1997a, 1997b, 1997c) now encourage us to ask of a given psychiatric classification or category which of its underlying values are defensible. These values are expressed in mental health norms that play a part in establishing the limits of mental disorder. They serve to fix the boundary between disorder and normal psychological variation.

Two moral values are involved in the DSM discussion of what makes a particular condition a mental disorder. Proposed as the criteria for disorder status are the disvalues or "negativities" of subjective distress or pain on the one hand and incapability or dysfunction on the other. The strength of these criteria is that they embody widely shared—perhaps even universal—moral values. States of human pleasure, happiness, or contentment are what philosophers call goods—goods, some think, desirable in themselves. Displeasure and suffering are not to be equated with a want of happiness or pleasure (one may be without unhappiness yet not quite happy). Nonetheless, happiness, pleasure, and contentment constitute at least part of the valued good corresponding to the disvalue we place on suffering. Capability is also such a good. We disvalue incapability because we find capability desirable—desirable in itself as an expression of autonomy, as well as instrumentally valuable in bringing about other goods.

Although they are explicit and agreed on and play a very central role in warranting the disorder status of numerous conditions, these values receive little attention in the DSM discussions. In the introduction to the DSM-IV it is noted merely that each of the mental disorders included is "conceptualized as a clinically significant behavioral or psychological syndrome or pattern that occurs in an individual and that is associated with *present distress* (e.g., a painful symptom) or *disability* (i.e., impairment in one or more important areas of functioning) with a significantly increased risk of suffering death, pain, disability, or an important loss of freedom" (p. xxi; my emphases).

Unspecified in this passage, and in later references to the role of distress and disability, are two things. First, this claim about present distress is ambiguous. Is the distress a symptom in the way that present distress is a symptom of several mood disorders (such as depression) but not of others (such as those marked by what the early psychiatrists used to describe as *la belle indifférence*)? Or is it occasioned by other symptoms (as when incapacitating or abhorrent compulsions cause their sufferer distress, for example)? Only in the second case, notice, would we naturally say that the distress was over or about the disorder, although in each case the distress may be said loosely to be due to or resultant from the disorder.

Also left unresolved—although it is not an issue pursued in the present discussion—is the relation these conditions bear to the ascription of mental disorder. That suffering or incapability could be regarded as singly sufficient for mental disorder is unlikely. But each condition, or one, or neither, may be necessary for mental disorder, and they may or may not be jointly sufficient for it.

Given the importance of the reliance on norms embodying happiness and capability outlined above, these values require more careful analysis. Such an analysis, which is sketched in what follows, suggests that it is important to problematize even these most agreed-on and widely accepted criteria for mental disorder.

Concerning pain and distress: we can identify different kinds of suffering (or pain/distress/unhappiness). In particular, there seem to be asymmetries between what are rather confusingly distinguished as physical and mental suffering. Psychological states of distress serve as criteria for attributions of mental disorder, and justifiably so. It is not that nonphysical pain does not exist or that it does not warrant attributions of mental disorder. But nonphysical pain—and particularly this role it plays in grounding our attributions of mental disorder—cannot be understood merely by appeal to the model of physical pain as medical symptom. Required is a careful account of the nature of "nonphysical" pain and a separate model of how such suffering relates to disorder status.

Concerning incapability: if incapability functions as a criterion for mental disorder, it does so in different ways depending on the symptom or disorder in question. At least two models of incapability are required to encompass the different disorders included in the DSM taxonomy, and the adoption of each model violates the DSM-IV goal of achieving an atheoretical and particularly a nonetiological classification.

Two recommendations emerge from the general injunction that we more fully understand the fundamental mental health norms of capability and happiness. First, the DSM would better serve its goal of providing an explanation of disorder status by acknowledging the disanalogy between sensation pain and emotional or "mental" suffering. It is not on analogy with sensation pain but as a separate kind of suffering that such distress enters in as a mental health norm and serves as a criterion for mental disorder, and this point could be made more clearly and strongly.

Second, it would be helpful if the DSM acknowledged the differing models of incapability on which it relies. Once these models of incapability are distinguished, it will be important to infuse the text with this recognition. Each of the disorders described in the manual might usefully be accompanied by an explicit identification of the kind of incapability involved.

The practical implication of the following discussion is thus clear. The features identified in this analysis of the DSM values of capability and happiness deserve brief, conceptually clear, and frank acknowledgment in subsequent manuals.

▪ ▪ Distress

Other theorists have directed their attention to the critical notion of distress or suffering. Most notable of these is perhaps Russell, who argues that to treat distress as a symptom involves both a failure to apply and a misapplication of the medical model. A symptom, she points out, is "defined . . . as a manifestation of a pathological condition," yet "because in most cases no underlying pathological condition is substantiated, the declaration that aspects of thinking or behaving referred to can be regarded as *symptoms,* must be treated with caution." The authors of the DSM "want to avoid the vexing problem of etiology, but they run the risk of conceptual incoherence in their talk of symptoms. It does not make sense to talk of symptoms in the absence of even conjectures about what the symptoms are symptoms *of* " (Russell, 1994, p. 247).

Russell's critique may be warranted. Certainly distress alone could not serve to confer disorder status; as was remarked earlier, it is not alone a sufficient condition. Much distress is entirely normal, so to treat distress as a criterion of mental disorder is to imply that some other condition—the presence of an underlying disease entity, perhaps—is met. Moreover, I later put forward a view about the incapability criterion for mental disorder which closely parallels Russell's suggestion that a risk of incoherence accompanies attempts at a definition of mental disorder as theoretically unencumbered as the DSM's authors would wish. But my concern here is with a different implication of treating distress as a "symptom."

Strong analogies undeniably link the "physical" or identifiably organic pain we suffer when injured, diseased, or ill, on the one hand, and the "mental" or emotional pain and distress associated with mental disorder, on the other. In the context of medical psychiatry, psychological disorders are often construed on a preexisting medical model (it is this, we saw, to which Russell objects). Whether it is right or wrong, this construction leaves psychological disorders as logically secondary, or derivative, so that the terms *pain, distress,* and *suffering* associated with mental disorder seem to be employed in a secondary or metaphorical way, derived from or parasitic on the more primary model in which ordinary sensations of pain are symptoms of bodily disorder. My arthritis produces pain literally understood; my depression, while equally or more painful, brings pain in some more extended sense. This interpretation is implied in the passage quoted earlier, where "painful symptom" is offered as an *example* of "present distress." That passage is obviously the offspring of one in the DSM-III-R, whose meaning is somewhat clearer: each mental disorder is there said to be "associated with present distress (a painful symptom)" (1987, p. xxiii). The parenthetical paraphrase serves to indicate that the distress is equated with rather than merely exemplified in a (sensation) painful symptom. (The difference is important. When such insight is present, the insight that a person has mental disorder of any kind is likely to engender distress and suffering in that person, but only some mental disorders such as depression have distress and suffering as *symptoms*. Alternatively put: depression gives rise to a primary distress, while having a depression or any other disorder might give rise to a secondary distress in addition.)

The logical priority of one sense of pain over another is not an issue for us here. But what we must ask is, How close are the analogies, whatever the logical priority? For several reasons, "not very close" seems to be the right answer to that question. There are asymmetries between what are distinguished as physical and mental pain and suffering which bear on the question of how satisfactorily we really understand the distress criterion for mental disorder.

Let us clarify terminology. As philosophers of mind insist, the state of "physical" pain is a quintessential phenomenological state: to speak of someone's suffering such pain is to presuppose conscious awareness and an experiencing mind. (An important disclaimer is necessary here to avoid misunderstanding. This separation of sensation pain from emotional pain offers a conceptual, not an empirical, analysis. For this theory of pain, the stimulation of physiological pain centers without conscious awareness of painful sensation would not be described as the occurrence of "pain.")

Because all pain is in this sense "mental," it is misleading to speak of only one of the two forms of pain we are interested in as mental pain. Let us instead use the terms *sensation pain* and *emotional pain*. When I suffer from a blow to the head, it is sensation pain; when I feel the worthlessness and despair of depression, it is emotional pain.

The distinction between sensations and emotions is a technical philosophical one whose terminological appropriateness here will become apparent. But first, another disclaimer is necessary, lest my overall point be misunderstood. Distinguishing these two uses of the notions of pain, distress and suffering, does not require us to distinguish physical from mental disorders, nor does it imply such a distinction. An unequivocally "physical" disease (cancer, say) may give rise to emotion pain, either because its sufferer is distressed over the illness or because the illness causes a depressive mood state; similarly, a "mental" condition such as a somatoform disorder may be associated with sensation painful symptoms, such as back pain or gastric pain.

The disanalogies between sensation pain and emotional pain can be explored in two different though related steps. First, sensation pain and emotional pain differ qualitatively in several significant ways, despite the obvious parallels between them; second, because of this, they can also be seen to differ in the presuppositions and assumptions implicit in the appeal that is made to them as indicators of disease or illness.

It would be a mistake to underestimate the analogies between sensation pain and emotional pain: after all, the same words—*pain, suffering, discomfort, distress, hurt*, and so on—span the two states, and this bespeaks immensely strong analogies. Nonetheless, there are important asymmetries here.

The first asymmetry was introduced earlier, when it was pointed out that only some pain is naturally spoken of as about or over a disorder. Emotions (such as emotional pain) are said by philosophers to be intentional, whereas sensations (such as sensation pain, but also itches, tickles, tingles, giddiness, throbbing, nausea, etc.) are not. This means that emotions are about or directed toward (intentional) objects. My emotional pain is over or about something or other, as my sadness is about the loss of a friend. Being intentional, emotions (including emotional pain) presuppose other beliefs such as the belief, in the previous example, that my friend has gone. The object of an emotion may refer to the same thing as the cause of a sensation. Thus my suffering (emotional pain) over or about a diseased body part, an ovary, for example, is distinct from but nonetheless focused toward the same diseased ovary that causes my sensation pain. But these pains are distinguishable: the ovary is object in the first case and cause in the second. My suffering over or about the ovary (say, a sense of bodily integrity violated, or a fear that disease will destroy other organs as well) depends on and is intrinsically bound up in a particular web of beliefs—about my body, the future, my values and ideals, and so on. We would not identify it as an emotion felt over my diseased ovary unless that particular web of beliefs were present. In contrast, the diseased ovary may cause sensation pain without my holding any beliefs at all; and if it prompts beliefs—about the pain itself, its location, duration, intensity, and likely cause—then these are not bound in with the pain in the same internal or conceptual way as are the beliefs about its object with emotional pain. The pain is caused by the ovary and thus rightly designated "ovarian pain" even if I mistakenly believe it to be caused by appendicitis.

A feature of this intentionality is that emotions permit a second-order ranking in that they may themselves be the objects of further emotions (Nordenfelt, 1996). Thus, while my state of dejection *is* a feeling of sadness, I may also feel sad *over* my state of dejection, regretting, for instance, how it bothers my loved ones or prevents my completing tasks. Sensations can be the objects of emotions. (I feel sad about my arthritic pain.) But sensations do not themselves take objects; they are not about or over anything beyond themselves.

The ovary example suggests another feature distinguishing emotions from sensations. Sensations are localized; emotions are not. There is an identifiable place where we feel sensation pain (even when, as after a fall, I might insist that I feel pain all over my body), but no such place where we feel emotional pain. True, emotional pain may be accompanied by somatic sensations, a sinking feeling in the stomach or a lump in the throat. William James even urged that emotions could be reduced to sensation or to an awarenss of sensation. But neither psychologists nor philosophers since have shared this notion that such reduction is possible without remainder: instead, pace James, we insist that there are two distinct things, the emotion (pain) and its accompanying sensations (the sinking feeling).[1] (Some emotions are perhaps nothing over and above their cognitive components, but the emotion of suffering is usually treated as possessing phenomenological content beyond its cognitive constituents.) Another feature distinguishing sensations from emotions is that sensations are always occurrences, mental or psychological "events" that take place at a particular time and have a particular finite duration. Emotions are sometimes occurrences, but not always. Thus, while it is unfailingly appropriate to ask when and for how long a sensation occurred, emotions sometimes elude occurrent analysis. Emotions are often more like dispositions to act or feel, rather than occurrences, and cannot be pinned down in the same way. This point may be illustrated if we think about attributing sensations and emotions to a person who is asleep. "She is sleeping and she is in great pain in her lower back" is nonsensical as a claim about sensation pain: unless she is now conscious of the pain, and thus conscious, we do not say she is in pain. On the other hand, "She is sleeping but I know she is still resentful (an emotion) over the slight" sounds acceptable because resentment may be analyzed dispositionally. "She resents" often means: she will feel resentment given certain conditions (she is awake and thinking about the source of her resentment, to name two such conditions).

We can sum up these differences: emotions are intentional, involving belief, nonlocalized, and not always requiring of analysis as occurrences.

Not all pain fits neatly into the categories of sensation pain and emotional pain distinguished here, a point illustrated by painful moods and psychosomatic pain. Nonetheless, the basic distinction and clear paradigms of each kind of pain remain, despite the presence of borderline and ambiguous cases.

The affective states sometimes categorized as moods are said by some theorists to be without an intentional object; commonly offered examples are free-floating anxiety and forms of pervasive and apparently nondirected depression. Moods may be genuine borderline cases. (Although many moods can be shown to fall into one category or another or to be compound states comprising emotional and sensation elements.)[2]

The case of psychosomatic pain also challenges the sharp division drawn here between sensation pain and emotional pain. Psychosomatic pain is expressive of meaning, we want to say, and thus it may be quasi-intentional. Again, the presence of psychosomatic pain does not explode the basic distinction between sensation pain and emotional pain; it merely shows that there are unclear, borderline cases that do not fit neatly into those two categories. (On the other hand, it may be pointed out that psychosomatic pain merely *represents* the emotion attributable to its sufferer. Thus person P consciously or unconsciously experiences emotion X, and P's sensation pain represents emotion X rather as a work of art may be said to stand as a symbol of some emotion. The work of art is not intentional, and no more is the psychosomatic pain, but each is the product or outcome of an intentional state.)[3]

To reiterate: that there are ambiguous and or genuinely borderline cases does not detract from the conceptual distinction between the two kinds of pain, and it is a distinction that needs to be clarified and acknowledged.

Now let us see how these dissimilarities explain the differing assumptions implicit in the appeal to distress or pain as indicator of disease or illness.

First, it will be helpful to explore the assumptions implicit in medical contexts in which ordinary organic disorder gives rise to painful symptoms (sensation pain). Masochists aside, people's dislike of pain and wish to avoid it (the motivational assumption known as the pleasure principle) create expectations about how they will behave when they experience painful medical symptoms: complaining of them, wanting to be rid of them, cooperating (at least to some degree) in their removal. These expectations are also related to some more purely epistemic assumptions on which clinical medicine rests. It is assumed that people can often be fairly accurate reporters of their symptoms. Like cases of masochists, cases of referred pain are obvious exceptions, and so this claim must not be over-stated. Nonetheless, it does seem to be assumed that people are not only motivated to convey their symptoms accurately for the reasons just out-lined but often capable of doing so.

Some of the asymmetries between the two sorts of pain identified ear-lier seem to prevent our accepting these assumptions as readily when the symptoms involve emotional pain. Reporting many other psychological symptoms (of which emotional pain is merely one) seems a much less straightforward and reliable process than reporting sensation pain. Some of this is epistemic and relates to the reportorial authority accorded the subject of sensation pain; some is motivational. My reports on my sensa-tions often go unchallenged; they are to be treated, philosophers say, as in-corrigible claims. But this epistemic authority is considerably weaker with reports of emotions. Emotional pain talk often refers to longer-term items, to states and dispositions—standing conditions rather than particular, datable moments of sensation suffering, as we saw. And emotional pain talk is more complex because emotional pain comes with a more complex and extensive cognitive web about the intentional object of the pain. Think of the person whose suffering (emotional pain) results from her false be-lief that the diseased ovary spells her doom, when in fact she will live a long life. Think of the person who mistakes her despair over her divorce for de-spair over her cancer. Doubtless because of these differences (emotional pain more often involves complex standing conditions), we seem more prone to error, exaggeration, and distortion in our reporting of emotional pain.

In addition to these differences there may be another. First we have the various strategies of "defense," or self-deception. From Freud's writing on, much theorizing shows how we repress, deny, or distort emotional pain we suffer. Moreover, we seem to do so in ways that come "naturally"; self-deception over emotion pain is a kind of second nature. With training, some people are able to reduce or deny sensation pain also, by using med-itation, imaging techniques, breathing exercises, self-hypnosis, and the like. But these skills do not appear to come so easily; unlike self-deception about emotional pain, they are not natural tendencies. A counter to this position might rest on the claim that we are the frequent recipients of (sen-sation) pain–inducing stimuli and by an analogous mechanism we also deny, repress, and prevent those stimuli from entering consciousness ex-cept when there are strong adaptive reasons for doing so. This is certainly a possible and even a plausible position, but notice that it rests on the re-ductionist program eschewed at the outset of this discussion. If *pain* is collapsed to mean "the stimulation of physiological pain centers," then indeed it may be true to say that we are the frequent recipients of pain-inducing stimuli whose conscious presence is repressed. But this not only presupposes reductionism; it also requires a meaning of *pain* contrary to customary usage.

At its simplest, this capacity to repress, deny, or distort emotional pain through self-deception results in conversion into physical symptoms; at its more complex, it is believed to result in other mental states and behavioral responses too diverse to count. I do not mean to adhere to a strictly Freudian economy here, but let us use the Freudian term *mechanisms of defense* to describe the multitude of ways people can avoid their emotional pain. (Nor are these mechanisms a Freudian discovery, of course. The recognition that we seek to hide painful emotions from ourselves antecedes Freud.) Together with these mechanisms or *means*, we have the *end* in some version of the pleasure principle: we naturally strive to avoid emotion pain.

My point is that unless we are especially trained, the presence of sensation pain together with the pleasure principle will be likely to direct us to seek medical help (or at least to want to seek help—for it is clear that practical considerations such as cost might still prevent a pain sufferer from taking the step dictated by his or her practical reasoning). In contrast, precisely because we can often satisfy the pleasure principle by engaging some mechanism of defense, the motivational assumptions differ with emotional pain, and the pain together with the principle does not as reliably direct us to seek medical help).

People do often bring emotional pain to medical attention, of course, and I do not mean to suggest that the defense mechanisms work, or work without burdensome psychic cost. But these mechanisms at least appear to present the emotional-pain sufferer with an alternative route to a satisfaction of the pleasure principle. And because of this, uncertainty is cast on the general status of the sort of reports its sufferers make about their emotional pain. The motivational and epistemic presuppositions about the relation between symptom and clinical knowledge of that symptom identified above (that people are usually motivated to convey their symptoms accurately and are often capable of doing so) cannot be adopted in psychiatry with the same confidence they are in nonpsychological medicine.

By drawing attention to some of these asymmetries between sensation pain and emotional pain when these are viewed as criteria for attributing disorder, I do not mean to dismiss or diminish the criterial force of the more nebulous, and publicly elusive, emotional pain. States of emotional distress are very widely accepted criteria for attributions of mental disorder, and they are, in my view, justifiably so. Rather, I wish to point out that any clarity thought to derive from the set of analogies between the two sorts of pain may be illusory, for places where the analogies seem to break down are precisely where they would have to be strong for us to rely on the force of the one to accept the other. It is not that emotional pain does not exist or that it does not warrant attributions of mental disorder. But in using emotional pain as a criterion for or indicator of mental disorder status, which we want to do, we cannot assume that people are in any uncomplicated way (1) usually motivated to convey their symptoms accurately and (2) often capable of doing so. Emotional pain and this role it plays in grounding our attributions of mental disorder have to be better understood, and they cannot be understood merely by appeal to the model of sensation pain as medical symptom.

Given what we know of emotional pain, what assumptions will enable us to regard it as a criterion for mental disorder? Certainly there remains the primary truth underlying the pleasure principle: people usually dislike pain and want to avoid it. But at least two other assumptions seem to be implicit in what has been said thus far. The first is that for severe (enduring and intense) emotional pain, the mechanisms of defense are insufficient, either in not working or in exacting so great a psychic cost as to be self-defeating. Freud believed this, I believe this, and most who accept the notion of depth psychology probably believe it. It is not particularly controversial; my point is only to insist that it be made explicit as an assumption. The second assumption, which is also, I suggest, fairly innocuous, is that therapeutic intervention with sufferers from emotional pain can improve their ability to communicate their symptoms effectively—that is, to recognize, name accurately, and describe their emotional pain. (Notice that what form of therapy this requires remains open. Insight-producing psychopharmacological intervention may work, as may the administration of drugs as "readiers" for some form of psychotherapy.)

My concern is that these assumptions (that people dislike pain, that the mechanisms of defense are inadequate in the face of severe emotional pain, and that therapeutic intervention can improve the ability to communicate emotional pain symptoms) be made explicit in discussions of emotional pain. The goal of a theory-free diagnostic classification associated with earlier DSMs would militate against adopting or acknowledging assumptions such as these, it is true. But such a goal is now widely discredited: today, we seem required to ask not whether to accept theoretical assumptions but which theoretical assumptions to accept. And I suggest that this pair of depth-psychological assumptions are both innocuous and useful.

From this analysis of pain and suffering as a symptom of mental disorder, it emerges that we have even to problematize one of the most agreed-on and widely accepted criteria for mental disorder, emotional suffering. To do so, I must again emphasize, is not to challenge or unseat the mental health norm of happiness. It is merely to require that the distinction between emotional and sensation pain and the two assumptions required for using emotional pain as a criterion for mental disorder be acknowledged.

An alternative course, however, is available to the authors of the DSM. It was pointed out earlier that the key passage from the introduction to the DSM-IV (p. xxi) reads ambiguously. Either distress is very strongly indicative of mental disorder while being neither necessary nor sufficient for it, an interpretation I have presupposed in the preceding discussion, or it is necessary but not sufficient for mental disorder. In this second interpretation, we can attribute mental disorder status when incapability is added to the presence of suffering (emotional pain) over or about the disorder or its effects. Each is necessary, but neither alone is sufficient for disorder status. This interpretation avoids the introduction of the special model of emotional pain as symptom outlined above. On the other hand, this interpretation places heavy emphasis on the notion of incapability, a notion that brings its own set of difficulties.

▪ ▪ Incapability

Incapability, too, is problematic as a criterion for the attribution for mental disorder, although, like distress, it is widely, and I believe rightly, accepted as a warrant for treating something as a mental disorder.

Many have explored the nature of the disability, incapability, incapacity, or dysfunction identified as a criterion for mental disorder (for a recent, comprehensive review, see Svensson, 1995), and I restrict myself to a few comments here, illustrated by particular disorder categories.

A word first on the distinction between these several terms (*incapability, incapacity, disability, dysfunction*). Although they appear to be used interchangeably in the DSM-IV, these several terms have been shown to carry distinct assumptions, implications, and connotations (Boorse, 1975; Kendell, 1975; Fulford, 1989, 1994; Wakefield, 1992a, 1992b, 1993; Griffiths, 1994; Lilienfeld and Marino,1995; Svensson, 1995). I favor the term *incapability* because of its more powerful invocation of the set of value norms associated with *autonomy, agency,* and *capability.* As others have shown (e.g., Fulford, 1989, 1994), the notion of *illness,* with its explicitly evaluative overtones, in certain ways better fits mental disorder than the ostensibly descriptive *disease*, and illness concerns not failure of function so much as failure of action, or agency. Moreover, there are several conceptual difficulties associated with the project that attempts to define *mental disorder* as a reflection of dysfunction (Fulford, 1989; Lilienfeld and Marino, 1995). So at risk of occluding some conceptually important differences or advantages associated with the notion of mental disorder as dysfunction, I focus my attention on the terms *incapability, incapacity,* and *disability,* defined as hindrances, apparently located in the person, to the normal exercise of capabilities, capacities, and abilities, respectively.

One point I wish to make is that the DSM's continuing attempts to offer an atheoretical classification by avoiding etiological assumptions interfere with the appeal to a want or lack of capability in offering criteria for mental disorder. This is because certain features of the notion of incapability pick up conceptual strength only with the acknowledgment of an "anchoring etiology" (the expression comes from Margolis, 1994). I illustrate this point below (in the first subsection) with reference to the category of personality disorder.

A second point(see the second subsection), illustrated here by reference to hedonic mood states such as mild mania, is that to get full strength out of the incapability concept, some mental disorders also appear to require adherence to nonetiological features of a thoroughgoing disease model. This suggests that at least two sorts of models underlie the attribution of disorder status to the range of conditions currently so designated by the DSM. One is a more theoretically spare deficit model, the other a more theoretically encumbered disease or illness model. (Each presumably falls under the broader category of "medical models," since nonpsychiatric medicine embraces both defects and deficiencies [e.g., congenital blindness, low intelligence] and diseases or illnesses [cancer, tuberculosis].)

Incapability, Personality Disorders, and the Need for an Anchoring Etiology

Goals made explicit in the introduction to the DSM-IV seem to encourage us to avoid, if possible, a full medical model of mental disorder, with its etiological assumptions and seemingly ontological presuppositions—about the organic or structural origins of the condition and about its progressive course. We find some of these medical assumptions and presuppositions in Reznek's definition of an illness (for our purposes here, the terms *illness* and *disease* are used as equivalents) as an abnormal, irreversible, harmful process (Reznek, 1987); others of these assumptions and presuppositions are more explicit in traditional biological-medical accounts of mental disease or illness such as Ludwig's "any debilitating, cognitive-affective-behavior disorder due primarily to known, suggestive or presumed biological brain dysfunctions, either biochemical or neurophysiological in nature" (Ludwig, 1975).

Although to adopt a medical model may be to go from the frying pan into the fire, as medical psychiatry's many critics have suggested, I argue here that not all the disorders included in the DSM allow us to avoid such a model successfully if we take seriously this notion of incapability. We may be left with an uncomfortable choice: embrace and explicitly acknowledge the medical model; reject the incapability criterion for mental disorder; or declassify some of the alleged disorders currently included in the DSM.

Functional deficit disorders of a nonpsychiatric kind, such as blindness or aphasia, seem to offer us a model of incapacitation which avoids the more encumbered disease model. There is some thing, some capability or function, that the person with a functional deficit cannot exercise, and that incapability warrants the disorder status of the person's condition. Typical deficit disorders include blindness, low intelligence, or aphasia, robbing their sufferer of the power to see, reason well, and speak, respectively. Certain symptoms associated with mental disorders can be identified as reflecting incapability in this rather strong sense, where the analogies with ordinary physical defect are very strong. Organic disorders and brain damage both prevent functioning in this way when, for example, they affect memory capability.

This model is not always easy to apply, especially, perhaps, when we are talking about psychological abilities. It is often difficult to identify and isolate the skill or capability that is absent or deficient because of the amorphous or complex nature of that skill. Aphasia and low intelligence are the easy cases, for being able to speak is a rather discrete ability, and being able to reason well has been trimmed, isolated, defined, and measured so that it can be tested. But many abilities are not so easily defined and isolated. We might call this *the problem of nondiscrete functions*. (For a discussion of this problem in another context, see Braude, 1991, pp. 180–87.) This difficulty remains true, however, even in relation to disorders and conditions resulting from known organic disease and injury. In his neurological studies Damasio struggles to portray the characteristic emotional good judgment in which his patients are left deficient, which is a complex mix of dispositional states, affective habits and responses, and cognitive skills each present in innumerable contexts of everyday functioning (Damasio, 1994).

I do not mean to underestimate the problem of nondiscrete functions, but it is not the limitation of the deficit model which is my focus here, since it is shared with the organic disorders. A more basic difficulty distinctive to the class of mental disorders is that at least some conditions designated as mental disorders apparently elude this rather strong notion of incapability.

The personality disorders are in one respect close to the sort of permanent defects which the deficit model of incapacitation best exemplifies, as their position in the DSM's organization suggests: they are long-term unchanging character traits, not diseases or illnesses in the usual sense. They are not processes, to be understood only longitudinally: they do not have a course, as proper diseases such as cancer and tuberculosis do. Nonetheless, there are difficulties if we try to apply the deficit model to them.

Take the case of antisocial personality disorder. Whatever it is which we say the patient suffering these conditions cannot do (and the task of defining these is not insignificant in either case, because of the problem of nondiscrete functions), the sense of "cannot" is problematic. Let us, for the sake of argument, introduce a want of capability in regard to entertaining other-regarding beliefs, attributed to the antisocial character in a recent discussion (Fields, 1996). (Other-regarding beliefs focus on other people's needs and states as distinct from one's own.) Intelligence deficit is a paradigm of the sort of incapacitating disability fitting the deficit model of incapacitation, as we saw above. But the example of intellectual deficit reveals the disanalogy between incapacitating disabilities as they have been understood thus far and the inability to form other-regarding beliefs. Like most who take intelligence tests, persons of low intelligence want to do well. But they cannot. In contrast to those diagnosed with antisocial character disorder, who give every impression that they are unwilling but able (to form other-regarding beliefs), persons of low intelligence are willing but unable, *prevented* from scoring well by their intellectual deficit.

As long as a person *seems* to act voluntarily, we have no particular reason to suppose that something prevents him or her from acting as he or she wished or intended. This presumption of normal volition is our customary, widely used default position concerning human agency and seems not unreasonable. It is a position, indeed, on which many of our cultural practices and institutions appear to rest. Yet if we adopt the presumption of normal volition, we must admit that the deficit model of incapacitation does not readily apply to personality disorders or perhaps also to a number of other mental disorders at the less severe end of the spectrum.

Following Reznek, Fields (1996) defines a mental illness as an abnormal, irreversible, harmful process and argues that, because it is not a process, sociopathy is not a mental illness. But here the issue of anchoring etiology enters the analysis. Reznek's account is etiologically unencumbered: mental illness neither results in nor derives from underlying organic abnormality or malfunction. In a more widely shared view associated with traditional medical psychiatry and the medical model, however, mental disorders, like physical diseases, are taken as evidence of underlying, organic deficit, abnormality, or malfunction. What I have elsewhere called a presumption of organicity is even attributed with functional disorders such as the personality disorders the nature of whose organic deficit or malfunction remains unknown (Radden, 1985, 1996a, 1996b). At least in this etiologically encumbered analysis of mental illness or disease, if not in Reznek's, then, if the antisocial character's behavior was judged to stem from a mental illness or disease, it would be the symptom of an underlying disease entity, itself some deficit, malfunction, or abnormality. Though not without certain conceptual difficulties (Radden, 1985), such a disease entity would go some way at least toward explaining and grounding the hypothesized incapacity or incapability in terms of which the behavior was characterized. This would be a causal explanation, with the antisocial behavior arising out of an incapability (over forming other-regarding beliefs, for example) in turn resulting from the underlying, abnormal state or condition, or deficit.

Although it is one way to understand the antisocial character's behavior, this cannot be Fields', however, because of his allegiance to Reznek's alternative etiologically unencumbered account of mental illness. Instead, Fields adopts what is the standard classification of antisocial character: it is a trait-based character disorder. When antisocial character disorder is portrayed as a trait-based disposition, however, there is no further explanatory level to ground and support the hypothesized incapability. Like normal variations of personality type, trait-based dispositions are nothing more than observed regularities of apparently voluntary response.

The dilemma alluded to above has particular application here. Some would classify antisocial character as a mental disease (certainly the history of psychiatry has reflected such classification). To do so is to violate the DSM's explicit goal of avoiding etiological assumptions, but it at least allows (through application of the presumption of organicity) that the antisocial character suffers an incapacitating condition on analogy with the standard cases of deficit disorder. A second choice would be to reject the incapability criterion for this particular mental disorder category. Certainly incapability as a criterion for mental disorder is presented in a disjunctive set: a condition warrants disorder status by exhibiting suffering *or* incapability such as, recall, to increase significantly the risk of suffering "death, pain, disability or an important loss of freedom." The suffering criterion is inapplicable here—there is not clinical evidence to support the view that antisocial character disorder results in greater than normal suffering. (To the contrary, the lack of suffering such emotions as regret and remorse is a noted feature of this syndrome.) Finally, the third choice must be to declassify some of the alleged disorders currently included in the DSM: in its favor it can be said of this alterative that these personality disorders, which include antisocial character, have long been targeted as "borderline" cases that some would be prepared or even eager to drop from the lexicon.

Cross-sectional Models of Incapability and Hedonic Mood States

Until it becomes more pronounced, mild mania is a puzzle and raises another sort of problem. There is not always and perhaps not even usually a readily identifiable incapability in the manic patient—rather the reverse: the hypomanic phase is associated with energy, creativity, and often agreeable mood states. What serves to distinguish the incapability of mania is something different. The manic state of mind is often an indicator of more serious later incapacitation. (When it is not, its disorder status must be questioned; see below.) While not always themselves disabling, hypomanic states are harbingers of the incapability accompanying the psychotic and extreme states likely to come. This "harbinger" notion of incapability embraces a longitudinal rather than a "time slice" or cross-sectional conception of disorder. In doing so, it more closely adheres to the traditional notion of disease or illness associated with ordinary medicine. We are again drawn not toward the decifit model but toward the complete disease model here—in this case, to the feature that a disease has a course, only understood and identified through longitudinal study. That is, if we regard mild mania as rightly accorded disorder status, then we can appeal to its reflection of incapability only by adopting the more encumbered disease or illness model.[4]

Some mild mania does not progress to severe mania and thus submit to the kind of resolution outlined here. Of course, the harbinger model of incapability will be inapplicable here, and the real concern over finding a warrant for the condition's disorder status remains and is pressing, as others have recognized (Nordenfelt, 1994; Seedhouse, 1994).

There are two incapability models, I am suggesting, that of deficits and that of diseases or illnesses. Functional disorders rarely require the disease incapability model (mild mania is the exception) because they *are* functional: they reflect some incapacity of functioning at the present time and thus only require a "time slice" type of analysis such as is required for deficits. But on the other hand, as we have seen illustrated by the case of personality disorders, functional disorders cannot be treated as analogous to the case of ordinary deficits unless assumed to have some vertical depth, that is, an anchoring etiology. Yet to adopt this description is to get closer to the traditional disease or illness model of incapability.

In differentiating these two ways (this was not intended as an exhaustive study, and there may be more ways as well) in which incapability is ascribable to mental disorders, I hope to have made the case that there are at least two distinguishable models for how incapability warrants disorder status. This is messy and complicated. Nevertheless, it may be that it is nothing worse and that once the separate models are acknowledged and the disorders identified as belonging to the one or the other model, the call for a brief, conceptually clear, and frank acknowledgment of the role of capability as a mental health norm will have been satisfied.

▪ ▪ Recommendations for the DSM

Without the two additions suggested here the DSM is vulnerable to several criticisms. A failure to acknowledge the dissimilarities between different forms of suffering and between the several different kinds of incapability, it might be said, invites conceptual confusion. Moreover, if these different kinds of distress and incapability are assumed to warrant disorder status, it might be said to be on the basis of false analogy. And finally, a failure to explain and justify these different models leaves the disorder status of some syndromes without proper warrant, thus inviting the charge of unjustified "medicalization" over their inclusion in the DSM.

Acknowledgments

In preparing these ideas I benefited from comments and suggestions made by many people: members of PHAEDRA (Jane Roland Martin, Susan Franzosa, Ann Diller, Barbara Houston, Jane Farrell Smith, and Beatrice Kipp Nelson); participants in the Annual Meeting of the Nordic Network for Philosophy, Medicine and Mental Health, especially Jenni Bullington; colleagues in the Philosophy Department at the University of Massachusetts: Mitchell Silver, Robert Rosenfeld, Nelson Lande, Lawrence Foster, and R. K. Shope. I am also grateful to John Sadler; members of the audience at the conference "Values in Psychiatric Nosology," held at Dallas, Texas, in December 1997; and Harold Pincus, whose incisive commentary led to significant revisions of this material.

Notes

1. This leaves the curious case of non-Western depression (characterized only in terms of bodily sensations such as weakness and dizziness) as one not of emotional pain but of sensations, some of them painful. Whether such conditions are reasonably equated with the emotional states identified in the West as depression will depend on the disorder model presupposed.

2. Apparently objectless affective states have been treated in several different ways. One way would use them to challenge the exhaustiveness of the distinction between emotions and sensations. Another way insists that moods are sensations: thus the pervasive and nondirected mood of feeling "blue," which is sometimes misleadingly cast as depression, is actually a dimly recognized pervasive bodily sensation. Alternatively, some theorists treat moods as emotions, that is, intentional states, whose objects, though present, go unrecognized by their subject because they are pervasive (thus, all my experience is what my depressed mood is over or about) or because they are hidden (they are unconscious). To maintain the distinction between sensations and emotions, one could employ each of the three alternatives outlined here. Depending on the particular states under discussion, it is sometimes plausible to say that it is really a sensation (this is true with some forms of anxiety), sometimes that it has a vast object (as in some forms of ennui), and sometimes that its object is unconscious (as with certain states of dread and pessimistic anticipation).

3. This analysis of nonintentional forms of representing is consistent with Freud's work but incompatible with that of phenomenologists such as Merleau-Ponty, as the following passages illustrate: "The great strength of the intellectualist psychology and idealist philosophy comes from their having no difficulty in showing that perception and thought have an intrinsic significance and cannot be explained in terms of the external association of fortuitous agglomerated contents. . . . Bodily experiences force us to acknowledge an imposition of meaning which is not the work of a universal constituting consciousness, a meaning which clings to certain contents. My body is the meaningful core which behaves like a general function, and which nevertheless exists, and is susceptible to disease" (Merleau-Ponty, 1945, p. 88).

4. The question asked here—why mild mania has disorder status—has been approached somewhat differently. Moore, Hope, and Fulford (1994) have asked why we should treat mild mania. But while its answer will have implications for matters of treatment, the first question is primary (Nordenfelt, 1994).

12

Why Criteria of Involuntary Action
Are Value Laden

CHRISTIAN PERRING, PH.D.

Much work has been done (especially in the present volume) on the ways that values do and do not enter into the practice and theory of psychiatry and the rest of the mental health profession. Here I argue that values are involved in the classification of mental illness not just in the assessment of the undesirability of the condition or connected behavior but also through the classification of the behavior as involuntary. That is, to say whether a person freely chooses to perform an act is not always a purely neutral descriptive fact. At least sometimes, deciding whether an act is voluntary or involuntary requires adopting an evaluative stance.[1] This is especially true in controversial cases of mental illness.

My claim will not be at all controversial for those who see psychology and psychiatry as thoroughly socially constructed and value laden. Indeed, social constructionists will probably view my claim as meager. My project, which is not intended as a critique of psychiatry, is largely in reaction against social constructionists, whose claims I see as overly broad and unsubstantiated. But I do not take on the social constructionists here, at least in the direct sense.

▪ ▪ Other Models of Illness

I do not review all previous theories of psychiatric classification, but it is worth spending a little time explaining how this chapter goes beyond what other theorists have already argued. Some have maintained that we can have a purely scientific and value-neutral classification of disease and illness (Boorse, 1975, 1976). Others have contended that values do in fact structure our classification of illness and that, while it might be possible to give a scientific, value-neutral classification, this would not fit with our practices and would not well serve the purposes of medicine (Veatch, 1973; Engelhardt, 1996; Culver and Gert, 1982; Reznek, 1987; Fulford, 1989, 1991, 1994; Lennox, 1995; Agich, 1997). These latter theorists have won the day, in my opinion, but they have largely overlooked the issue of voluntariness.[2]

▪ ▪ Involuntariness of Illness

Many theories of illness are mute when it comes to the issue of voluntariness of symptomatic behavior.[3] Those theories that do address the issue agree that the symptomatic behavior is only partially voluntary. For instance, Fulford describes illness as "failure of action" (1989, chap. 7; 1994, p. 222). Voluntariness is not an issue for most physical illnesses, because it is so clear that their symptoms are not chosen. One does not choose to have a runny nose when one has a cold, or a fever when one has the "flu," for example. One does have a choice about how to treat the illness and even in how to react to it. Some people with bad colds soldier on refusing to succumb, whereas others retreat to their sofas, cover themselves with blankets, and get their families to bring them hot drinks. But those reactions to the illness are not themselves symptoms of the illness.

It is, of course, more difficult to separate out symptoms of mental illness and reactions to it. However, the symptoms cannot be freely chosen. This should be reflected in the official definition of illness or disorder. Consider the definition of *disorder* in the introduction to the DSM-IV (which was also used in the DSM-III and DSM-III-R).

> Each of the mental disorders is conceptualized as a clinically significant behavioral or psychological syndrome or pattern that occurs in an individual and that is associated with present distress (e.g., a painful symptom) or disability (i.e., impairment in one or more important areas of functioning) or with a significantly increased risk of suffering death, pain, disability, or an important loss of freedom. In addition, this syndrome or pattern must not be merely an expectable and culturally sanctioned response to a particular event, for example, the death of a loved one. Whatever its original cause, it must currently be considered a manifestation of a behavioral, psychological, or biological dysfunction in the individual. Neither deviant behavior

(e.g., political, religious, or sexual) nor conflicts that are primarily between the individual and society are mental disorders unless the deviance or conflict is a symptom of a dysfunction in the individual, as described above. (American Psychiatric Association, 1994, pp. xxi–xxii)

This definition contains no statement that the syndrome must be involuntary, but it does say that the syndrome must be a manifestation of a dysfunction. This is a vague phrase, of course, in quasi-technical language that does not seem to have very specific meaning. It is probably motivated by a desire to adopt a quasi-biological concept of disease, but this is by no means explicit. What does seem clear, though, is that the main idea behind this definition is that the syndrome must be, on the one hand, bad for the person suffering from it and not autonomously chosen by that person and, on the other, still arising from internal psychological conditions rather than, say, being compelled by another person. The worry being addressed is that psychiatry should not be medicalizing free expression of character such as political deviance or individual quirks.

The need to specify that mental disorder is involuntary comes out in many diagnostic criteria. Here are a few examples from the DSM-IV. Substance dependence requires that "there is a persistent desire or unsuccessful efforts to cut down or control substance use" (American Psychiatric Association, 1994, p. 181). In bulimia nervosa, there is "a sense of lack of control over eating" during the binge (p. 549). In pathological gambling, there are "repeated unsuccessful efforts to control, cut back, or stop gambling" (p. 618). In obsessive-compulsive disorder, the person engages in repetitive behavior that he or she "feels driven to perform in response to an obsession" (p. 423).

However, many criteria of mental disorders also include what seems to be intentional behavior. Here are some examples. Anorexia nervosa includes "refusal to maintain body weight at or above a minimally normal weight for age and height" (p. 544). Substance dependence requires that "a great deal of time is spent in activities necessary to obtain the substance . . . , use the substance . . . or recover from its effects" (p. 181). But this does not mean that the behavior is really voluntary. In these two cases, it seems that the intentional behavior is not really freely chosen because it is the result of craving in the case of substance dependence and intense irrational fear of gaining weight in the case of anorexia.[4] Presumably the same is true of impulse disorders such as kleptomania, pyromania, and trichotillomania (the recurrent pulling out of one's own hair resulting in hair loss). Each is char-

acterized by an increasing sense of tension before the behavior and grati-
fication or relief after the behavior (pp. 612–21). These are also aberrant
episodes not representative of the sufferer's desires at other times. Presumably this is also the reason why manic episodes are not expressions of
autonomous behavior, that is, they do not represent the person's true desires.

In schizophrenia and psychotic disorders, the explanation of behavior
of people with these disorders is especially complex and controversial. But
even if the bizarre behavior of the sufferer may not be explained by cravings and he or she may not have made any efforts to stop the behavior, it
is still possible that the person's actions may still not be freely chosen. For
example, people who hear voices telling them to do things sometimes say
that the voices made them do it. It is hard to evaluate the reasonableness
of such claims, but it is worth considering what our reaction to the case
would be if the voices were real, that is, if a real person were saying the
things the voices said to the patient, including making threats. We might
well count the resulting behavior of the patient as reasonable or at least co-
erced.[5]

Maybe personality disorders are the most troublesome category of
mental disorder for the view that all behavior symptomatic of mental disorder is involuntary. Here, again to generalize, the person's behavior does
not occur in aberrant episodes but is deeply ingrained in the person's character. The person is not delusional and does not (generally) suffer from irresistible cravings or fears. I do not explore the case of personality disorders here, but they clearly deserve greater scrutiny.[6]

I have just argued that in most of the accepted mental disorders we
have today, there is a reasonable justification for thinking that the symptomatic behavior is in a significant sense involuntary.[7] To summarize, I
found three ways in which we can count a form of behavior as involuntary:

1. It is the result of an irresistible craving or overpowering fear.
2. It is the result of an aberrant and temporary desire external to a person's true personality.
3. It is the result of a delusion.

▪ ▪ Controversial Diagnoses

It would be fair to say that diagnostic criteria in psychiatry are more
controversial than in any other branch of medicine. Sometimes the con-

troversy is about whether a condition is really undesirable. For instance, some people point to hypomania as a condition in which a person can have large amounts of energy and feel very good, or they point to schizophrenia episodes as spiritual, rather than pathological, events (Jamison, 1995; Farber, 1993). But in much of the controversy surrounding the classification of mental disorders, the disputants agree that the conditions in question are undesirable. The debate is over whether they should be seen as involuntary or as a natural part of life. I will consider some examples, although almost any kind of mental illness will illustrate my claim clearly.

Schizophrenia

In the 1960s several theorists proposed that schizophrenia is not so much an illness as a rational reaction to schizophrenogenic families. Ronald Laing was the best-known proponent of this view (Laing, 1959; Laing and Esterson, 1964). Laing himself was influenced by existentialism, which promotes the view that all behavior is freely chosen. Insofar as he was denying that schizophrenia is an illness,[8] it was not on the ground that the schizophrenic condition is desirable. Laing did not encourage people to try living as schizophrenics (even if he was enthusiastic about the use of hallucinogens to open the mind). Although coming from a very different perspective, Thomas Szasz has also argued that schizophrenics are not ill, that they are merely experiencing problems in living (Szasz, 1960). Laing tends to put the responsibility for the condition on society, while Szasz is a rugged libertarian who advocates personal responsibility, but both men want to put the behavior of schizophrenics on a par with that of ordinary people. Their views are now often dismissed as ridiculous, partly because of the greater knowledge we have of the brain but mostly because of the intuition that people with schizophrenia have been afflicted by something external to them and their lives are not freely chosen.

Alcoholism

The view that alcoholism is a disease has won much popular endorsement over the past couple of decades in the United States.[9] Part of the reason for this was the discovery that there is a genetic element that predisposes some humans to become alcoholics. Whether or not a condition is genetic would seem to have no relevance to its value or disvalue, but it is relevant to whether or not drinking is a choice. Presumably the public thought that a person's genetic predisposition to alcoholism made his or her drinking less of a free choice.[10] But there are some people who reject the view of alcoholism as a disease, and their reasoning tends to be that it cannot be a disease because alcoholics have control over their behavior and simply are too selfish or self-destructive to live responsibly (Peele, 1990; Peele and Brodsky, 1991; Fingarette, 1988).

Depression and Dysthymia

According to the 1994 National Comorbidity Survey (reported in the *Archives of General Psychiatry*), 10 percent of all Americans have had a major depressive episode in a twelve-month period, and 19 percent would undergo an often disabling mood disorder during their lifetime. The DSM-IV reports similar statistics and also says that the point prevalence of dysthymic disorder is about 3 percent and the lifetime prevalence is about 6 percent. Some have questioned the use of depression criteria that yield such large percentages (Shorter, 1997, chap. 8). The objection is to the classification of unhappiness as an illness. But unhappiness is certainly undesirable, and surely it is not freely chosen, for who chooses to be unhappy if a better alternative is available? So on what grounds is it thought to be not legitimately an illness?

The behavior associated with depression tends to be more inactivity than activity: a depressed person is often unable to socialize, interact well with family, work productively, or even care for him- or herself. One possibility is that people think that, although mild depression is not desirable, it is a normal part of life and we should not expect to be happy all the time. If this is the reasoning behind the controversy about whether mild depression should count as a mental disorder, then it has nothing to do with voluntariness. Another possibility is that people think that depressed people have gotten themselves into a rut of selfish and self-defeating behavior and should just snap out of their funk.

We should note, though, that many in the public see depression as a character weakness, and this raises the question what attitudes the public have toward such weakness. Being weak is something that one cannot change immediately, although maybe by going through difficult experiences one can strengthen one's character. So, if a tendency to depression is a character weakness, this seems to be a case in which people are held responsible for their behavior even when it is not thought to be under their direct and immediate control.[11]

▪ ▪ Insufficient Criteria of Voluntariness

Having discussed several controversial cases of mental illness classification and shown how the controversy often centers around the voluntariness of the associated behavior, I now want to investigate how to determine voluntariness. In a previous section I spelled out how the actions associated with some mental illnesses could be counted as involuntary. (An action is involuntary if [1] it is the result of a delusion or if [2] it is caused by a desire that is overpowering or [3] external to the person's true self.) However, I now argue that these are not sufficient criteria for involuntariness.[12] Many actions share the same features and yet are not considered involuntary.

First I concede (if only for the purposes of this chapter) that there can be a neutral descriptive fact as to what *knowledge* a person has relevant to performing an action. I am not basing my argument on the case of delusions and so am conceding that it is possible that there can be some neutral descriptive facts about involuntariness. When a person does not have the facts, or has false beliefs, his or her freedom or autonomy is reduced. This is not a large concession, since this condition only applies in cases of delusion.[13]

My argument is based on those cases in which an action is judged involuntary on the grounds that it is caused by an overpowering or external desire. My contention is that whether or not a desire is overpowering, or is external to a person, is not a neutral fact, and is not determined by neutral facts, because the psychological facts that describe a person are insufficient to indicate whether he or she performed the action involuntarily. Our classification of an action as voluntary or involuntary must inevitably, if it is to be rational, partially depend on values.

It is worth noting that it is not a necessary requirement of voluntariness that the agent have a conscious experience of voluntariness or trying to perform the action. We do not pay much attention to most of the actions we perform, and make no conscious effort to accomplish them, yet this does not show that they are involuntary. Furthermore, it is unlikely that the fact an action is accompanied by a conscious experience of choice in the performance of it guarantees its voluntariness. There seem to be cases in which people are wrong or even self-deceived in thinking their choices are voluntary. Actions of people acting under delusions or people given posthypnotic suggestions might be the best examples here.[14] People regularly believe that they are acting autonomously, when other people in a good position to judge see those actions as being controlled by others.

When is a desire overpowering? When a person is not able to resist it, we might say. But how do we distinguish between a strong desire and an overpowering desire? Presumably, a desire can be strong but not overpowering, that is, a person can have the strength to resist even a strong desire. We can make these distinctions conceptually, but when it comes to actual cases, our intuition is much less clear. Does the fact that a person has tried to give up smoking but failed tell us that his or her desire to smoke was irresistible? No—she might simply not have tried very hard to resist. Does the fact that there is a physiological component to nicotine addiction show that it involves irresistible desires? No—obviously sometimes the desires must be resistible or else no one would have ever given up smoking. On what grounds do we judge that a desire to watch one's favorite TV show is not overpowering while an alcoholic's desire to drink is? The inner phenomenology of the two cases does not give us a conclusive difference, even if we had some way of directly comparing the two cases. It will also not decide the issue to ask a person whether or not a desire was overpowering. Even supposing we get a sincere reply, these are the sort of cases which invite self-deception, and so the agent cannot be the ultimate authority about whether or not he or she could have acted otherwise.

Even more difficult to judge is when a desire is external to a person, such as in personality changes associated with manic states and dissociation. How do we decide which desires are representative of a person's "true self"? It is not sufficient that they be out of character. For instance, when a person loses inhibitions under the influence of alcohol and does something out of character, he might see himself as doing something he has wanted to do for years but was too shy to try. Or else he may say that he does not know what came over him, that he wasn't himself. Again, his word on the issue cannot be final because people will be very tempted to tell the story in a way that reflects well on themselves and so will alter the truth either deliberately or through self-deception. Some psychological theories suggest that people live most of their lives as a "false self," even if those people don't realize it themselves (Winnicott, 1965; Kohut, 1977). So it may happen that a person has a revelatory experience and a dramatic shift of character, yet instead of this being judged a move away from the true self, it is seen as a move toward it. The purely descriptive psychological facts about a person will not by themselves decide which actions are authentic and which are inauthentic.[15]

▪ ▪ The Role of Values in Deciding the Voluntariness of Irrational Behavior in Mental Illness

In real life, where to draw the line between voluntary and involuntary action is often unclear, arbitrary, and dependent on prejudices or values. For example, consider the history of thought about homosexuality or the distinction between antisocial personality disorder and being a nasty person. However, the mere fact that people let their values affect their judgment does not show that our classification of the behavior has to be value laden. Often in debates over disputed forms of behavior, we wish that people would be neutral rather than prejudiced. My claim is that judgments of involuntariness *rationally need* to be value laden, rather than based on purely neutral descriptive facts.[16]

Suppose the argument of the previous sections is correct, and we do not have clear value-free criteria for judging when an action is involuntary. It does not automatically follow that the judgment made is value laden. It might instead just be arbitrary. It is certainly true that arbitrary elements have some influence on the classification of illnesses. History is often determined by random events. Furthermore, the judgment in question might also not be based on any value judgment concerning the *person being evaluated,* but only factors *external* to that person. For instance, psychiatrists might want to lower the thresholds for determining mental illnesses such as depression or sexual deviance not because of any value-laden judgment about the behavior involved but simply because they see this as a way to get more patients and make more money. So, for my argument to succeed, I need to show that, at least sometimes, determinations of involuntariness both are and rationally need to be determined by a value-laden view of the agents.

Given that there is so much indeterminacy concerning involuntariness, those making the decision have considerable discretion. One of the factors to take into account is the consequences of their decision. If it would be good or bad for society, for the psychiatric profession, or for a disadvantaged group within society if a certain kind of condition was classified as a mental illness, then this is a morally relevant factor in deciding whether to so classify it. Since deciding if a condition is an illness is often directly linked to deciding whether the associated behavioral symptoms are involuntary, the consequences of the decision are relevant to the classification of the behavior as involuntary. So issues of welfare and fairness should enter into the decision of classifying a form of behavior as involuntary. This is a clear sense in which the classification is value laden.

There are other ways, however, in which the classification is value laden. This is clearest in judgments of externality.[17] I have already indicated the indeterminacy of the boundaries of the true self. In deciding whether a form of behavior is internal or external to the self, the shape of the self as recognized by psychiatry is being made more definite. This sends a message to the public about what is officially sanctioned. Again, there is a consequentialist element to this, since the classification will have an effect on the public view of what is normal. But this is not the only evaluative element: also relevant is the intrinsic value of the self to be promoted. To illustrate this, suppose that psychiatry widened its view of the boundaries of the self so that manic behavior was not, as it is now, seen as external to the self. It might not be good for the stability of society as a whole, but one might nevertheless argue for such a reclassification on the grounds that it allows us a more playful and spontaneous view of being. Such a view is taking a stance on value and is also relevant in the classification decision.

Finally, to illustrate the value ladenness of the classification of overpowering desires, take alcoholism. Psychiatry could decide not to classify alcoholism as a mental disorder and instead say that it is just irresponsible behavior.[18] This might have a bad effect on society, since it would mean that alcoholics would be denied all the help that they can get from medical insurance and government programs.[19] But independent of the total societal effects of this classification, there is an issue of whether psychiatry should endorse a view of the self as being unable to control drinking. A clue to the social values relevant here might involve examining the differences between Europe and the United States. The United States could be claimed as, on the whole, more puritanical, so the threshold criteria for alcoholism are considerably lower than in Europe.[20] That is, what is considered normal drinking in many European countries is classed as alcoholism in the United States. In deciding between a low and a high threshold, psychiatry should take into consideration what should count as a worthwhile sort of life, and this again is a value-laden factor if ever there was one.

▪ ▪ Conclusion

I have given a rational reconstruction of our concept of illness, concentrating on the role of the judgment of involuntariness, which is especially important in mental illness. To summarize briefly, for a condition to be an illness, it must be judged to be a disvalue for the person with the condition and also involuntary. But there is considerable indeterminacy in both the concepts of disvalue and involuntariness, which leaves much room for discretion on the part of those doing the classification. In making the decision, they need to look at both the effects on society and the model of health they want to promote. To judge a condition involuntary, they must say it is either based on delusion, is the result of an overpowering desire or emotion, or is the result of a desire or emotion that is in some sense external to the person. So in deciding what counts as a mental illness, the classifiers need to judge what model of the self to promote in at least three dimensions: what counts as a delusion, what counts as an overpowering affect, and what counts as external to a person.

I end with two observations. First, this model does not adequately cover all cases of illness. For instance, as we saw earlier, personality disorders seem to result in behavior that meets none of the criteria of involuntariness. We might conclude that it is wrong to classify personality disorders as illnesses or disorders, or we might conclude that we have more than one concept of illness/disorder. It is not my purpose here to make recommendations about which concepts to adopt, since I am limiting myself to an explication of concepts. However, and this is my second observation, once a thorough explication of our illness concepts is available, we will be in a better position to evaluate them and maybe decide to construct new ones. Some will find it unsatisfactory for so much arbitrariness and so many implicit value judgments to be involved in our psychiatric nosology. Psychiatrists are put in the position of having to look as if they can make clear descriptive judgments of involuntariness when in fact much of the time many normative factors are being smuggled into those judgments. It is no wonder that the official diagnostic criteria for mental disorders are rather vague and underplay the issue of involuntariness. We might want to explore new ways of characterizing disorders that depend much less on involuntariness criteria (and maybe this is what is starting to happen with cases such as personality disorder). Alternatively, we might want to be much stricter in our classifications of involuntariness, which would result in far fewer psychiatric conditions being classified as disorders. To make such decisions we will have to understand and evaluate the larger role of psychiatry in society.

Notes

1. As will transpire, there are ways in which the judgment can be made without taking an evaluative stance. What I mean here is that in order to make the judgment of involuntariness for certain kinds of actions in a reasonable and responsible way, we have to take an evaluative stance.
2. There has, of course, been some discussion of involuntariness. It is Fulford's work that pays most attention to the issue of action; Culver and Gert (1982, chap. 6) also devote a chapter to volitional disabilities, and Edwards (1981) defines mental illness as lack of rational autonomy. Agich (1994) discusses closely connected issues with reference to antisocial personality disorder, and there has been a good deal of discussion of the voluntariness of alcoholism and addiction (see below). For completeness, I should explain and discuss these writings in more detail. However, space does not permit this here.

3. I would argue that those theories implicitly assume that symptomatic behavior is involuntary, because common sense and practice require this, as I show concerning the DSM-IV definition of *mental disorder*.

4. Whether the craving or fear is strong enough really to take away all the sufferer's freedom is an important question that I will leave unanswered here.

5. But not always. Sometimes a person's reaction to a delusion would be unreasonable even were the delusion real. See Elliott (1996, chaps. 6 and 7).

6. See Elliott (1996, chaps. 4 and 5) for a thoughtful and interesting discussion of related issues.

7. For the purposes of this chapter, I am equating freedom, voluntariness, and autonomy. A more sophisticated discussion would find useful distinctions between these qualifies. See Berofsky (1995, chap. 1).

8. I am unsure whether an interpretation of Laing requires this conclusion.

9. See my paper "Addiction and Freedom" (unpublished manuscript) for a more detailed discussion of the issues here.

10. I argue against this inference in "Addiction, Self-Defeating Behavior, and Mental Illness" (unpublished manuscript). For a useful overview and critique of various models of alcoholism and addiction, see Heyman (1996), although I have strong reservations about his positive model of addiction, as my peer comments indicate.

11. Some might argue that this is evidence that Western folk morality has strong Aristotelian elements.

12. A general argument for this is that the notion of voluntariness is generally supposed to be all or nothing, even though most people would acknowledge that it comes in degrees. If it does come in degrees, then the decision about whether a condition of the gray area of voluntariness will have to be resolved by extra considerations, and these are bound to be partly pragmatic.

13. Two parenthetical comments. First, I may be conceding too much here. Nearly all agents have some false beliefs, and all are ignorant about something. Because of the holism of beliefs and desires (e.g., Davidson, 1984), it is very hard to draw a boundary around sections of knowledge and say that all and only the knowledge in that section is relevant to the action being chosen, so any piece of knowledge may be potentially relevant to any action. Thus, judging that one person had all relevant true beliefs while another lacked relevant knowledge in making a decision is not so cut and dried as I suggest in the main text. It may well be that judgments of value creep into assessing whether or not a person had all the relevant knowledge in performing an action. However, this is a speculative argument and would require some concrete examples in order to be convincing. Second, I have blithely assumed in the main text that delusions can be equated with false beliefs. I am aware of the problematic nature of such an equation. Nevertheless, even if delusions are not merely false beliefs, they still reduce a person's autonomy.

14. However, the philosophical thought experiments in the free-will literature seem to prove the same. For example, if a neurosurgeon has hooked up my brain so that he or she can control my choices, doesn't this mean that my actions are involuntary even if they seem to be voluntary?

15. This assumes there are such things as purely descriptive psychological facts of hu-

man behavior. Many would say that any rich description will be laden with value. If so, this would help to confirm my main thesis.

16. I am assuming, of course, that there is a significant distinction to be made between descriptive and evaluative judgments, even if there is a large gray area between the two. I do not intend to take any position about whether there are any such things as *evaluative facts.*

17. This discussion of externality is unfortunately brief. There is a large literature on authenticity, the real or true self, the ego, inauthenticity, the false self, and the id. Although much of the literature is psychoanalytic, one of the most important influences on my thinking on this topic is Harry Frankfurt (1976, 1987, 1988), although I doubt that Frankfurt would endorse the view for which I argue here.

18. For a more detailed argument for this, see my "Addiction, Self-Defeating Behavior, and Mental Illness."

19. Of course, alcoholism does not get full status as an illness in the United States because it is explicitly not covered under the Americans with Disabilities Act. If it were regarded as a full illness, alcoholics would get more help than they do.

20. I don't know whether this difference is reflected in official diagnostic criteria, although I would expect it to be. Rather, my claim is based on the different societal attitudes toward alcohol, and I would expect these to be strongly reflected in physicians' implementation and interpretation of official diagnostic criteria. I hope to do some further research of the literature which will back up my expectations here.

Part Four

Personal and Collective Interests

13

The Hegemony of the DSMs

MICHAEL ALAN SCHWARTZ, M.D., AND
OSBORNE P. WIGGINS, PH.D.

> *It is . . . important to guard against becoming addicted
> to any particular theory: we must not let ourselves be
> caught in a mental prison.*
>
> Karl R. Popper, *The Myth of the Framework: In Defense
> of Science and Rationality*

THE DSM HAS COME to dominate clinical practice and research in American psychiatry (Tucker, 1998; Kendell, 1988). Indeed, we think it permissible to speak of "the hegemony of the DSM" throughout the field of mental health. If we ask why it has achieved this degree of hegemony, the authors and proponents of the DSM are likely to answer that it has achieved this because it is scientifically based (Guze, 1992; Lieberman and Rush, 1996; Pincus and McQueen, Chap. 2 in this volume). Its scientific approach allows the DSM to hone and secure its categories on the basis of ever-growing data. Of course, the initial reason for constructing a manual like the DSM is the clinical need for such a manual by every medical specialty: in their day-to-day clinical work doctors need well-established lists of diagnostic categories. And, like all of modern medicine, these categories must be as scientifically secure as possible. Hence the requirement for strict science follows from the more basic clinical requirement inherent in any medical specialty, the requirement to define the disorders or diseases with sufficient precision. Because this clinical need underlies and drives the scientific investigations, the science is at any given time only as good as it can possibly be *at that time;* that is, the science is always imperfect, incomplete, and unfinished. And yet, at any given time, it is necessary to be as scientifically rigorous and comprehensive as possible. Hence the authors and proponents of the DSM will argue that it deserves its hegemonic status because it, better than any alternative, fulfills the clinical and scientific requirements of psychiatry as a medical specialty: it provides a manual of diagnostic categories which fulfills the clinical need, and it does so on the basis of the best and most extensive scientific evidence available (Pincus and McQueen, Chap. 2 in this volume).

Because they are scientifically based and subject to ongoing scientific revision, the categories of the DSM can serve both psychiatric research and clinical practice. They serve research by rendering classifications and selections of populations reliable and uniform. And they serve clinical practice by (1) rendering diagnosis more reliable, (2) sharpening and stabilizing the language of all the mental health fields, and (3) facilitating communication with patients and third parties, such as insurance companies. It is for advantages such as these, we think, that in their chapter in this volume (Chap. 2) Pincus and McQueen repeatedly emphasize the scientific methodology followed in designing the DSM-IV. They refer to "data" and "evidence" and allude to the systematic and unbiased recording of observations, "understanding of rules of evidence," and "comprehensive and systematic searching, extracting, arraying, documenting, assessing, and integrating of all the published literature." The DSM-IV merits its hegemonic role because its scientific credentials are far superior to those of any other classification system currently available in psychiatry. To return to our question, then, why has the DSM achieved its hegemony in psychiatry, the answer we receive is framed in scientific terms: we hear about the careful collection and analysis of data, the unswerving reliance on controlled studies and empirical research, the development of rating scales, and so on. Furthermore, because the DSM is firmly based on the best and most extensive evidence available, it furnishes a uniformity of categories with which clinicians, researchers, patients, and third parties can reliably communicate with one another.

One might, on the other hand, claim that the hegemony of the DSM has been achieved by other means. One might use, not scientific, but political terms to explain this hegemony. Political concepts such as "power," "authority," "regulation," "control," "ideology," and even "coercion" come to mind. We might say that the DSM dominates present-day psychiatry because the American Psychiatric Association has endorsed it and consequently given it the highest stamp of legitimate authority in the field. Because of this authority bestowed by the APA, the DSM exercises enormous power over the thoughts, decisions, and practices of clinicians, researchers, and students. Other economic and political forces, such as third-party payers and granting agencies, put pressure on psychiatrists to use the DSM categories exclusively.

Now the proponents of the DSM might respond that this political authority and power, although real, have nevertheless been derived from nonpolitical sources, namely, the scientific and clinical success of the DSM. Because the DSM is scientifically convincing and clinically helpful, it has been accepted by these other "forces" and has thereby gained dominance of the field. No one can then legitimately object to the political power exercised by the DSM: this political power is dependent on and always subject to correction by a politically neutral authority, scientific proof and clinical efficacy.

But does the scientific proof currently available really justify the political dominance that is supposedly derived from it? Just how extensive is the scientific support for the DSM-IV? Does this scientific evidence truly justify the exclusion of other categories in psychiatric diagnosis, treatment, and research? We maintain that it does not justify such exclusion. As emphasized by Gary Tucker (1998, p. 160), the diagnostic practices of psychiatry "are nowhere near the precision of the rest of medicine." Therefore, other categories and approaches should not be excluded, not because these other categories and approaches enjoy strong scientific support, but rather because our scientific knowledge is so limited in psychiatry that no conceptual scheme deserves to dominate the field. And because our genuine knowledge exhibits very serious limitations, psychiatric approaches should be more open, inclusive, and multifaceted than they have become under the dominance of the DSM.

If our knowledge in psychiatry is as limited as we say, then it certainly remains desirable to extend this knowledge. It seems to us, however, that the hegemonic authority of the DSM could retard the advancement of psychiatric knowledge as much as it may further it.

The hegemony of the DSM could retard the advancement of psychiatric knowledge by (1) restricting the acceptable scope of conceptualization and theorizing. Researchers will become less and less willing to allow themselves to imagine long-range projects unless they fit neatly into DSM criteria. Bold new conceptions of mental disorders which significantly deviate from DSM categories could encounter strong opposition within the psychiatric community simply because of their deviance. Hence, it seems unlikely that researchers would be willing to invest considerable amounts of time in projects that inevitably involve fending off such opposition. (2) The hegemony of the DSM could limit the range of acceptable evidence to the kinds of evidence clearly related to DSM criteria. Evidence that has no pertinence to DSM categories is likely to go unnoticed and unexamined because it does not appear to pertain to anything. And (3) the hegemony of the DSM could limit the range of fundable research projects. Psychiatric research that significantly departs from DSM criteria may become unlikely to be awarded funding and internal and external support.

Moreover, the hegemony of the DSM could restrict the range of clinical conceptualization and treatment because (1) clinicians will increasingly see themselves as having no other choice than to adhere to the DSM criteria, (2) we shall enter a time in which the DSMs have become so thoroughly accepted as the "gold standard" in the conceptualization of mental illnesses that it never occurs to clinicians to think outside their range, and (3) in the case of conflict between DSM criteria and the practitioner's clinical judgment, the practitioner's judgment will almost inevitably be set aside. This will make it less likely that new clinical insights can occur and, even if they do occur, that they will be deemed credible. And (4) even if clinicians remain able to conceive of mental disorders differently than those in the DSM, third-party payers are almost certain to deny them reimbursement for treating such disorders.

In order to consider this point, let us construct a simple thought experiment. Imagine that the psychiatry of 1890, after decades of sorting through a wide range of professional opinions and conducting field trials, had developed its own classification manual. And imagine that this manual had become as thoroughly developed, widely accepted, and highly respected as the DSM-IV is today. Now Kraepelin and Bleuler come along, and they define in their own ways what is today known as schizophrenia. Insofar as their approaches are unexpected and novel in terms of the "conventional wisdom" of the day, which has now been codified in a manual, how much success, we wonder, could they or any other innovator have had in obtaining a broad hearing in such a professional environment? Large numbers of psychiatrists would probably have paid no attention to them. When one way of conceiving mental disorders has been accepted and employed as the "official view" of an entire field and profession, radically different ways of conceiving "the same" items will encounter resistance from the entire field.

If, then, the scientific evidence favoring the DSM-IV cannot support its hegemony in the field, what does? The hegemony obtains its primary support from the assumption that the DSM approach, its basic way of thinking, is the truly scientific one. If the DSM approach is the truly scientific one, then the fact that this approach has not yet yielded sufficient results to justify its hegemony means only that we need to continue to apply this approach so that in due time it will inevitably yield those results. Even many psychiatrists who feel deeply dissatisfied with the DSM find themselves unable to criticize its assumed conception of science. The reason it is difficult to criticize this conception of science is that it seems to be one that securely undergirds the rest of medicine with its firm, effective, and growing knowledge. This indeed seems to be the main aim guiding the construction of the DSM: psychiatry must come to resemble the rest of medicine in its clinical practice (i.e., diagnosis and treatment) and research methods. The basic axiom at work here is the following: psychiatry is a medical specialty, and therefore the approach psychiatry should take is the scientific and pragmatic approach taken so successfully by the rest of medicine. To deny that the DSM approach is the most promising one, then, seems to entail the denial that psychiatry is a part of medicine and consequently similar to medicine in methodology and subject matter.

Our contention is, however, that even though psychiatry is a medical specialty, it is a quite peculiar one. In psychiatry it is much more difficult to distinguish normal conditions from abnormal ones than it is in the rest of medicine. In other words, it is not clear that the conditions with which psychiatry is concerned are diseases. This uncertainty regarding whether mental disorders are mental diseases does not simply result from our current ignorance regarding the etiology of these disorders. Even if we knew the etiology of all the mental disorders, this would not tell us whether any of them are diseases. Indeed, even if we knew a precise brain mechanism that produced each of the mental disorders, this would not tell us whether these disorders are diseases. All we need do is assume that every reality has a cause, and we know that every mental disorder has a cause or set of causes whether we currently know exactly what it is or not. A disease entity is not distinguished from a nondisease entity by the fact that the former has an etiology and mechanism and the latter does not; every entity has an etiology.

In addition, psychiatry has another peculiarity that makes it difficult to view the field as one medical specialty like others. There are many more psychological, social, and cultural variables that affect the nature, manifestation, and course of disorders in psychiatry than in the rest of medicine. The rest of medicine can function relatively well—although here, too, we would express serious reservations—through reducing the patient to an organism that is suffering from certain biological dysfunctions. Psychiatry, however, needs to view mental problems in terms of how they alter the very personhood of the patient. These ways of altering personhood can even sometimes turn out to be creative and productive. Whether they do turn out to be so depends, of course, on other components of the person's character, opportunities, and influences; they depend, in other words, on the total makeup and life history of the individual who has the mental problems. Kay Redfield Jamison, in her book *Touched with Fire: Manic-Depressive Illness and the Artistic Temperament* (Jamison, 1993), has documented numerous examples of great artists who suffered from manic-depressive illness. Granted, these artists suffered much; but their personalities, shaped through the mental disorder, perceived and created visions that revolutionized and advanced our culture (Jamison, 1993).

Avoiding complexities of this kind, psychiatry has downplayed the task of trying to conceptualize the multifaceted reality of a human being coping with a mental disorder and by default has fallen back on implicit notions of normality and abnormality closely tied to prevailing standards of social conformity. Physicians, patients, and their families can all agree on these assumptions regarding normality, abnormality, and successful treatment because they are taken for granted in our shared culture. Consequently, a man has been "cured" of his mental difficulty if his boss and co-workers attest that he is performing his job more efficiently and his wife says that his outbursts of anger at her have subsided. A child has been "successfully treated" for her behavioral problems if her teachers report that she is concentrating on her assignments in school and her parents note that she is now playing placidly with her siblings at home. Other modifications of the patient's behavior can be disregarded if, according to people in her surroundings, she is to their satisfaction conforming to normal social expectations. There is no need to examine critically what has happened to this person if "everyone is happy" with the outcome. Such is the utilitarianism that defines "success" in present-day diagnosis and treatment.

The difficult task of conceiving adequately the profound complexity of human life in the grip of mental problems has been replaced by the far more achievable program of establishing reliable criteria for psychiatric diagnosis. But once establishing criteria with demonstrated reliability is the definition of success, it becomes easy to oversimplify the use of these criteria. Indeed, such oversimplification is almost unavoidable when economic pressures lead to nonpsychiatrists making psychiatric diagnoses. In the hands of nonpsychiatrists, DSM categories can be used as simple algorithms requiring yes or no responses. "Are you depressed?" "Yes." "Do you have trouble sleeping?" "Yes." "Have you lost your appetite?" "Yes." In an economic environment in which doctors are permitted only fifteen minutes or less to see each patient, this kind of simplified diagnosis can even seem to constitute an advance. After all, doesn't this mean that psychiatry is becoming more like the rest of medicine in which a quick urine test for hyperglycemia can allow any medical person to diagnose diabetes? Inside the realm in which the DSM reigns, all of this can appear to be a great medico-socio-economic good.

Because the DSM aims at rendering psychiatry more like the rest of medicine, it appeals to those who deem such resemblance desirable. Those who deem the resemblance desirable are, accordingly, likely to applaud the hegemony of the DSM in the field of psychiatry. We submit, however, that, although the DSM as a large-scale project deserves to be pursued, the hegemonic status it has achieved poses certain dangers. It poses a danger in particular to the advancement of psychiatric insight and discovery. Rather than the monolithic approach that results from viewing psychiatry as needing to follow as closely as possible the methodology and procedures of the rest of medicine, we think that psychiatry, at least in the present stage of its development, needs to remain far more open and receptive to a plurality of methods and conceptual schemes (McHugh and Slavney, 1983). It needs to remain open and receptive because (1) its present categorical and knowledge base is not as firm as it may appear with the reign of the DSM, (2) alternative modes of thought might fruitfully revolutionize our way of viewing mental disorders, and (3) the human being who has a mental disorder is a far more complex reality than can be conceived within the DSM framework. This need for pluralism (McHugh and Slavney, 1983) does not rule out projects such as the DSM-IV. It rather implies that this project should not be automatically deemed the one to furnish the main manual for psychiatry. The DSM-IV could be viewed as one approach among others, needing to prove its utility and accuracy in an ongoing contest with these other approaches. This contest fails to occur today, not because of the firm scientific basis of the DSM-IV, but because of the hegemony discussed above. In the future psychiatry could become a discipline significantly different from what it is today, and not, as some people think, because the brain turns out to be "where all the action is." But this different-looking future, we have maintained, could be needlessly postponed in an era dominated, as thoroughly as it is today, by the DSM. In this regard we can call to our aid Karl R. Popper's provocative statement: "I hold that orthodoxy is the death of knowledge, since the growth of knowledge depends entirely on the existence of disagreement" (1994, p. 34).

Let us take just one example of the lack of pluralism in today's psychiatric environment. The time-honored discipline of psychopathology has fallen into neglect, because the DSM emphasis on reliability and operationalization as methods for categorizing disorders simplifies their defining characteristics. These methods use norms that are fixed in advance and which predefine what is to be measured by imposing forced-choice options on the patient. Unless the patient's experience just happens to fit into these pregiven measurements, it is passed over. And even if the patient's experience does fit on the scale, it is captured only in the simplified terms provided by the criteria. This approach may prove useful to many because of its precision and ready transformation into data, but such a Procrustean method may also preclude the possibility that the patient's experience can be vividly conceptualized and understood. However helpful this clarity and exactitude may be for biological psychiatry, they remain far from adequate for psychiatry as a whole.

In this manner, the methodology sponsored by the DSM project renders the pathological states of the patient's psyche inaccessible. By placing all the methodological emphasis on reliability and operationalization in the determination of symptomatology, the DSM remains faithful to its favored positivistic methods, but in doing so it rules out other methods that would facilitate a thorough investigation of mental pathology. If the methodology of the DSM achieves hegemony, then these other methods are not simply other; they instead become "unscientific," "illegitimate," and, of course, "unreliable." But if the range of acceptable approaches became sufficiently open to encompass those methods that are needed if we are to know what is going on in the minds of mental patients, then we would have a psychiatry that, in addition to including the DSM, would include supplementary viewpoints.

In addition to the need to reopen the field of psychiatry to a plurality of approaches, conceptual schemes, and methods, there is the need to maintain vigilance regarding the uses to which the DSM has been put in an era of its hegemony. The DSM has been employed in the past in ways that are highly questionable. Indeed, these misuses have aroused such concern that the entirety of page xxvii of the DSM-IV has been reserved for a "Cautionary Statement" that warns against some of them (American Psychiatric Association, 1994). We have mentioned above the oversimplified use of DSM criteria, and at least one sentence in the "Cautionary Statement" in the DSM-IV seems aimed at preventing such misuse. By recognizing this misuse and warning against it, the authors of the DSM-IV have taken an important step toward placing their manual in the proper light.

And certainly this oversimplified employment of the DSM is a consequence that the authors of it never intended. We would like to contend, however, that the fact that this misuse is a consequence of the DSM which its authors never intended does not entail that they are not now responsible for taking extensive actions in order to prevent continuing misuse.

It may seem absurd to say that those people who participated in producing the DSM should be responsible for the ways in which other people utilize it. After all, how could the creators of the volume be responsible for every use that is made of it and equally of its misuses? The answer to this question is that people who, of their own free will, set themselves up as the authors of a volume do so in order to achieve certain ends. But when one voluntarily acts in order to achieve certain ends, one is also responsible for ensuring that other, undesirable ends do not result from it. If the action were not freely taken, the moral responsibility would not extend this far. But in this country at least, no one who participates in the creation of a manual of a large professional organization does so out of necessity. As Hans Jonas (1984, pp. 90–108) has helped us recognize, by freely assuming this responsibility, one takes on a status and role that one need not take on and which consequently bears a responsibility that other people need not bear. It will not do to plead that the misuse was not intended by the authors and that no one can be held responsible for all the unintended consequences of his or her actions. Lack of responsibility for the unintended consequences of one's actions would hold only if one could not have foreseen these consequences; and such lack of foresight can exist only before the misuse has occurred or before one knows about it. Once the unintended misuse of one's product has occurred and one knows about it, one is obligated do whatever is in one's power to prevent the continued or repeated misuse.

We conclude from the above ethical considerations that the architects of the DSM are responsible for the known misuses of this manual, although, of course, these misuses are ones they never intended. But now that the misuses have occurred, are known, and continue to occur, the authors are obligated to do everything they can to prevent further ones. And since, moreover, the DSM has been adopted as the official manual of the American Psychiatric Association and the authority of the APA stands behind it, this organization is also obligated to prevent further misuse. Such obligations are not adequately discharged by inclusion of a "Cautionary Statement" in the DSM-IV. This cautionary statement is certainly necessary, but it is not sufficient if it fails to prevent continuing misuse. Actions that extend beyond this verbal disclaimer should be taken.

Throughout this chapter we have expressed doubts concerning the desirability of what we have called "the hegemony of the DSM." But by criticizing this hegemony we do not want to disregard what in our first paragraph we cited as the "clinical need" to which the DSM was designed to respond: doctors' need for established lists of diagnostic categories in their day-to-day work. This clinical need, we think, is entirely legitimate and should be addressed adequately. We simply contend that because of the current limits of psychiatric knowledge the DSM pretends to a precision and complexity in its classifications which are neither scientifically justified nor practically necessary. We would recommend a diagnostic manual that more faithfully reflects the present limits of psychiatric knowledge. In this manual the categories would be few in number, and they would have the logical virtue of what in other publications we have called "ideal types" (Schwartz and Wiggins, 1987; Schwartz, Wiggins, and Norko, 1989). That is to say, they would be general concepts with broad coverage. The categories should be viewed as flexible; they should be adjustable in order to be useful for a wide variety of purposes. They should be so general as to remain open: they should lack specificity so that clinicians and researchers could fill them in with whatever specificity they needed. The tentative and provisional nature of the categories should be acknowledged and recognized so that the features of the disorders they indicate would not be reified or essentialized.

We conceive, then, of a psychiatry in which uniformity of diagnosis, communication, and research exists on the basis of the modest manual we have described above. Within such a psychiatry the DSM project has an important and continuing place. But other conceptual and methodological approaches also have important and continuing places. In this pluralistic field much discussion, controversy, and counterargumentation exists. One approach encounters and responds to criticisms from other approaches; and one approach, reshaping and reformulating its position, deals objectively and publicly with critiques from within its own ranks. The marketplace of ideas is open, and the participants are competing with one another for the sake of truth and reason.

Here again we believe that Karl Popper is helpful: "A discussion between people who share many views is unlikely to be fruitful, even though it may be pleasant; while a discussion between vastly different frameworks can be extremely fruitful, even though it may sometimes be extremely difficult, and *perhaps* not quite so pleasant (though we may learn to enjoy it)" (1994, p. 35).

■ ■ From 1963 to 1980 to 2000

In 1963, Karl Menninger recommended that classification systems be abandoned altogether and that psychiatric diagnoses be replaced by formulations (Menninger 1963). This antidiagnostic stance was inspired by the desire to be as scientific as possible. At that time, however, psychoanalytic conceptions dominated the field of psychiatry; and indeed they exercised a hegemonic power not unlike that of the DSM today. Within that dominant psychoanalytic framework, "being scientific" meant seeing past a superficial symptomatology to the "real" underlying psychic mechanisms and to formulations regarding the psychodynamic workings of those mechanisms. Today a different framework dominates psychiatry. It is a positivistic one that is antithetical to underlying mechanisms when they are psychodynamic but friendly to underlying mechanisms when they are neurological. The advent of this new framework for psychiatry was heralded by the publication of the DSM-III in 1980. And the DSM-III and its successors have also been inspired by the desire to be as scientific as possible.

The danger inherent in both Menninger's and the DSM's stances is not, we think, that they advocate different conceptual and methodological frameworks. And the dangers certainly do not consist in the striving of such approaches to be as scientific as possible. The danger emerges when one rises to hegemonic authority and power, when one succeeds in dominating the field of psychiatry and excluding other approaches. The danger arises from monism. Against this monism we have advocated a psychiatric pluralism, a pluralism in which the various methods and perspectives of psychiatry can coexist and compete with one another.

14

....

What Patients and Families Look for in Psychiatric Diagnosis

LAURA LEE HALL, PH.D.

ALTHOUGH I AM trained as a neuroscientist and have worked as a policy researcher in the biomedical and psychiatric fields, my comments here are intended to reflect the views and perspectives of the members of NAMI (the National Alliance for the Mentally Ill)—168,000 members representing people with severe mental illnesses and their families. To give you some perspective on NAMI, about 75 percent of the members are family members (a little more than half of whom are moms), and almost 25 percent are consumers (people with severe mental illness). If you look at diagnosis, approximately 65 percent of the membership come to NAMI because of a diagnosis of schizophrenia or schizoaffective disorder; 15 percent or so come because of bipolar illness.

The chapters of this book contain relatively few descriptions of the illnesses of which we speak. While most readers are likely aware of what we are talking about, I have come to believe that professionals' deliberations can, through no ill motive or intention, lose sight of the profound significance of the illnesses at hand. We should not forget that 10 to 15 percent or more of those with schizophrenia and severe mood disorders will end their lives by suicide. Suicide is also a significant risk with some other illnesses, such as severe panic disorder and borderline personality disorder. Remember also that schizophrenia, bipolar illness, obsessive-compulsive disorder, and other illnesses typically emerge as people are just beginning their adult lives or earlier and often persist chronically, interrupting education, career, and some of the core experiences of human adulthood—

marriage, having children, having a decent place to call home. As many as 50 percent or more of those with the most severe mental illnesses depend primarily on a family member for their everyday care; 85 percent of those with the most severe illnesses are unemployed. Because of lack of treatment and services, many individuals with these chronic and severely disabling illnesses are homeless (estimates suggest one-third of homeless people have a severe mental illness), and an estimated 10 percent of those in jails and prisons have these severe diseases. So, despite our treatment advances, the picture of severe mental illness in our country is one of tragedy and suffering. As we speak of values in psychiatric diagnosis, we are duty bound to remember always that the plight and well-being of these individuals are affected by our work and decisions. These human beings and their families must be our primary value and concern.

So, patients and their families in a personal way are the focus of this work. But, of course, medicine and psychiatry are also political. What we call "psychiatric illness" directly and indirectly shapes the policies and perceptions of mental illness, and this indirectly affects individuals with these diseases and their families. Although diagnostic classification and nosology are clinical issues, we cannot neglect or ignore the fallout of our work on society.

▪ ▪ What Do I Mean?

At a victory party celebrating passage of the first federal legislation requiring equal annual and lifetime limits for mental and physical disorders in private health plans, the chief sponsor of the legislation, Senator Pete Domenici (R-N.Mex.), commented that he wished that the mental health and scientific community would agree to a definition of serious mental illness. His remarks reflected his desire to improve the circumstances of individuals with serious mental illnesses, such as his own daughter. Also reflected is the fact that persuading some of his colleagues of the moral imperative of ending discrimination against people with mental disorders can be difficult when mental illness encompasses everything from schizophrenia to criminal activity to fractious personalities and other deviances and distresses.

This theme was also exhibited during the legislative sojourn of the Americans with Disabilities Act (ADA). Disability stemming from mental disorders is, in fact, covered by the ADA. But at various times during the congressional debate over the ADA, people with mental disorders were vulnerable to exclusion because of the lampooning of certain diagnoses. The final result illustrates these struggles as the ADA excludes certain diagnoses—transvestism, transsexualism, pedophilia, exhibitionism, voyeurism, and others.

A variety of policies and social commentaries reflect similar concerns, be it the question of overmedicating children who are too active, commitment of pedophiles and sexually violent predators to mental hospitals, or frank DSM-bashing, a recurring sport for some editorial writers and authors. I do not want to join the ranks of the DSM-bashers, but how can I, as a lobbyist or communicator in the media, write about mental disorders as classified by the DSM when it includes such things as pedophilia, voyeurism, and narcissistic personality disorder on par with schizophrenia, manic-depressive illness, autism, and obsessive-compulsive disorder?

The consequences of such a nosology are damaging to the mental health profession, exposing the field to ridicule. For people with serious mental illnesses and their families, it is ever more profound. Every effort to advance public policies that affect people with these illnesses is hamstrung by a nosology that does not make clear the distinctions between diagnoses in terms of seriousness and what are largely agreed on to be illnesses. The director of the National Institute of Mental Health, Dr. Steven Hyman, recently acknowledged this very concern in a letter to the editor of the *Wall Street Journal* Hyman, 1997).

> Neither researchers nor well-trained health-care providers nor patients and families confuse the tally of people with schizophrenia, depression and manic depressive illness, crippling panic attacks and life-threatening anorexia nervosa with the much larger population who meet criteria for every condition listed in the Diagnostic and Statistical Manual of Mental Disorders (DSM-IV). That volume . . . provides a definition of conditions . . . about the gamut of problems and illnesses that distress as well as disable people. . . . With the exception of a handful of diagnoses, a DSM listing by itself suggests little about severity or of need for professional help. . . . Poking fun at the American Psychiatric Association's classifications . . . is bound to generate confusion at the expense of the small percentage of our population who desperately need treatments of proven effectiveness for real medical illnesses that affect the brain.

A crucial desire of many patients and family members facing serious mental illness is a nosology that distinguishes serious illness. In other words, they would like to see psychiatric classification put the primary value on the most serious illnesses.

I have reluctantly dipped my toe in the forbidding waters of psychiatric nosology, where many more expert than I have waded, been submerged, and even survived. But despite the incomplete nature of our scientific evidence about mental disorders and the political and professional tensions that surround the issue of psychiatric diagnosis, the needs of individuals with the most serious illnesses must predominate. Access to treatment is greatly influenced by this.

It may be no surprise that as a representative of NAMI I would advocate the value of most serious illnesses first. But I do understand that medicine, in general, concerns itself with more than serious, disabling, and chronic illnesses. At the very least, less severe illness comes to the attention of physicians who must decide if it is something benign, self-limiting, or of relatively small consequence, or if the presenting symptoms signal something of more significant clinical consequences in the present or down the line. A classification system will never supplant the need for well-trained health care providers who can, by virtue of clinical training and judgment, distinguish the serious from the less serious condition—the condition warranting treatment versus those that may not. Can't we look to our classification system to distinguish better what is illness and serious illness from what are distressful experiences and deviations from the norm?

One cannot address the issue of diagnostic classification from the perspective of patients and their families without acknowledging the impact and experience of "labeling." Having a diagnosis—especially, perhaps, a psychiatric diagnosis—is an intimate experience. It often becomes a part of an individual's identity. To attach a diagnosis to an individual's patterns of emotions or psychic experiences of self speaks to the very value of an individual's personhood. So many consumers have spoken in disgust at how a diagnosis is used in practice to reduce every thought or emotion that an individual has to simply being diseased. Many consumers are reluctant to reveal the presence of a mental illness because all that they do or express so often is dismissed as illness. The positive aspects of a person which may even be related to illness are denied. Our words and labels matter, beyond guiding treatment.

I have had something of a personal experience with concerns about labeling, making this a consideration more than an academic or professional one. My daughter Isabella has a genetic abnormality. Now I have every hope that this will make little difference in terms of her health. But I have to admit that the words used to describe her difference were difficult for me. I cannot bring myself to say *genetic defect*. Even *abnormality* grates on my sensibilities. My daughter is a beautiful, wonderful child, and whatever her genotype and ultimate phenotype, she is to me always a beautiful, wonderful person. Words matter.

I do not think that the impact of labeling is unique to mental disorders (although it may be more insidious because of the stigma attached to these disorders), nor do I think the answer is not to classify, since a diagnosis is so important for effective treatment. Certainly as a parent I want to see the best science has to offer available to my child. My only point is that words matter.

I guess I would offer the simplistic advice that we must be certain that a diagnosis does not become a synonym or adjective for a person. There must be zero tolerance for such terms as *schizophrenics* or *schizophrenic patients,* for example. Such diagnostic labeling is not only pejorative to many consumers and families, but it also implies that individuals *are* their illness, that their diagnosis is their destiny. Given the fact that mental disorders afflict the very machinery of a person's psyche, that they are stigmatizing illnesses in the society, and that our diagnostic system and knowledge is so incomplete, labeling as such must be avoided.

Avoiding labeling does not mean avoiding sound diagnosis. A reluctance to pin a diagnosis on individuals, especially children, given the limitations of our science and the implications for stigmatization and discrimination that may follow, is understandable. But not receiving a proper diagnosis can also have negative implications. Without the right diagnosis how will the individual ever be guided to effective treatment? When I informally surveyed several dozen NAMI members in preparation for the conference that led to the development of this book, I frequently heard about how important the right diagnosis proved to be for them or their loved one. It proved to be the gateway to effective treatment and understanding.

This informal survey of NAMI members raised a few other observations that are relevant here. There proved to be a general sense that the diagnostic system (the DSM), in terms of the serious illnesses that NAMI members experience, can work. That is, the criteria for diagnosis, when properly applied, generally led to a clinical intervention that proved effective and made sense in light of their own understanding of what was happening.

This is not to say that there were no problems—finding experienced clinicians who could make a proper diagnosis; inadequate emphasis on early or prodromal symptoms; and insufficient attention, at lease in practice, to accompanying physical symptoms as well as to family history information and other biological markers. The members I interacted with understood that no biological measures are wholly indicative of a specific disorder. However, some information about biological variables appears to be helpful in some situations. Certainly, explanation of the state of our knowledge about the biological underpinnings of mental illness and other research-derived facts such as phenomenology and treatment options for a disorder help many patients and their families better understand what is happening. I get the sense that consumers and families are able to handle the incompleteness and complexity of our diagnostic enterprise if relayed in a competent way. We should not forget that patients have a long history of interacting with medical science which is complicated and does not have all the answers. We should not pretend it is otherwise.

My survey is not a rigorous or statistically sound one. But these "results" at least suggest that more surveys of patients and families could provide useful information and feedback on issues concerning the classification of mental disorders.

So what kind of questions would NAMI members at least like to see more attention given to in the future versions of the DSM? As I noted, I think the field has some serious contemplation to do to distinguish better between, on the one hand, what is appropriately called illness and, on the other, distress, behavioral differences, and deviance. This matters enormously in a political sense. I do not pretend to have the answers or suppose that distinguishing medical illness from nonmedical illness is straightforward or easy, but I question if we really have raised the bar high enough. Every behavioral difference or deviance, every distress is surely not best conceptualized as an illness. Every disorder listed in the DSM does not have the same level of evidence or historical foundation as a diagnostic entity. Can't that be better elucidated in the DSM? Every classification does not have the same risk of serious, clinical outcome. Every listing does not enjoy the same level of consensus in terms of it being an illness. Now I do not mean to suggest that every illness necessitates treatment—that is not true in any part of medicine. But it is profoundly important that we be extremely discerning in terms of what we call illness—mental illness.

I would strongly endorse continued adherence to a science-based approach in our consideration of psychiatric diagnosis. Phenomenology, course of illness, epidemiology, and treatment information need to be the cornerstone to ongoing consideration of nosology. It will not answer all the fundamental judgments about what is illness and what is not, but it is necessary to be taken seriously in modern medicine.

I would also caution against philosophy taking wing without strong anchoring in scientific knowledge. Mind/brain musings have long been a favorite topic of philosophers, but the fact is that we are learning quite a bit about the brain and, even as we dismissed notions of black bile causing melancholia, we can be sure that cherished views of the mind will be challenged and supplanted, often in unexpected ways, by the accrual of scientific knowledge. We must welcome the insights of science and have our philosophy address the issues arising from science.

Having said that, I think that it is undeniable that biological research will ultimately transform our approach to diagnostic classification. How much it can do so now is basically an empirical question. Biology will not answer all our value issues, but it will influence profoundly how we diagnose mental disorders. We should, in my view, be focusing on how the data to date speak to the diagnostic system. Biomedicine is a powerful source for improved treatment and destigmatization of mental disorders, showing that mental disorders are not a reflection of evil or moral turpitude. I know this raises issues even as it answers some. But we clearly must ready ourselves for the contribution of biomedical research to our definition of mental illness.

Finally, I would caution against a segregation of mental disorders from physical disorders. Even the terms hark back to an outdated divide between mind/brain and body. We should be careful to acknowledge that mental illnesses are brain disorders but that people are more than their diseases.

Valuing people with serious illness—whether mental or physical—and their families is a principle that must inform all of medicine. I hope my comments provide some useful thoughts on the values of people with serious mental illness and their families for the purposes of psychiatric nosology.

15

Softened Science in the Courtroom: Forensic Implications of a Value-Laden Classification

DANIEL W. SHUMAN, J.D.

A LAWYER ADDRESSING values in psychiatric classification bears a heavy burden. The legal system's goals, values, and methods appear to have little, if anything, in common with the mental health profession's goals, values, and methods. Lawyers lack adequate education and training in psychiatric diagnosis, research, or treatment to offer expert assistance in shaping a diagnostic nomenclature. What could the law possibly contribute to or learn from a discussion of values in psychiatric nosology that would justify granting it a voice in this debate?

Perhaps some understanding of the role of the law can be gained by asking the question in a slightly different form: What is the legal relevance of the DSM? From the vantage point of the drafters of the most recent editions of the DSM, one might assume that the DSM exists solely for the benefit of researchers and clinicians and has no legal relevance. Yet this assumption has not always been shared by the DSM's drafters. Although the DSM-I contained no reference to its use in the courts, the DSM-II optimistically anticipated its use "in consultation to the courts" (American Psychiatric Association, 1968, p. viii). Reflecting apparent displeasure with the DSM-II's use "in consultation to the courts" over the ensuing decade but without any explanation of the basis for the shift, the DSM-III contained a warning that its use in legal settings "must be critically examined in each instance within the appropriate institutional context" (American Psychiatric Association, 1980, p. 12). This cautionary language has been strengthened in each subsequent DSM. The DSM-III-R had a special page for a cautionary statement noting that "inclusion here . . . does not imply that the condition meets legal or other nonmedical criteria for what constitutes mental disease, mental disorder, or mental disability. The clinical and scientific considerations involved in the categorization of these conditions as mental disorders may not be wholly relevant to legal judgments" (American Psychiatric Association, 1987, p. xxix). And the DSM-IV notes explicitly that when it is used "for forensic purposes, there are significant risks that diagnostic information will be misused or misunderstood. . . . In determining whether an individual meets a specified legal standard . . . additional information is usually required beyond that contained in the DSM-IV diagnosis" (American Psychiatric Association, 1994, p. xxiii).

Notwithstanding the more recent efforts of the drafters to uncouple the DSM from forensic practice, the DSM has been used extensively in civil and criminal litigation, both with and without expert guidance. Expert witnesses addressing mental or emotional issues in a broad spectrum of cases ranging from workers' compensation and tort claims, criminal responsibility and sentencing, to domestic relations regularly rely extensively and explicitly on the DSM. Lawyers and judges utilize it as a metric to assess offers of expert mental health testimony. And the DSM has been incorporated in substantive legal standards, such as the disability regulations of the Social Security Act, to give it immediate legal authority (Shuman, 1989).

The DSM has not only become a staple presence of civil and criminal litigation, it has transformed that litigation as well. For example, the recognition of the diagnosis of post-traumatic stress disorder in the DSM-III transformed tort litigation resulting in a host of new claims tied to the diagnosis (Shuman, 1995). And the recognition of the diagnosis of post-traumatic stress disorder transformed criminal trials resulting in a host of new defenses such as battered woman syndrome and Vietnam veteran post-traumatic stress disorder tied to the diagnosis (Shuman, 1994).

The DSM is now regularly used unadulterated in forensic contexts notwithstanding its cautionary statements or observations. Indeed, there is little reason to expect these cautionary statements to have much forensic impact. Lawyers are ethically and legally obligated to advance the lawful interests of their clients. Within the framework prescribed by the legal system within which they operate, it is appropriate that lawyers scour relevant professional landscapes to discover theories or practices that support their client's claims or defenses. If we found ourselves thrust into the judicial system with our life, liberty, or fortunes hanging in the balance, would we want our own lawyers to do any less? Concomitantly, courts must screen the admissibility of evidence based on these wide-ranging theories and practices. As courts struggle to assess the validity of a barrage of claims and defenses that purport to rely on the mental health profession's understanding of litigants' mental and emotional conditions, it is unrealistic to expect the judicial system, making decisions on which lives and fortunes turn, not to seek out all possible bona fide sources of guidance. When one source of guidance bears the imprimatur of the preeminent organization of American psychiatrists, it is hardly surprising that lawyers and judges turn to the DSM.

Thus, the legal relevance of this debate becomes clearer. While the law cannot and should not have the capacity to dictate the decisions of private, nongovernmental entities about the organization and articulation of a psychiatric classification, the legal use of the DSM provides concrete evidence of some of the consequences of different approaches to this classification system. Although the courts are not the intended audience of the DSM, the legal system nonetheless provides a visible canvas on which its changes are illustrated. The role of values in psychiatric nosology matters to the law and ought to matter to those who, as responsible citizens, create this psychiatric diagnostic nomenclature, as some answers will have a very different impact on its forensic use than others.

▪ ▪ What You Might Want to Know about the Role of Science in the Courts: The Shifts in the Last Decade

The legal system seeks to ascertain truth, without unnecessary expense or delay, in proceedings that are justly determined. An important element in this process designed to achieve these goals is the parties' selection and presentation of witnesses who describe their perception of some relevant event, leaving it to the fact finder (i.e., the jury in the case of a jury trial, otherwise the judge) to draw any appropriate inferences or opinions from these perceptions to the ultimate legal issues. Of course, in some instances, this presentation of lay or fact witnesses will not be adequate to reach an informed decision, as the significance of facts will not be comprehensible to a lay judge or jury without some specialized assistance. Yet the decision to admit specialized assistance through expert testimony presents courts with a perplexing decision.

Expert testimony is admitted because the judge or jury lacks specialized knowledge on an issue. The fact-finders are thus dependent on the expert; it is not their field. The extent to which the judge or jury ought reasonably to depend on the expert's opinion is a function, among other things, of the validity of the theory that underlies the expert's specialized knowledge. If the expert's opinion, cloaked in professional jargon largely unintelligible to the lay public, is based on the assumption that one plus one equals three or that the sun rises in the west, the resulting opinion will be worthless and should not support a finding in the case. The fact-finder's lack of technical sophistication, it is often feared, either will prevent understanding of the flawed assumption or will require a substantial, and unjustified, lengthening of the trial and added costs to reveal the flawed assumption. (Shuman, 1994, pp. 6–7)

Likely reflecting the absence of established bodies of relevant research, the earliest recorded judicial approach to scrutinize the admissibility of expert testimony in the sixteenth and seventeenth centuries focused exclusively on the qualifications of the witness, without independent scrutiny of the validity or the reliability of the science of the methods and procedures underlying that testimony (Chapin, 1880; Faigman, Porter, and Saks, 1994; Osborn, 1935). This approach carried forward through the nineteenth century. In retrospect, the decision that most clearly reflects a shift in this approach is the well-known decision of the District of Columbia Court of Appeals in *Frye v. United States* (1923). *Frye* involved the admissibility of a predecessor to the polygraph which measured systolic blood pressure, and it articulated the now well-known *general acceptance* test that deferred to the judgment of the scientific community to guide the courts in the admissibility of novel scientific evidence: "Just when a scientific principle or discovery crosses the line between the experimental and demonstrable stages is difficult to define. Somewhere in this twilight zone the evidential force of the principle must be recognized, and while courts will go a long way in admitting expert testimony deduced from a well-recognized scientific principle or discovery, the thing from which the deduction is made must be sufficiently established to have gained general acceptance in the particular field to which it belongs" (pp. 1129–30).

Ultimately, *Frye* did much to transform judicial scrutiny of scientific testimony. Perhaps the most significant aspect of *Frye*'s role in shaping judicial scrutiny of scientific expert evidence is its movement of the analysis away from qualifications as the sole test for admissibility. The *Frye* court acknowledged the unchallenged qualifications of the expert who offered the test results. Nonetheless, it imposed an additional level of analysis on the admissibility decision which focused on the quality of the underlying science the expert offered. To assess the quality of the underlying science, the court chose the test of general acceptance in the relevant scientific community. In courts applying the *Frye* test, witness qualifications are a necessary but not a sufficient condition of admissibility.

Ironically, as *Frye*'s importance grew, the Federal Rules of Evidence, promulgated in 1974 as an effort to codify and reform a disparate body of evidence case law, which often seemed skewed to exclude evidence and keep the jury in the dark, did not contain a single reference to *Frye*. The Federal Rules of Evidence instead appeared to permit expert testimony by a qualified expert merely if it would "assist the trier of fact to understand the evidence or to determine a fact at issue" (Fed. R. Evid., 1974, p. 702). This silence about *Frye* led to a debate in which its proponents and opponents claimed that the silence proved alternatively that *Frye* had been retained or rejected.

One decision that might have offered some insight into this question was the Supreme Court's 1983 opinion in *Barefoot v. Estelle*. The expert testimony at issue in *Barefoot* was the clinical opinion testimony of a psychiatrist offered by the prosecution in a capital sentencing proceeding that turned, in part, on the risk that the defendant posed to others if not executed. The psychiatrist testified that, based on his experience, whether or not Barefoot was confined, if he was not executed there was "a one hundred percent and absolute chance" (p. 919) that he would commit future acts of criminal violence. In response to a challenge to the trial court's admission of this testimony and the jury's imposition of the death penalty, the American Psychiatric Association, which filed an amicus brief in the case before the Supreme Court, presented a review of the research concluding that "even under the best of conditions, psychiatric predictions of long-term future dangerousness are wrong in at least two out of every three cases" (pp. 920–21). Rejecting the constitutional challenge to Barefoot's state court conviction, the United States Supreme Court upheld the admissibility of this evidence, without imposing any threshold scrutiny beyond relevance, making the sweeping pronouncement that "the rules of evidence generally extant at the federal and state levels anticipate that relevant, unprivileged evidence should be admitted and its weight left to the fact finder, who would have the benefit of cross-examination and contrary evidence by the opposing party" (p. 898).

The next guidance that the Court provided on the standards for the admissibility of scientific expert testimony occurred in its 1993 decision in *Daubert v. Merrell Dow Pharmaceuticals, Inc. Daubert* involved a tort claim filed in federal court alleging that in utero exposure to Bendectin, an antinausea drug manufactured by Dow, had caused the plaintiff's limb reduction birth defects. Unlike *Barefoot*, in which the prosecution's challenged expert testimony was not legally required for the judge to submit the decision about the imposition of capital punishment to the jury, for the plaintiff's case to be permitted to go to the jury in *Daubert* it was necessary for the plaintiff to produce admissible expert testimony linking the defendant's drug and the plaintiff's injury. The defendant objected to the plaintiff's expert testimony, asserting, among other things, that *Frye*'s general acceptance test governed the admissibility of this expert testimony and that it could not survive such scrutiny. The defendant asserted that it was generally accepted that only human epidemiological research should be used to establish a causal link between Bendectin and human limb reduction birth defects and, of thirty published epidemiological studies, none found such a link. In response, the plaintiff offered the expert testimony of well-credentialed chemists and biostatisticians with appointments at prestigious academic research institutions, who sought to link the plaintiff's limb reduction birth defects to Bendectin using animal studies, pharmacological studies comparing Bendectin with known teratogens, and reanalysis of the published epidemiological studies. The trial court accepted the defendant's general acceptance argument, struck the plaintiff's experts, and granted summary judgment in favor of the defendant; the court of appeals affirmed the decision, and the Supreme Court agreed to review it.

If the Supreme Court's logic in *Barefoot* governed, the plaintiff's proposed evidence, although contradicted by the existing research, nonetheless should have been admitted because it was relevant, and its weight should have been left to the fact finder to sort out through cross-examination and contrary evidence by the opposing party. If *Frye* governed, the trial court and court of appeals decisions should have been affirmed. The Supreme Court, however, articulated a new standard under the federal rules that required federal courts to consider the scientific validity of the reasoning underlying the testimony and the propriety of applying it to the facts of this case, and it remanded the case to the court of appeals for consideration in light of the new standard. The Court also rejected the suggestion that *Frye* had been incorporated into the Federal Rules of Evidence. Instead, it required the federal courts to make their own "preliminary assessment of whether the reasoning or methodology underlying the testimony is scientifically valid and of whether that reasoning properly can be applied to the facts in issue" (p. 590). Relying heavily on Karl Popper's notion of falsifiability as the talisman for the scientific enterprise, the pragmatic considerations the Supreme Court outlined to use in this assessment included a consideration of whether the underlying theory or technique can be and has been tested, whether it has been subjected to scrutiny by others in the field through peer review and publication, whether the error rate and standards for controlling it are acceptable, and the degree of acceptance within the scientific community.

Why might the Court treat these two cases so differently? One inescapable consideration in this disparate treatment is the difference in the experts' methodologies. The expert in *Barefoot* presented his opinions based on his experiences as a clinical practitioner and did not purport to rely on research-based information. Conversely, the experts in *Daubert* offered to present research-based, scientific testimony. That is not the only significant difference between the cases, but the language of these opinions strongly supports the conclusion that the methodologies underlying the testimony provide the critical distinction. *Daubert* discusses the scientific method and many of the major works addressing it and attempts to incorporate these in the standard for admissibility. *Barefoot* does not discuss the scientific method or articulate a test that addresses the validity of the research underlying the expert's conclusions, let alone how it was applied in this case. *Barefoot* and *Daubert* send very different signals about the standards for the admissibility of expert evidence. These decisions posit implicitly, and numerous state court decisions posit explicitly, that courts should scrutinize expert testimony derived from clinical opinion differently than expert testimony derived from scientific research. Yet they offer no explicit explanation as to why this distinction exists, let alone how it should be applied in varied fact situations.

This distinction is unsound both as a theoretical and as an empirical proposition. If differential scrutiny of expert testimony relying on scientific research and clinical opinion is based on the assumption that there is less risk that jurors will be in awe of clinical-opinion–based testimony than scientific-research–based testimony, the empirical evidence is not supportive. The research indicates that jurors make expert specific and not categorical assumptions by class or type of expert (Shuman, Champagne, and Whitaker, 1996). Moreover, if the theory underlying this distinction is that jurors routinely accord expert testimony relying on scientific research greater weight than expert testimony relying on clinical opinion, it fails to explain how jurors are any better able to assess the validity of clinical-opinion–based testimony.

Although courts have not routinely been rigorous in scrutinizing the scientific basis for the methodology underlying clinical opinion testimony, they have generally been more willing to engage in rigorous scrutiny of clinical opinion testimony when aspects of the scientific process are explicit, even in the case of behavioral or social science evidence (Shuman, 1994). So, for example, when an expert offering a clinical opinion relies on a particular test or syndrome, courts have been more willing to invoke their rigorous standard of scrutiny. And, in certain kinds of cases (e.g., recovered repressed memory claims), courts have been increasingly demanding of even clinically based testimony (*State v. Hungerford*, 1995).

The popularity of competing attitudes about protecting versus informing jurors shifts over time. The courts took a relatively restrictive approach to the receipt of expert testimony prior to the adoption of the Federal Rules of Evidence in 1974, fearing that an uneducated, naive jury might abdicate its decision-making responsibility to the expert. Accordingly, expert testimony was generally admissible only when the issues were wholly beyond the ken of the fact finder. The Federal Rules of Evidence reflected a relaxation of these traditional approaches premised on greater confidence in the intelligence and sensibility of jurors. The current attitude reflects a shift toward greater restrictiveness, proceeding on the assumption that experts who either are unqualified or utilize unreliable methods and procedures have frequently persuaded unsophisticated or unprincipled juries to reach unjust results. In part, this shift is fueled by politically based attacks on the use of experts to advance the business and insurance industries' tort reform agenda and, in part, by judicial and scientific attacks on abuses in opinions advanced as expert scientific testimony. Thus, even as *Daubert* has been adopted in an increasing number of states, its larger significance, particularly for psychiatric and psychological evidence, is as "part of a trend in both state and federal courts toward more demanding level of scrutiny requiring scientific support or validation for the assertions made by mental health professionals in forensic settings. This trend is even seen in states that have chosen to apply the 'general acceptance in the relevant professional community' test instead of *Daubert*" (Greenberg and Shuman, 1997, p. 55).

▪ ▪ The Implications for the DSM and Strategies to Address Values in Psychiatric Nosology

The Choices

In their starkest terms, the choices placed on the table by this book are to externalize and make explicit the value choices in the DSM or to avoid externalizing value choices and make science the dominant value in psychiatric nosology. Viewing this choice from the perspective of the legal system as a consumer of the DSM, I am profoundly ambivalent about this choice and its forensic consequences, seeing cause for celebration and concern in each, and much uncertainty.

Deconstructing the DSM

Neither law nor science is value neutral, and, as the values of these two disciplines often lack congruity, it is important to recognize these differences explicitly to acknowledge their incongruence and, where possible, to embrace their congruence. Deconstructing the DSM by externalizing its value choices has the potential to assist the legal system to understand more fully the boundaries of psychiatric and psychological information and to achieve a better fit for interdisciplinary collaboration by using that information more appropriately. And, what could be bad about that?

One risk of acknowledgment of these value choices in the DSM is that as courts apply more rigorous scrutiny to the admissibility of scientific evidence, deconstructing the DSM has the potential to persuade courts to reject testimony that relies on the DSM as not sufficiently scientific, ironically preferring pure clinically based testimony, not grounded in methods or procedures that have been subjected to rigorous testing. It is one thing to assert that psychiatrists and other mental health professionals lay claim to the scientific high ground. It is quite another matter for psychiatrists and other mental health professionals to lay claim to a moral high ground. If the entirety of DSM, and not merely a conclusion here or a judgment there, is understood to be infused with value choices, particularly where those values may not be those of mainstream America, then courts may be more inclined to reject testimony grounded in diagnostic categories in favor of clinically based testimony resting on untested theories and procedures, which courts have naively not subjected to the same degree of scrutiny.

This preference could have a serious consequence for the accuracy of expert testimony, as well as judge and jury decision making. An expert offering an opinion about a defendant's competence to stand trial, for example, might rely on an empirically tested structured interview and screening instrument or the expert's untested clinical intuition about the defendant's competence to stand trial. There is a large body of social science research examining the accuracy of clinical (i.e., in this example the clinical intuition) versus actuarial decision making (i.e., in this example the structured interview or screening instrument). One of the most consistent findings of this body of work is that the actuarial method of judgment and decision making outperforms the clinical method (Dawes, Faust, and Meehl, 1989). Moreover, that research reveals that there is no correlation between confidence in one's clinical opinion or decision and the accuracy of that opinion or decision; nor can lay decision makers distinguish between the two (Dawes, 1994; Meehl, 1954). Thus, a rule of admissibility which accepts clinical decision making but hesitates to accept actuarial decision making that relies on the DSM because of its explicit value orientation would likely contribute to greater error in trial court fact finding.

Of course, one may ask, Is this such a bad result? It is unlikely that drafters of the DSM, who have sought to limit its forensic linkage, would be troubled by a result that increases the likelihood that the legal system will be more cautious in using the DSM. But would this result benefit the quality of the information that courts receive from psychiatrists and psychologists?

This likely depends on the answers to a panoply of questions for which we have no empirically defined answers. Is psychiatric and psychological testimony clarified or confused by the use of psychiatric diagnoses? Do diagnoses help litigants to deal with their mental health problems, or do they provide litigants with additional incentives to reframe their injuries for legal ends? Would psychiatric and psychological testimony unadorned with diagnostic labels be more or less valid/reliable?

Making Science the Only Value Legitimate for Discussion in Psychiatric Nosology

The most likely forensic impact of making science the exclusive concern in psychiatric nosology is on the quality of evidence presented. It is difficult to develop rational arguments in opposition to the efforts of scientists and the courts to raise the bar for the assessment of the quality of information presented as scientific expert testimony. Making science the dominant value in diagnostic nosology seems likely to enhance the quality of science underlying psychiatric and psychological evidence.

There are however, some unexpected risks to improving the scientific content of the DSM. One such risk is an increased forensic usage of and deferral to the DSM and its unexplored value judgments. For better or worse, a solution that demands the ignoring of values in psychiatric nosology and a closer linkage between the DSM and research might encourage even greater forensic use of psychiatric and psychological evidence and greater willingness of the law to defer to its implicit, incongruous values. Highlighting the scientific basis for the DSM and minimizing its values seems likely to increase use of the DSM as a forensic mantra, without addressing its forensic failings (Shuman, 1989).

Will It Really Make a Difference in Court?

In large part, however, whether any change in the articulation of the values implicit in the DSM will really make a difference in court turns on how well the legal system is doing now in deconstructing the DSM and psychiatric nosology. The question begs an empirical response, yet the only evidence is anecdotal. Where values are fairly obvious and testimony common, there is some evidence that the legal system often gets it. Trial lawyers quickly learn that the DSM is subject to a vote and that the exclusion of homosexuality as a disorder was not preceded by any body of scientific research but rather changing attitudes of those voting on the change (Bayer, 1987, 1981).

Where values are less obvious and the topic of testimony less frequent, it is less clear how well the legal system does. Several factors within the legal system may contribute to this situation. One is the resources of the party to finance thoughtful (i.e., expensive) research and discovery, and the other is the rules that govern pretrial discovery. Civil tort cases generally tend to involve litigants who are relatively closely matched financially. Poorly financed litigants do not usually make it into the tort arena. To pursue tort claims, plaintiffs' lawyers must be well financed, as these cases are expensive to litigate and generate fees, if at all, often years after they are instituted. Given the costs and the risks of litigating these cases, plaintiffs' lawyers rarely pursue medical malpractice or products liability claims involving potential damages of less than $50,000 to $100,000, and then only when the defendant is insured against this risk or has sufficient nonexempt assets to satisfy a judgment. Such defendants generally have the financial wherewithal to explore and raise challenges to plaintiffs' experts.

In contrast, most criminal defendants are indigent and represented by court-appointed counsel (Green, 1993). Although there is a constitutional obligation on the part of the government to provide expert assistance to the defense counsel to make meaningful the Sixth Amendment guarantee of effective assistance of counsel (*Ake v. Oklahoma*, 1985), appellate courts have been wary to interpret this requirement expansively. Thus, most criminal litigation lacks the scrutiny of experts common to much civil litigation.

This difference in the scrutiny of experts and the methods and procedures that underlie their opinions is also exacerbated by differences in pretrial discovery rules in civil and criminal cases. Civil litigants are entitled to extensive disclosures about the experts an opponent will present and to depose those experts (Shuman, 1994). Criminal litigants are generally entitled to less extensive disclosures about the experts an opponent will present and are rarely entitled to depose them (Shuman, 1994). Thus, the differences in civil and criminal litigation suggest that the opportunity to deconstruct the DSM and its role in forensic assessment varies widely across the legal system.

▪ ▪ Conclusion

Courts struggle to be more informed, critical consumers of expert testimony. Yet, wedded to the adversary system in which the parties select both the lay and expert witnesses they wish to present, courts reach decisions about issues beyond lay competence based on competing partisan experts selected because their testimony assists that party. Thus, for the benefit of both the courts and the professions whose public persona stature is often significantly shaped by judicial appearances, it is important that responsible professional bodies engage in rigorous independent analysis of the relevant research to provide a benchmark against which partisan presentations can be judged.

The DSM is an opportunity for psychiatrists and other mental health professionals to provide the courts with such a benchmark. To ask whether science or an exposition of the values underlying that science is more important to the courts is to set up a false dichotomy. Both are important, and neither can be neglected if the mental health professions are to provide useful guidance to the courts.

....

16

Speaking across the Border: A Patient Assessment of Located Languages, Values, and Credentials in Psychiatric Classification

CATHY LEAKER, PH.D.

THIS CHAPTER ADDRESSES the problem of the marginalized subject within psychiatric classification. It argues that the DSM-IV as a now institutional fixture in psychiatry functions according to a model of segregation and exclusion: that certain groups are disenfranchised with respect to not only speech but also knowledge. The primary group excluded from full participation in psychiatric classification is that most affected by it: the patients.

Against this model of exclusive authority, I posit bell hooks's fantasy of a "revolutionary effort which seeks to create space where there is unlimited access to the pleasure and power of knowing, where transformation is possible" (1990, p. 145). I claim that such an effort demands the inclusion of multiple and dissenting voices. As such, I approach this problem from three separate but interrelated subject positions, all "autobiographical" and each of which shapes my methodology. Those three positions are patient, cultural theorist, and writer. I use my own diagnosis of borderline personality disorder to illustrate the dilemma of the prohibited margin. My primary method is a close analysis of the language used in the clinical and popular literature of psychiatric nosology. My method is informed by my training in critical theory, implicitly the work of Michel Foucault and explicitly that of postcolonial, deconstructivist, feminists such as Gayatri Spivak, but I am careful to dissociate my own work from a reductivist antipsychiatry because my ultimate goal is dialogue, not diatribe.

Ultimately my argument is simple: quality in future classification must be based on a language that is responsible not only to the needs of science (legitimate or otherwise) but also to the many constituencies, including patients, affected by that language. Simple though it is, however, it is also unfortunately utopian, given the present establishments, constitutions, institutions, and industries of psychiatry. bell hooks's fantasy of "unlimited access to the pleasure and power of knowing" remains precisely that: a fantasy. Thus, concrete and specific suggestions to psychiatric nosologists are difficult to articulate; indeed, the difficulty of such articulation is indicative of the problem. I can only advocate (more or less vaguely) a (more or less radical) change in conceptual approach to psychiatric classification: that dialogue and inclusion replace exclusion and prohibition as the core values of the DSM, that alternative voices be both invited and invoked within its deep structure.

▪ ▪ The Image of the Border

Let me begin by presenting my credentials, or rather, in this context at least, my lack thereof. After reading some of my earlier work on psychiatric classification, Ted Brown, a medical historian at the University of Rochester, told me, "You'll never get the medical community to take you seriously without empirical data." Nevertheless, I am not including any empirical data. And there may well be other reasons why the medical community will not take me seriously. I have not written this chapter as a clinician or as a technically trained expert in psychiatric research. My skills, training, and fourteen years of experience in the field are decidedly elsewhere. Or are they? One of the most benignly memorable moments in Woody Allen's *Everybody Says I Love You* was the generic Woody Allen character's discussion of his career dilemma: "I couldn't decide whether to be a therapist or a writer," he explains to his former wife and her husband, "so I compromised, I became a writer and a patient." While one can hardly hope to improve on Woody Allen, either in wit or in neurosis, I would amend his remark in my case to "I became a writer, a grad student, and a patient." And it is in these three capacities that I approach and confront the issues this book aims to address. Moreover, it is precisely these noncredentials that entitle me to write in a discursive enterprise in which I am an outsider or, at best, a border dweller.

The image of the border is particularly resonant for me because my own diagnosis is borderline personality disorder, and most of my critical research has focused on this "severely dysfunctional form of personality organization whose clinical presentation is intimately connected to the interpersonal context in which the patient is observed" (Gunderson, 1989, p. 1387) and which furthermore presents "one of the biggest challenges for both the novice and experienced therapist" (Goldstein, 1993, p. 172). My point in revealing this, and drawing it out further in the later parts of this chapter, is *not* to prove somehow beyond the shadow of a doubt that "I'm not a borderline . . . ," for that would, of course, be "classic borderline behavior"; indeed, for the purposes of this book, I'm more than willing to declare, as it were, "Ich bin Borderliner" (though I hope it will become clear that I use that term in a different sense than does the DSM). My point in representing myself this way is to again raise the issue of credentials and of credibility; it is worth considering that of all the autobiographical details I could offer about my "self," this one might most strain readers' credulity with regard to the contents of this chapter. To confess to a borderline diagnosis as a point of introduction to the readers, psychiatrists among them, is likely to cast my critique—to put it mildly—in a certain "the lady doth protest too much" light; it might well be assumed that, to use the language of the DSM-IV, I am appearing here in my (deluded) "righteous avenger of past mistreatment" mode, the necessary antipodes of my "needy supplicant." Nor is my having been designated an individual with borderline personality disorder likely to increase my popularity. Aside from the off-the-record discourse surrounding this condition, we have the words of J. Christopher Perry and George Vailliant, who in Kaplan and Sadock's authoritative *Comprehensive Textbook of Psychiatry* point out that "their character traits are unlikely to endear themselves to mental health professionals" (Perry and Vailliant, 1989, p. 1352); indeed, claims Benjamin (1993), citing Groves, "the physician's troubled reaction is an important diagnostic sign for BPD" (p. 114).

I am not bringing any of this up to avenge past mistreatment or even to prove Kaplan and Sadock wrong by endearing myself to a very large group of mental health professionals; I want simply to interrogate credentials and credibility on the one hand and incredulity and (virtual) disenfranchisement on the other—and to challenge orders and disorders of entitlement as well. What criteria—endearing or otherwise—entitle an individual to speak about psychiatric diagnosis, and more important, what "criteria" systematically and systemically silence another individual? How and where and by whom and against whom is the border drawn? This question is at the heart of my research, my methodology, and my advocacy.

▪ ▪ Credentials, Credibility, and Segregation

In the case of the DSM-IV and psychiatric nosology, that question, "Who is entitled to speak," metastasizes into the even more politically totalitarian "Who is entitled to know?" In a very real sense, attempting to enter into the discourse of psychiatry is like cracking a code, breaking into a file of classified information, crashing a party at a private club, emblazoned with the sign "Members Only." Consider, for example, the "Cautionary Statement" that concludes the introduction to the DSM-IV (American Psychiatric Association, 1994); in what amounts to a kind of "Don't try this at home" disclaimer, the editors of the DSM write: "The specified diagnostic criteria for each mental disorder are offered as guidelines for making diagnoses, because it has been demonstrated that the use of such criteria enhances agreement among clinicians and investigators. The proper use of these criteria requires specialized clinical training that provides both a body of knowledge and clinical skills" (p. xxvii). Notably left out of the agreement between clinicians and the dubiously named "investigators" is, of course, the patient, who presumably (except in the rare case of a Kay Redfield Jamison) does not have access to specialized clinical training. But I would argue that there is more at stake here than a simple question of "proper use," guerdoned by a body of knowledge and clinical skills; the "Cautionary Statement," I would suggest, has less to do with Caution than with, if you'll forgive the term, Power. Gayatri Spivak, a literary and postcolonial theorist at Columbia University, argues in her brilliant essay "Explanation and Culture: Marginalia" that "what inhabits the prohibited margin of a particular explanation specifies its particular politics" (1987, p. 106). If, as seems reasonable, we understand the DSM-IV as an elaborate system of explanation, then patients' inhabitation of the prohibited margins of Credited Speech and Credentialed Knowledge might allow us to specify the latter's politics—at its worst—as that built on exclusion and discrimination, on separate and unequal segregation.

Stuart Kirk and Herb Kutchins, in *The Selling of DSM*, identify two primary functions of the DSM: it "sets the boundaries of the domain in which psychiatry claims expertise and exclusive authority . . . and equally important [the] DSM as a classification system asserts how knowledge should be organized and how it should be accumulated" (1992, p. 12). The patient, lacking the expertise and authority to participate in the "enhanced agreements" that determine her, is nonetheless the object of the expertise and of the knowledge that is organized and accumulated about her. This leads to a third function of the DSM: the exclusive authority to assert how knowledge should be dispersed. Thus, for example, John Docherty concludes his essay "To Know Borderline Personality Disorder" with a call for a "psychoeducational process" by which "friends, therapists and family members learn or are taught to cope with interpersonal and personal stress experienced and wrought by BPD patients" (1992, p. 338). At the upper end of this psychoeducation is the technical argot—recondite and abstruse—of research psychiatry, the contained site where knowledge is accumulated and shared among an elite community of experts. The information and explanations produced, then, form this "enhanced agreement," which is then filtered to clinicians—with the appropriate body of knowledge and clinical skills—and finally to the lowest end of the spectrum, a presumed extended community of caregivers. And lurking beneath the lowest end of the spectrum is the borderline him- or herself, who, though excluded from this particular psychoeducational process, is nonetheless conscripted into a different kind of psychoeducational process, for example, that of "cognitive-behavorial treatment." Thus, the patient is in the paradoxical position of being simultaneously locked into and locked out of the diagnostic process and, more broadly, the psychoeducational process. It is this paradox that I attempt to address, or more accurately redress, in my work.

Against the paternalistic model of expert and authoritative "agreement" generated by the DSM and its innumerable and well-marketed progeny, I again offer bell hooks's fantasy of "that revolutionary effort which seeks to create space where there is unlimited access to the pleasure and power of knowing, where transformation is possible" (1990, p. 145). My method for participating in this "revolutionary effort" is simply to advocate the value of multiple perspectives, particularly those of outsiders. For my own purposes, I would like to describe briefly the specific and constitutive perspectives and the conceptual strategies that each of my roles (patient, student, writer) offers me in my negotiation of the very dense and immensely thorny problems that classification and diagnosis present (on both sides of the couch). Philip Cushman poses as an alternative to the unified and united diagnostic gaze "a basic tenet of interpretive hermeneutics: the process of reading humans is not the same as reading persons as texts but more like standing behind them and reading over their shoulder the cultural text from which they themselves are reading" (1995, p. 23).

Let me illustrate this point by simply analyzing the goals of the conference that spawned this book, as stated in the "Call for Papers" according to what I might call the "Readers and Shoulders Method." The second goal of this conference is articulated in that document as follows: "to improve the quality of future classifications through an enhanced awareness of value issues." I choose this apparently straightforward goal precisely because of its obscured vagueness; the entire phrase is saturated with vagueness, but I want to focus on one specific provocative and enormously generative ambiguity: the word *quality,* a word that shifts in meaning depending on the reader and the shoulder in question. From the standpoint of many nosologists, I assume the *word* quality refers to "accuracy." Not coming from a scientific background myself, accuracy is hardly my golden calf; indeed, given my theoretical bias, the word *accuracy* is like a red flag to the proverbial (postmodernist) bull.

I read the word *quality* through the lenses of my three subject positions: patient, student, writer; in reality, of course, these roles do not represent distinct and separate selves but in fact constantly interpenetrate and shape one another. Thus, for each of these positions, quality is a function of "my" relationship to language and its effects; my rationale for this is based on the premise that, as bell hooks reminds us, "language is also a site of struggle" (1990, p. 146). Language may well appear not to be the most immediate concern, or site of struggle, as we "debate the virtues and liabilities of taxonomies for mental disorders" ("Call for Papers," 1997). And yet, given that Donald D. Goodwin and Samuel Guze reiterate in the fifth edition of *Psychiatric Diagnosis* that "classification has two functions: communication and prediction" (1996, p. xi), the issue of language, and bell hooks's claim with respect to it, must be a central one. Further, I would suggest that the communicative and predictive function of diagnosis within specific language choices, even and perhaps especially when it is carried on only within the clinical literature to which the patient has virtually no access, can have an iatrogenic effect. Thus, for example, when I finally gain access to Lorna Smith Benjamin's predictive communication that early emotional learning "sets the BPD on a course of ever-escalating symptomatology" and that "*My misery is your command* summarizes the BPD's plan for the therapy or the marital process," (1993, p. 121), or when she states that "for the BPD, anything that can go wrong has gone wrong" (p. 113), I as a patient, a student, and a writer feel compelled to intervene and intercede. Language—particularly in its guise as communication and prediction—is indeed a site of struggle; and admittedly, in each of my roles, I have a very distinct plan—only indirectly grounded in my so-called misery—in entering this struggle. Let me try to illustrate.

As Patient

Assuming, as we must, that it is quite a different operation to diagnose and to *be* diagnosed, I first want to outline the "being diagnosed" element in my work, not because it is the most important, but because it is the most marginal. Kirk and Kutchins (1992) use the following epigraph from Lewis Carroll's *Through the Looking Glass* to introduce *The Selling of DSM*: "What's the use of having names," the Gnat said, "if they won't answer to them?" "No use to *them*," said Alice, "but it's useful to the people that name them, I suppose." Kirk and Kutchins use the exquisitely disingenuous Alice to highlight the fact that naming is a privilege of power: there are thems and then there are *thems,* and naming the latter exclusively serves the interests and needs of the former (though significantly the Gnat—in all his buglike wisdom—allocates the power to refuse a name to *them*). I might argue, then, that the word *quality,* as read through the conversation of Alice and the Gnat, would demand a name that would be of some use to me or at the very least ensure that what is putatively "of use" to you is not *as a consequence* harmful to me, since the alleged usefulness of naming so easily slides into the worse than uselessness of name-calling. Further, if I might put the Carrollian dialogue into a Marxist paradigm (an admittedly odd maneuver), I would argue that diagnosis has an apparent use value for, and an obvious exchange value among, professionals but has little, if any, use value for me. This is partly because I am excluded from the system of diagnostic exchange by which names—in this case disorders—become, in effect, commodities; and patients become, via this process, alienated from their illness.

However, I don't have the space to develop a critique of the relationship between capitalism and the DSM-IV here (though I think there are real links), except insofar as the more or less insistent subtext of this chapter is about the ownership of language. I instead try to explain what I mean by a diagnosis having, or not having, a use value for me as the patient. Or to return to the words of the Gnat, "What might be in a name that I would not refuse to answer to it?" Sadly, at this point in my "psychoeducational process," I can only answer this question in the negative (and again I think that fact alone speaks volumes about the DSM-IV). The word *quality* for me as patient, then, means that language that is least pernicious to my own sense of self and, more important, least malignant in terms of others' response to that constructed "self"; both of these relate quality in the *representation* of disorder not to an accurate clinical description of my suffering, nor even (yet) to fundamental *improvement* of my well-being, but simply to a stasis, if you will, that if it cannot help it will at least not hurt.

I argue an improvement in quality in this respect would of necessity demand the participation of patients' voices *and* agencies at every level of diagnostic revision. If indeed it is necessary that "our" suffering be named, classified, differentiated from yours' and reduced to a limited linguistic, as well as numerical, code, it is only reasonable that "we" have some say in what gets written, represented, and subsequently codified about us. Neither case studies nor the Borderline-on-Display method adopted by so many popular texts on the issue permits us that "say," though they seem to; in the words of Janice Cauwels, "the case histories and descriptions included in this book represent my attempts to transcend diagnostic criteria and capture something of [the borderlines'] inner lives" (1992, p. 8) Yet, in both clinical and popular texts, there is a (re)presentational sleight of hand going on in which the patient's naming and framing precedes her "speech." Thus, though she seems to speak, these are merely other and more dubious mechanisms by which she is silenced. As such, neither case studies nor self-congratulatory empathic self-help texts provide a sense of inclusion but rather a sense of fear; as bell hooks says: "Silenced. we fear those who speak about us, not to us and with us" (1990, p. 152).

My own fantasy of inclusion of my voice is tied directly to my agency: to disrupt the frame and shape the name rather than allow the name to shape me. If I had to adopt a paradigm for the kind of exchange I am proposing, I would use one that would be familiar to you: that of the professional consultation. This might be implemented at the level of drawing out and drawing from patients' personal (though not necessarily emotional) narratives—not to shore up medical descriptions but to challenge them. bell hooks, in her essay "Choosing the Margin as a Space of Radical Openness" (one of her many compelling discussions of racism), refers to this process as "intimate intervention" and describes it in the following way: "Private speech in public discourse, intimate intervention, making another text that enables me to recover all that I am in language, I find so many gaps, absences in the written text. To cite them at least is to let the reader know something has been missed, or remains there hinted at by words—there in the deep structure" (1990, p. 147).

As patient, I would argue that "the quality of future classifications through an enhanced awareness of value issues" demands that the "something missed" hooks refers to be first recognized and then both invited and invoked in the process of revisioning, or to use again hooks's extremely resonant word, recovering the DSM, a particularly communicative and predictive written text. Quality, then, would institute a process that would contribute to recovery of the something missed and, as a consequence, to recovery of "all that I am [and am *not*]" and ultimately to recovery of my "health." That kind of intervention—which can *only* come from patients—is all the more necessary, at least from my perspective, because I remain doubtful as to whether patients' uncontaminated voices are in any way a part of the "deep structure" of the DSM in particular and psychiatric nosology more generally.

But how do we get to this "something missed"? Clearly it is not a mere matter of Oprah-like testimonials or indeed Ricki Lake–like confrontations. Still, both testimonial and confrontation are, I think, integral to intimate intervention, yet I want to focus instead on what lies beyond moments. My own writing and work, and the contribution I hope to make, come from that still rather nebulous "beyond." My belief is that that beyond—a space where the "being diagnosed" moves from reactive response to active engagement—can provide a means, indeed an actual method, of working through precisely those issues that the conference met to resolve. This still vague "beyond" space to which I refer can, I think, produce a "talking diagnosis" that might then recover the talking cure from an increasingly debased psychoanalytic context to one that is more inclusive, expansive, resonant, dialogic, and, for lack of a better word, democratic. Central to this process is movement, on the part of both the person who diagnoses and the one who is diagnosed.

Essentially, I would characterize this movement as one toward mutuality; true dialogue demands mutuality. This particular move can be something as simple (or as difficult) as a negotiated truce, or to put it more crudely, each party cutting the other some slack. I know in my own work, for example, a tendency to fall into a "Psychiatrist stupid; me smart" rhetoric, which is inaccurate, misguided, and "unlikely to endear me to mental health professionals." More important, however much psychiatric nomenclature may and does contain oppressive elements, there is no malicious intent behind it. Neither the advocacy and activism I am interested in nor the narratives I myself construct tell monolithic stories of oppressors and victims. Although I have undergone more than my fair share of turbulence during my years as a frequent flier in psychiatric air space, my point would be lost were I to present myself as a psychiatric survivor (much as I respect the importance of patient self-help groups). For one thing I'm not (I still continue to take medication and see a therapist regularly, and I still continue to wrestle with internal demons more or less pernicious). Moreover, such a construction is reductive and can only shut down dialogue rather than initiating it. Finally, it would not serve my agenda (and, like everyone else here, I have a distinct and palpable agenda) to reify this paradigm further for it merely perpetuates the fetish of an inherent antagonism that must be dismantled if I am to achieve anything. Though my work is informed by Laing, Szasz, Caplan, and others, I do not see myself participating in some sort of resurrected, monolithic antipsychiatry movement; indeed, I agree with sociologist Peter Miller when he claims that "what has been called anti-psychiatry has bequeathed to us a set of notions which hinders the process of critique" (1986, p. 14). More simply put, mounting a critique of the complex diagnostic system based on a premise of a Psychiatric Evil Empire whose sole mission is to stamp out deviance is both intellectually naive and politically short sighted.

If, then, my responsibility, as patient, in initiating mutuality is both to avoid excessive intellectual hubris and not to allow myself to fall into (splitting) binary narratives of power relationships (though the greatest mutuality *must even so not* elide the question of power), what move (if any) is demanded of physicians in this comedy of psychiatric Pride and Prejudice? I would argue that primarily physicians must learn to rehear and rethink patients' voices, particularly with respect to diagnosis. And again I will use a word the meaning of which depends on one's location: resistance. All too often, and I base this both on my own experience and on my reading, resistance is configured within psychiatric terms as denial, or in more magnanimous constructions, as a more or less high-level defense mechanism. In the case of the BPD diagnosis, that model is accentuated to the point where the patient's resistant voice is written out altogether and then written back in as complaint, since she is constructed, according to the DSM-IV, as simultaneously "a needy supplicant," "a righteous avenger [presumably without cause] of past mistreatment" (American Psychiatric Association, 1994, p. 651), and, in John Gunderson's phrase, "a help-rejecting complainer" (1984, p. 176). She is also, of course, extremely sensitive to criticism. All these qualities (criteria) communicate and predict, as Gunderson points out, "specific clinical dilemmas . . . that are important insofar as they suggest that the problems in treatment [including, we must presume, resistance or help-rejecting complaining] [are] not understandable as a misapplication of the concepts of either psychoanalysis or theraputic communities but reflec[t] something perversely troublesome within the patients themselves" (1984, pp. 2, 175).

For me, however, resistance, though it may well be perceived to be "perversely troublesome" by my skilled clinician, might be exactly that (healthy) impulse bell hooks alludes to when she discusses the personal imperative to recover all that I am in language. This always resistant impulse is all the more insistent when it is set up against a system that claims the authority to *uncover* all that I am (told I am) in language decidedly not my own ("perversely troublesome" comes immediately to mind). The process of uncovering is, in this sense, antithetical to the process of recovering. In making this claim, I do not want to take an antipsychiatry stance that would *exclusively* privilege the subjective experience; instead, the "value" I am embracing and advocating here is agency. Within the current structures and systems of psychiatric nosology there is little room for a patient's agency. I might again refer to the "don't try this at home" caution in the DSM. Patients are ironically excluded from the process of differential diagnosis and the decisions about subsequent differential treatment. The enormous gap here between *un*covering and *re*covering creates and reifies an ideology similar to that which Martin Luther King, in "Letter from the Birmingham Jail," mentions in his discussion of segregation and the relationship it sets up between the segregator and the segregated: "Segregation, to use the terminology of the Jewish philosopher Martin Buber, substitutes an *I-it* relationship for an *I-thou* relationship and ends up relegating persons to the status of things (1963, p. 484). There is, of course, something absurd, not to mention politically heinous, in a dorky white girl likening, or appearing to liken, contemporary psychiatric institutions to the pre–civil rights South. Let me be clear that, in referring to segregation, I am not in any way adopting a kind of "Jim Crow: c'est moi" posture. Still, King's allusion to Buber has some relevance here. The DSM—not only at the level of concept but also at the level of language—without question (in my mind at least) does indeed relegate persons to the status of things or, more accurately, of numbers. This is so even despite the DSM-IV's careful and well-intentioned prescription that "a common misconception is that a classification of mental disorders classifies people, when actually what are being classified are disorders people have. For this reason, the text of DSM-IV (as did the text of DSM-III-R) avoids the use of such expressions as 'a schizophrenic' or 'an alcoholic' and instead uses the more, accurate , but admittedly more cumbersome, 'an individual with Schizophrenia' or 'an individual with Alcohol Dependence'" (1994, p. xxii).

This is all well and good and even high minded, but in the day-to-day setting of the inpatient or outpatient treatment facility, there is a very slippery (and sloppy) slope between naming disorders that people have and naming people. As the authors of the DSM-IV themselves acknowledge, the former is quite simply "more cumbersome."

But even in the unlikely event that the cumbersome phrasing of the DSM-IV were to be mandated in every treatment center, the *I-it* would prevail. Surely one of the most fundamental differences between an *I-thou* relationship and an *I-it* relationship is that the former ideally distributes agency and voice equally whereas the latter does not. The difficulty in borrowing Buber's powerful paradigms is that the *I-it* relationship that is thus necessarily established between diagnoser and diagnosed is quite often obscured by the more or less "real" *I-thou* that can be developed between therapist and client. Nonetheless, because the *I-it* is part of the systemic, institutional, and "public" psychiatric apparatus, it always already overrides the *I-thou* of the private therapeutic space. Although it is an integral part of mental health care, the particular and specific therapeutic relationship is cordoned off—segregated, as it were—from the larger discourses of communication and prediction which maintain and mandate it. This is true to the point where the very real integrity of the *I-thou* is so compromised by the *I-it* by which it is prescribed that the former becomes little more than an operative fiction. If this is true of the therapeutic relationship, it is all the more true of the patient within that relationship, who in most instances is entirely excluded from the discourses that name her, given the standard practice of not disclosing a given diagnosis to a patient (and even when she is told, she is not so much a participant as an appropriately "blank-slated" pupil). As pupil, she is virtually unable to challenge what she is being taught because she has so little access to the professional discourse, to the language, that explains the larger medical (and social, political, and economic) implications of that diagnosis. This exclusion, I would argue, does indeed amount to a segregation between patients and professionals at every level of institutional psychiatry; that segregation is only spuriously bridged by the intimate space of psychotherapy, a space that, not incidentally, participates in the patient's separate and unequal "education."

As it is currently constituted and implemented, the DSM-IV's central guiding principle—despite its prescriptive references to "individuals"—is that of *I-it* and therefore that of segregation. Following his reference to Buber, King writes: "Hence, segregation is not only politically, economically and sociologically unsound, it is morally wrong and sinful" (p. 484). Although I am personally uncomfortable with the religious and, to a lesser degree, the moral language with which King concludes his point, I would reiterate that psychiatric classification as currently practiced, based as it is on segregation, is indeed politically, economically, and sociologically unsound. I would also add that it is *medically* unsound. Certainly it prevents the mutuality I referred to earlier. As such, it must be resisted, and indeed "Letter from the Birmingham Jail" was written both to justify and to advocate civil disobedience. Let me stress here that by resistance, or even disobedience, I do not necessarily mean what you would understand as "noncompliance," or more specifically the refusal to enter treatment or take medication (the dynamics of psychopharmacology are not at issue here); rather, I mean resistance as a refusal of the structures of diagnosis as they are presently configured and a demand both to enter the process and, when necessary, to change its terms. Resistance in this sense does not signify disorder but rather a profoundly ordered initiative both to recover all that one is in language and, in so doing, to restore one's status in an *I-thou* relationship that is systemic as well as personal. Thus, speaking now from the standpoint of a patient too long segregated from her own treatment and alienated from her own illness, "the quality of future classifications" would recognize and then enact within their deep structure the "value" of resistance, recovery, and the *I-thou* relationship that would allow them. Given the demands on psychiatric nosologists and the hegemony (for better or worse) of the DSM, this may yet be too difficult, perhaps impossible, to achieve at the conceptual level, but it is possible, I think, to begin—only begin—to effect this change at the level of language. And this brings me to my own scholarship as a student of language, or to put it another way, to my "specialized clinical training that provides both a body of knowledge and clinical skills."

As Student

My sense of the word *quality* comes not simply from the standpoint of my training as a student of language but from my very specified political and intellectual development as a student with a distinct and distinctively chosen viewpoint. That is to say, my development as student has not granted me objectivity but rather more rigorously has situated my subjectivity within a charged ideological context: feminist, Marxist, postmodernist. Thus I approach my studies, my research, and my analysis of language through particularized cultural theories. As with my acknowledgment of patientness, particularly BPD patientness, this admission, too, predicts almost irresolvable conflict, since yes, this means I will be dredging up Foucault among others and yes, it means tossing around perhaps tired words such as power and ideology. Peter Miller outlines the near futility of a psychiatric/postmodernist "meeting of the minds" when he details the "coping mechanisms," as it were, of psychiatry on the one hand and cultural theory on the other, in the following way: "Whilst psychiatry comforts itself with propagandistic notions that it is developing and progressing towards sophisticated modes of treating, this critical sociology in turn comforts itself with the notion that what is emerging is an increasingly refined network of social control" (1986, p. 14).

Miller's image is not quite another demarcation of the Science Wars because each side remains contented, isolated, self-satisfied, and even smug—engaging with the enemy is hardly worth the trouble. Despite all the bombast and posturing, however, if there is a value to be found in the Science Wars, it would be in simply provoking such engagement and thereby invading the isolation, disquieting the self-satisfaction, and uncomforting the comfort. At its best, the humanities or the more trendy medical humanities can engage with the medical profession, not as "righteous avengers" in a long-standing family feud but as colleagues who are simply trained to ask different questions. No more. No less. And the facilitation and implementation of different questions can amount to a methodology for "improv[ing] the quality of future classifications through an enhanced awareness of value issues."

This is not to say that psychiatric nosology is not on some level unable to challenge its own assumptions. Indeed, Theodore Millon, in a somewhat disingenuously self-reflexive moment, offers the following caveat to his fellow "scholars":

> Scholars often find it useful to step back from their intense and close involvement in their subject, disengage themselves from its current themes and assumptions, and reflect on a series of philosophically naive yet fundamental questions such as:
> What is essential to the subject?
> What distinguishes it from others?
> What are the questions for which I should find answers?
> What observations and concepts have given the field its legitimacy as a science?
> Do these data and ideas limit and distort my thinking?
> Can the empirical elements of the subject be identified in a more efficient and reliable manner than previously?
> Can its central notions be defined more relevantly than heretofore?
> Might I formulate relationships among its elements in a more productive and coherent way than has been done in the past?
> (1986b, p. 639)

These questions are all well and good and in their own way necessary, though it is worth briefly noting precisely what "values" the questions unselfconsciously endorse and, indeed, reify: that is, observations, concepts, legitimacy, science, efficiency, reliability, productivity, and coherence. But if revisions of the DSM proceed solely on the basis of these questions and these values, there will continue to be a rather substantive "something missed," or perhaps something more or less willfully ignored, within the "deep structure" that constitutes its value system. This laundry list of, to use Millon's phrase, "philosophically naive yet fundamental" precepts suggests that what is required is perhaps not so much a step back as a step aside, a step over, a step across.

Such a step would require relinquishing, at least provisionally, the fiction of objectivity and putting in its place a complex network of shifting but deeply invested desires, discourses, and ideologies. The scholar-subject from a postmodernist, deconstructivist, theoretical position might pose alongside or against Millon's questions the following question, and here I'm quoting again from Gayatri Spivak's provocative "Explanation and Culture: Marginalia": "The trick is to recognize that in every textual production, in the production of every explanation, *there is the itinerary of a constantly thwarted desire to make the text explain.* The question then becomes: what is this explanation as it is constituted by and as it effects a desire to conserve the explanation itself; what are the 'means devised in the interest of the problem of a possible objective knowledge?'" (1987, p. 105; emphasis mine).

What precisely is this dense question asking? What is the "something missed" to which it is alluding? For Spivak, explanation is an ideological, cultural, and political exercise as well as an intellectual, pedagogical, or empirical one. Thus, she highlights the hidden "itinerary of a constantly thwarted desire" in the "production of every explanation." In the case of the DSM-IV, a medical- cultural text that provides explanation of mental distress as a means of communication and prediction, Spivak's question directs the gaze not to the explanations the text offers but to its desire to *make* and *conserve* explanations. Throughout *The Selling of DSM,* Kirk and Kutchins make the perhaps by now familiar argument that the itinerary of a constantly thwarted desire behind the reconstitution and subsequent revisions of the DSM is essentially a conservative (though not necessarily a "bad") one: to shore up the legitimacy or reliability of psychiatry as a science; in a more limited sense, given the status of the DSM, its desire might be "explained" simply as the not-so-thwarted (indeed, not-thwarted-at-all) desire to conserve the DSM as a self-sustaining commodity industry. If we accept their claim, as I do, the question we then need to ask is, as Spivak says, "What are the means devised" to operate this itinerary and how does that affect the "quality" of the classifications themselves? I would argue, following Kirk and Kutchins, that the means devised are precisely those I have already alluded to: ownership, exclusion, segregation. The obvious, at least to a Foucaultian model, extension of these means is Control. And precisely as the value of Control moves to the center of the diagnostic system, the value of Choice is pushed further and further toward its (prohibited) margins. In her discussion of all cultural explanations, Spivak argues that "explaining, we exclude the possibility of the radically heterogeneous" (p. 105). This seems to me particularly true of the DSM.

To illustrate the inverse relationship of Control and Choice within psychiatric diagnosis, I would like to return to the language of BPD. I begin by highlighting some of the metaphors that attempt to "explain" this disorder both to clinicians and to those more or less outside the profession. I have already noted the terms *needy supplicant* and *righteous avenger,* which appear in the DSM-IV. I would like to examine some of the other metaphors that appear in both the clinical and nonclinical literature, since, as Gayatri Spivak reminds us, "every metaphor is contaminated and constituted by its conceptual justification" (p. 115). As an aside, while I was researching this chapter, I came across a slightly different "explanation" of metaphor, this one coming from a psychiatrist "explaining" borderline patients' tendency to speak in metaphor: citing Kramer, Richard Chessick labels the use of metaphor on the part of patients as a "compromise formation . . . used to ward off anxiety by means of the mechanisms of displacement" (1993, p. 217).

Although I focus on Spivak's understanding of metaphor, it is perhaps useful to pit her political explanation of metaphor with Kramer's psychodynamic explanation in considering the most common metaphors used about BPD. In addition to the standard trope of "emotional hemophilia," Janice Cauwels offers the following insight into the "borderlines' inner lives": "Each borderline is like a burn victim alone on a flimsy raft in the middle of the ocean buffeted unpredictably and trying frantically to keep from being splashed" (1992, p. 372); my own personal favorite of the metaphors I've turned up is from *I Hate You, Don't Leave Me* (the title alone functions as a rather vexed and vexing metaphor) and describes BPD as "a kind of Third World of mental illness—indistinct, massive and vaguely threatening" (Kriesman and Strauss, 1989, p. 5). There is also the allusion, in several texts, to Alex Forrest, the Glenn Close character in *Fatal Attraction,* as the prototypical "individual with Borderline Personality Disorder" to the extent that the reference is in effect a metaphor masquerading as a clinically significant case study (indeed, the authors of *I Hate You, Don't Leave Me* actually go so far as to rewrite the script of *Fatal Attraction* to illustrate how Dan might have controlled Alex's erratic behavior and thereby saved the life of at least one bunny). This example of the elision between fact and fiction is all the more disturbing given that a sustained analysis of the film reveals that Alex functions as a deeply contaminated metaphor for far more than a personality disorder; that is to say, she is a vehicle for the film's misogynist impulses or "displaced anxieties."

All these metaphors suggest—to more or less ridiculous extremes—the borderline's utter inability to control herself and, as a presumably obvious consequence, to take care of herself in a manner not persistently, pervasively, personally, and interpersonally pathogenic. The conceptual justification for these metaphors is the need for psychiatry to intervene by to imposing Control, or as some of the clinical literature more delicately puts it, "containment." And the fact that BPD is reputed to be so difficult to control merely ups the ante. Thus, for Michael Stone, Control becomes a literal game of wits, or as he puts it, of "death-poker," in which "our [meaning the therapists he is addressing in his article] task is to play it better than they [meaning the patients who are presumably not reading the article]" (1993, p. 270). Earlier in the essay, Stone points to the need to "out paradox the borderline's paradoxical behavior" and explains the relationship between physician and borderline patient this way: "the situation approximates that of the detective and the prisoner, each trying to outfox the other" (p. 264). John Gunderson suggests the multiple means of outfoxing when he remarks that "no other patients so routinely require the full gamut of technical intervention" (1984, p. 180); Gunderson's point then becomes the conceptual justification for the most contaminated (and bizarre) metaphor I've encountered: "Borderlines lack the boots much less the bootstraps with which to pull themselves up" (Kriesman and Strauss, 1989, p. 152).

In psychotherapy, there can be a tendency—nurtured by patient, therapist, and clinical literature—for the patient to assume a kind of wounded bird role; borderlines, however, seem condemned to the status of bootless bird, unable not only to heal themselves but also to choose the "straps" that would allow them to pull themselves up in a culturally sanctioned manner. What's at stake, I think, in the image of the bootless bird (and the ideologically loaded and oh-so-Republican reference to bootstraps) is precisely the issue of choice. The borderline is persistently figured as an individual unable to make stable and consistent, and therefore appropriate and responsible, choices; three of the nine criteria listed in the DSM-IV address this fundamental deficiency. Of course, these criteria are not "explained" in terms of choice (because most of us, given the heritage of humanist individualism, value choice far too much to pathologize it) but rather as, to quote directly from Criterion 3, "markedly and persistently unstable sense of self (American Psychiatric Association, 1994, p. 654). Criterion 3 is further explained in the DSM text as "sudden and dramatic shifts in self-image, characterized by shifting goals, values, and vocational aspirations" (p. 651). It seems at least possible to me given the particular examples listed—career, sexual identity, values, and types of friends (p. 651)—that one man's identity disturbance is another woman's "consciousness-raising," her right not only to choose but to make multiple choices in response to her culture, personal development, and life situation. In diagnosing, then, we do indeed (whatever else we might do) exclude even the possibility of the radically heterogeneous and the radically and dynamically transformative.

So what can this brief and highly situated political reading of the DSM-IV, enabled as it was by Spivak's challenging questions, offer us in terms of strategies for "improving the quality of future classification through an enhanced awareness of value issues"? Recognizing the politics of explanation (and the relationships between margins and centers which constitute and are constituted by them) might allow a revision of classifications which, because it would be more "aware" of "value issues" (read: political investments), might be able to shift those investments in some way. Because, as a well-bred postmodernist, I believe that it is impossible for any text—scientific or otherwise—to be divested of its political and ideological underpinnings, I can't advocate that the quality of future classifications will depend on the extent to which they are apolitical. And given that my own politics are hardly disinterested, "quality" for me, in an idealistic world, would be a revision that shifts the ideological valence of future classifications toward my own ideological position. Realistically, however, I think it is possible to revise classifications so that there ideologies are more open ended, in which the central value is choice. This may well require a re-thinking of that "itinerary of a constantly thwarted desire to make the text explain" such that, even in the necessarily prohibitive act of explaining, we allow some room for the radically heterogeneous.

As Writer

My work as a writer is a development and extension of my "identities" of patient and student; indeed, I only officially became a writer after I entered graduate school and after I'd become a patient. As a writer, I appreciate the difficulty of an act of writing which must clarify *and* include. Writing by its very nature demands exclusion. And yet it is as a writer that I understand "improving the quality of future classifications" in its most idealistic, some might say naive, sense. Uruguayan author Eduardo Galeano writes that "the word has significance for those of us who wish to celebrate and share the certainty that the human condition is not a cesspool" (1976, p. 123). Sadly, I find this certainty shaken, and sometimes shattered, when I read through the pages of the DSM-IV or of the clinical literature that builds on it. And when it comes to the language and literature of the Axis II Personality Disorders, I am compelled yet again to refer to King's

"Letter from a Birmingham Jail," in which he wrote that "any law that up-lifts human personality is just. Any law that degrades human personality is unjust" (1963, p. 483).

For me, as a writer, there is something profoundly unjust about the way personality disorders are described and explained. Quality in future classifications would demand a relentless search for a more just language, a language responsible not only to the demands of science (legitimate or otherwise) but also to the many constituencies, including patients, who are affected by that language. And this is not merely a matter of changing words; I am not calling for a kind of Psychiatric Political Correctness or, as the Episcopalian version of PC would have it, "if you can't say something nice, don't say anything at all." What I am asking for is both more and less than that. Less in the sense that given the task of psychiatric classification you can hardly restrict yourself to saying only "nice" things. More in that I don't think the justice the Reverend Dr. King was talking about can be achieved by words alone; Galeano writes that "words are weapons and they can be used for good or evil; the crime can never be blamed on the knife" (1976, p. 124). Galeano's point is that words do not exist in a vacuum (or even in a cesspool); there are intentionalities, desires, ideologies, and powers behind them. So in order to find a just and responsible language, the dynamics of intention, desire, ideology, and power must be relentlessly examined. And here perhaps is where I fall into naive optimism: I *do* believe it is possible to write about—and even, if need be, diagnose—human distress in a way that is not degrading, that is responsible and just, but I think to achieve this, the very essence, or as bell hooks calls it, the "deep structure," of the DSM-IV and what it is about need to be rethought.

▪ ▪ Rethinking the DSMs

I don't have the answer as to how precisely to go about this process of rethinking. The suggestions I have offered are only partial ones, born of partial vision. I do believe that the rethinking has to occur on a collective level and a collaborative level. Although this chapter has been more conciliatory than anything else I have written on this topic, it has nonetheless been based in opposition, and I am well aware that my own metaphors are contaminated with my anger and my sense of urgency. However, Chicana writer Gloria Anzaldua, in explaining what she calls the "Consciousness of the Borderlands," discusses the problems of, in her words, the "counter stance," of speech that never moves beyond the reactive and the oppositional:

But it is not enough to stand on the opposite riverbank, shouting questions, challenging patriarchal, white conventions. A counter stance locks one into a duel of oppressor and oppressed; locked in mortal combat, like the cop and the criminal, both are reduced to a common denominator of violence, and, for this, it is proudly defiant. All reaction is limited by, and dependent upon, what it is reacting against, because the counter stance stems from a problem with authority—outer as well as inner—it's a step toward liberation from cultural domination. But it is not a way of life. At some point, on our way to a new consciousness, we will have to leave the opposite bank, the split between the two mortal combatants somehow healed so that we are both shores at once. . . . Or perhaps we will decide to disengage from the dominant culture, write it off all together as a lost cause, and cross the border into a wholly new and separate territory. (1987, pp. 78–79)

I am not yet ready, nor able, to disengage from the dominant culture—in this case psychiatry as represented by the DSM-IV—and I've had enough of shouting across the river (though sadly, it seems, a border dweller *must* shout to be heard—hence my polemic). The problem seems to be that in order to stand with you on *your* riverbank we must be invited, and, for me, the price of admission is still too high; as Spivak reminds us, "the putative center welcomes selected inhabitants of the margin in order to better exclude the margin" (1987, p. 107). I have no wish to be a selected inhabitant, a token borderline, until the terms of selection have changed.

So what options remain to, as Anzaldua puts it, heal the split? I hope that by using my experiences, training, and clinical skills with respect to language, and my deep sense of commitment and responsibility to the written word, I can be a representative of the something, or, more accurately, somethings, missed and an advocate for the "radically heterogeneous." By understanding, and speaking out, about the technical sophistication/mystification and multiple sites of investment in psychiatric diagnosis, I hope to expose gaps and fissures through which certain marginalized subject positions might interrupt, disrupt, and displace psychiatry's hegemonic authority to communicate and predict subjective experience. In activating and listening to that coalition of marginalized voices, moving in solidarity toward and with them, we might be able to talk together about and ease human suffering in a way that neither segregates nor degrades.

I'd like to conclude by addressing an irony that has infused this entire

chapter. Not to acknowledge it would be politically irresponsible and ethically dishonest. Though the point of this chapter has focused on margin-
ality and my own position as a marginal subject, to the point where I have
at least hinted that there is something "radically heterogeneous" about me,
there is a great deal more about me which is entirely too homogeneous, or
as the late comedienne Anna Russell once put it, "Homogenous. As in
milk." It may or may not have escaped your notice that most of the writers I have cited as valuable resources in my thinking about these matters—
King, hooks, Spivak, Anzaldua—are racial minorities and that their writing addresses, in large part, the institutional racism that "contaminates"
contemporary American culture. Although my status as patient, and, to a
lesser extent, as lesbian, and to a still lesser extent, as woman, makes me
"marginal" in some respects, I am nonetheless very much a part of the
dominant culture against which these writers are writing.

Everything that I have been able to accomplish or will be able to accomplish in my work in this area is founded on privilege: the privilege of
race and of class. Including covering the substantial cost of my monthly
medication, my family's wealth has allowed me more or less financially to
opt out of the DSM-IV and seek out and find a private therapist who not
only could use the word *ideology* in a sentence but also was willing to engage in just the kind of mutuality and dialogue to which I have been referring. My education, very much a function of my class and race, has enabled me to develop the critical skills to deconstruct my way out of the
DSM-IV (more or less) and to (begin to) locate and critique substantively
its "hidden itinerary of a constantly thwarted desire."

I am too well aware that not all patients—or "dysfunctional individuals"—have such good fortune and the freedom of choice and of possibilities it brings. It is that good fortune—coupled with the not-so-good (and
not so postmodern) fortune of intimate acquaintance with "mental illness" as daily, lived experience—which motivates my work. My own particular task in the collective endeavor I have alluded to is to bring my private speech into public discourse and in doing so to inhabit simultaneously
and publicly both the margin and the center. Once again Gayatri Spivak
provides me with a model for this kind of doubled speaking: "Since one's
vote is at the limit for oneself, the deconstructivist can use herself (assuming one is at one's own disposal) as a shuttle between the center (inside)
and the margin (outside) and thus narrate a displacement" (1982, p. 107).

I find the metaphor of the shuttle, or rather the shuttling, useful because I think the "displacing" work that I can do—given that I am indeed
lucky enough to be at my own disposal—is and will be a function of my

movement between ever-shifting margins and centers, between ever-evolving selves and silences: between the critic who is writing this and the woman who cowers in a corner of her bedroom too terrified to leave her apartment, between the postmodern girl who reads the DSM-IV as disturbing social/political text and the well-meaning friend who urges another woman to accept that she is bipolar and to please, please take her lithium, and finally between the silences that underwrite and legitimate "the rhetoric of science in psychiatry" and the silences that underwrite and legitimate the rhetoric of mythology in antipsychiatry.

17

Psychotherapists as Authors: Microlevel Analysis of Therapists' Written Reports

CAROL BERKENKOTTER, PH.D., AND
DORIS J. RAVOTAS, M.A., L.L.P.

THIS CHAPTER DEALS with the problematic consequences of the dominant influence of psychiatric classification in the practice of psychotherapy. It describes the processes through which a central activity in the natural sciences, classification, is instantiated in the writing practices of psychotherapists. The authors examined several psychotherapists' grammatical, lexical, and rhetorical strategies for writing their initial evaluations of their clients' problems using membership categorization device (MCD) analysis from ethnomethodology. Several therapists' written initial evaluations were analyzed for their use of microlevel categories and categorizations drawn from the clients' own (oral) representations and the therapists' professional repertoire of terms. From this microlevel perspective, the oral (client) material from the first session is recontextualized into the written record through the therapist's lexical choices and grammatical constructions, especially through his or her use of nominalizations. The resulting analysis suggests that clients' emic, contextually grounded expressions are absorbed into a monological account reflecting the therapist's professional interpretive framework. The therapist thus translates the client's concerns into a set of meanings compatible with the classifications of psychopathology of the DSM-IV. In this way, psychiatric nosology comes to bear on the therapist's situated record-keeping practices. The resulting written account supports a billable diagnosis, thereby fulfilling its institutional purpose. It fails, however, to serve another important purpose for many therapists, which is helping the therapist to guide the therapy process by providing a record of the client's perspective of his or her life-world.

The written texts of psychotherapy are a little-studied but important discursive site for understanding the therapist's processes of representation which serve both the collaborative psychotherapeutic activity of client and therapist and the institutional and professional requirements of the health care system. The therapist's practice of making notes and reports begins the work of drawing the individual clients into the systems of re-imbursement, health care, research, medical reasoning, and so on. Perhaps even more important, psychotherapy notes and reports are the avenue where the clients themselves may recontextualize their own perceptions of themselves.

Therapists' notes and reports are part of a cycle of talking and writing which psychotherapists engage in (Labov and Fanschel, 1977; Ferrara, 1994), and as such they refer to and summarize oral interactions between client and therapist. From a macrolevel perspective, therapists' records may be seen as artifacts circulating within a network of texts that make up the communicative economy of mental health agencies. Although they are constructed from the oral interactions of the therapy session, they are also linguistically connected to the powerful DSM-IV, a major interpretive code of the mental health profession.

The classification of psychopathology, as seen in the DSM-IV, is a sub-specialty of diagnostic nosology, the systematic classification of diseases. Nosology, as a branch of medicine, is concerned with defining diseases based on the common features of a variety of individual cases. Nosography, a related practice, deals with the hierarchical distribution of disease entities—species classified into orders and genera. Both diagnostic language and the act of symptom-based diagnosis in the context of an initial meeting with the therapist have become a matter of concern to many therapists (Wylie, 1995). This activity has the effect of *pathologizing* the client, that is, labeling the individual as an instance of a particular pathology (Scheff, 1984), thus reducing the complex, multidimensional problems that clients present in psychotherapy to a one-dimensional typification, a presenting mental disorder (cf. Soyland, 1994; Barrett, 1988; Harré, 1985).[1] This reification and its resulting objectification of the client has been the subject of a long-standing argument between psychiatrists who are concerned with the importance of standardization to research, prescriptive treatment, professional accountability, and other psychiatrists concerned with the reifying diagnosis. Members of other mental health disciplines, such as psychologists, often struggle with a similar conflict between positions. Nevertheless, the use of the DSM-IV (or its medical counterpart, the ICD-10, has become the sine qua non for mental health care professionals working for public agencies in the United States (cf. Bowker and Star, 1999).

Researchers interested in the rhetorical character of professional communities' discursive practices have investigated the persuasive power of the DSM-III-R on the reading and writing practices of health care professionals (McCarthy, 1991; Reynolds, Meir, and Fisher, 1995) and documented the political and social factors influencing the revision of the DSM-III-R. In a three-year study of the construction of the DSM-IV, McCarthy and Gerring (1994) observed the revising activities of one of the thirteen DSM-IV work groups (the Binge Eating Disorder Work [BED] Group). (The job of the work groups was to update the 250 categories of mental disorder.) These classifications were called Research Diagnostic Categories (RDCs) because they have been putatively identified and formulated through empirical research. By taping the BED Work Group members' discussions over three years, McCarthy and Gerring were able to document the political and social factors at work in affecting group members' changing views of the validity of this category. They observed a change in the arguments that the group was willing to accept in order to approve BED in the DSM-IV appendix as a new category requiring further research to substantiate it as a unique disorder (i.e., as distinct from bulimia).

In contrast to the way in which the Research Diagnostic Categories were seen to be contested knowledge claims during the period that the DSM's most recent revision was under construction, an earlier case study conducted by McCarthy (1991) shows the DSM classifications to be *black boxed* (Latour, 1987; Bijker, Hughes, and Pinch, 1984) for the psychiatrists who routinely use them in writing up psychiatric assessments and other reports. By "black boxed," we mean that the conditions of production of knowledge which involve contesting claims, political maneuvers, and power brokering are obscured from view with the publication of each successive edition of the DSM. In other words, knowledge that was tentative and contingent in one context (the writing and revising of the successive editions of the DSM and ICD) becomes part of a community's stock of knowledge once it has been stabilized in the published text. The DSM can thus be seen to be a forceful rhetorical construction, black boxing controversies, asserting the dominance of psychiatry over psychology and related fields, and maintaining authority through institutional necessities and responsibilities. Psychotherapists, though impelled by the needs of their clients, are also impelled by professional and institutional obligations and responsibilities to fit those needs into the activities of a professional world structured around DSM-related activities.[2]

The study reported here builds on the work of McCarthy (1991) and McCarthy and Gerring (1994) by examining at the lexical and grammatical level the influence of the DSM-IV as a powerful classificatory system or coding scheme (and genre) on psychotherapists' discursive practices. Specifically, we were concerned with the written texts that describe therapists' initial evaluation of their clients' problems, often called the "Psychosocial Assessment." This text is developed from information that the therapist has gathered in an initial interview (first encounter) with the client. The purpose of the psychosocial assessment is to present a clinical picture of the client's difficulties which supports the therapist's summative formal diagnosis (taken from the most recent DSM or ICD). It is also a record of the initial oral interactions between client and therapist which the latter will use as a memory jog for ongoing care. Like other paperwork genres, the psychosocial assessment is used for reimbursement purposes; however, it is also read by other agency personnel and can be subpoenaed for use in court.

The psychosocial assessment interview is very important to the client's role and identity because it is constructed in the lexicon of the psychiatric profession. Barrett, for example, has described the ways that the written psychiatric assessment functions in the "induction of a patient into a career of mental illness" (1988, p. 292). Harré, in a study of patients' files in the psychiatric department of a hospital, examined the written communication between psychiatrists and general practitioners and observed that "a complaint, originally written out in the language of the patient[,] was retranscribed into an 'official' language . . . of psychiatry. Thus 'feeling miserable' may be described as 'displays low affect' to reflect the situational requirements of scientific objectivity embodied in the jargon of psychiatrists" (1985, p. 179).

Soyland, in a related study of case conference discussions (the oral summaries of patients' presenting problems made by members of a psychiatric hospital team), contended that studies of the language of clinical psychiatry reveal much about the situated production of knowledge in psychiatric units of hospitals. He argued that "the case conference, like the admission interview analyzed by Barrett, is a site at which the psychiatric discipline exerts its power to create a patient's identity" (1994, p. 115; see also Hak, 1992; Hak and de Boer, 1995; Soyland, 1995, for a review of related literature).

Use of the psychiatric nomenclature that appears in therapists' psychosocial assessments and other written documents reflects the successful efforts of a group of research psychiatrists in the 1960s and 1970s to standardize clinical diagnosis and its reporting.[3] Initially during the 1960s and 1970s, the efforts to systematize the classifications of psychopathology reflected the interests of a relatively small group of academic psychiatrists; however, since 1980, the year that the DSM-III appeared with its research-based diagnostic classifications, the use of an authorized, systematic diagnostic nomenclature has become mandatory among not only psychiatrists and physicians but also the other professional groups working in the mental health industry, including psychologists, family therapists, nurses, and social workers. Indeed, the DSM has become the lingua franca of the mental health professions (Wylie, 1995).

Many therapists, however, have found the pathologizing nomenclature of the DSM to contravene their therapeutic aims to help clients seek solutions to problems and rebuild a sense of personal agency (see, for example, Freedman and Combs, 1996; White and Epston, 1990).[4] Nevertheless, whether or not the therapist wishes to include a diagnosis in the psychosocial assessment, a DSM- or ICD-based diagnosis must be included in order for that therapist to be reimbursed by a third-party payer. Moreover, the various sections of the text must present information in a way that will "argue" the case for and build to the diagnosis at the end of the document. Toward this end the organizational headings of the psychosocial assessment (such as "Presenting Problem," "Personal History," and "Medical History") constitute narrative elements that lay the groundwork for the diagnosis.

▪ ▪ Microlevel Analysis of Therapists' Processes of Representation

We now turn to an analysis of the microlevel descriptors that therapists use to construct the client within the categories defined by their psychiatric nosology, the DSM-IV. To do so we examine their processes of discursive representation. Because we were not examining the oral interaction in the initial interview, our analysis in this study was confined to therapists' written texts. Our concern, therefore, was with the only information available to readers of therapists' reports, readers not privy to the oral interaction and who therefore have no basis for comparing what was actually said in session with the written report that follows. What is it about the lexicon, syntax, and grammatical constructions in the written records which makes it possible for readers from different professional communities (other therapists, psychiatrists, physicians, insurance company reviewers) to make the inferences they do?

To answer this question we adapted Sacks's (1972, 1995) concepts of membership categorization devices (MCDs) and category-bound activities (CBAs), originally used to examine the "inferencing" activities carried out in oral interactions, to our examination of therapists' notes and reports. Sacks sought to characterize what he called "some very central machinery of social organization" (1995, p. 40). He observed people getting to know each other through the asking of questions that enabled them to draw from stores of inferences, for example, "Where are you from?" "What do you do?" From these observations he speculated that people routinely describe individuals vis-à-vis "families" or category sets such as race, gender, age, class, occupational group, mental status, and so on. These category sets he called "membership categorization devices," suggesting that our use of such devices activates implicit common, cultural norms shared with others in the same culture or community of practice.

Sacks developed a number of "hearers' rules" to flesh out his concept of membership categorization devices. Two of these are relevant to our discussion here:

- The "economy rule": If a member uses any single category from any membership categorization device to describe some population of persons (e.g., use of the term *daughter* from the collection "family," or "Borderline Personality" from "Personality Disorders"), he or she can be recognized to be doing *adequate reference* to a person (1972, p. 333). Other features or characteristics of that particular category ("Borderline Personality") are implied by such descriptors as "Mary is *manipulative* in the group session."
- Category-bound activity: Certain activities are, through social typification, attributed to or bound to certain categories: hence, "babies *cry*," "anorexics *starve themselves*," "schizophrenics *hallucinate*," "borderlines *manipulate* other people." Many stereotypes are thus predicated on speakers' or writers' references to category-bound activities and the inferences that may be made from such references.

The same client might be described by a therapist-writer in any one of the following ways: as (1) "a survivor of sexual abuse"; (2) "a local school teacher and mother of five"; (3) "an obese woman with bulimia"; or (4) "a twenty-four-year-old Native American woman with a depressed affect and a somewhat unkempt appearance." Each of the above descriptions carries a different set of associations and functions to frame the subject within a particular category set. In other words, each of the above categories is "heard" (or read) by listeners or readers as deriving from some *collection of categories.* In the example above, "local school teacher and mother of five," the category "mother" belongs to the larger MCD "family"; "teacher" belongs to the MCD "occupation."

Sacks (1972) suggests that the only way to bypass MCDs, CBAs, or other category-bound descriptors is to contradict explicitly the activity or quality that is associated with the category by implication. For example, in the sentence "My aunt is ninety-two years old, but she ran in a marathon last year," the clause "but she ran in a marathon last year" is intended to contradict the category-bound activity of being sedentary. Without this disclaimer, the sedentary nature of a ninety-two-year-old would be inferred, thus backgrounding (or ignoring entirely) other major aspects of this particular ninety-two-year-old's life.

This process of inferencing can be observed in therapists' use of diagnostic reifications. When a therapist speaks or writes, "The client is a *Borderline,*" other therapists *hear* that this person is manipulative and clingy, fears abandonment, has self-destructive tendencies, and is unable to maintain intimate relationships. Thus the term *borderline* functions as an "adequate reference" that supplies the hearer of the professional community with a description or "clinical picture" of the client which serves to objectify and, we would argue, pathologize the person. In fact, the reification of diagnostic categories is so ubiquitous that even with an explicit contradiction of the above descriptors (i.e., "She has a supportive relationship with her husband"), many therapists would be skeptical (i.e., "Her marriage only *appears* to be supportive").

Although MCD analysis has been used primarily in the analysis of oral genres (see Hester and Eglin, 1997, for a review of these studies), it has also been used in the analysis of written genre conventions, such as newspaper headlines (Hester and Eglin, 1997, pp. 35–46). We believe it to be useful as well for enhancing our understanding of the microlevel representational activity in therapists' written reports, keeping in mind that what occurs at the microlevel is shaped by the genre in which it appears. Like Harré (1985), we found therapists' written reports of oral interactions filled with the vocabulary and nominalized constructions of a formal professional register that Harré described as "file speak" (p. 178). An MCD analysis of this vocabulary and these constructions revealed how the client's densely contextual "raw material" (Hak, 1992) became recontextualized and reified in the written report into the therapist's nominalized psychiatric categorizations. Often these nominalizations were cast in the terminology used in the DSM-IV to describe symptoms of various mental disorders.

▪ ▪ Background of the Study

Our examination of therapists' written practices is part of a larger study that includes linguistic and rhetorical analysis of five therapists' written initial evaluations as well as interviews with the therapists regarding how they wrote their reports. The majority of the data were collected at a community mental health center of a rural community in the Midwest. One of the authors (Ravotas), who is a clinical psychologist, was previously employed by the mental health center and possessed an intimate knowledge about the practices and requirements within that setting. The therapists who were interviewed and have supplied their written texts are Ravotas's colleagues. They represent a spectrum of approaches to therapy.

Additional interviews and written texts were supplied to the authors at the "Narrative Ideas and Therapeutic Practice" psychotherapy conference in Vancouver, British Columbia, Canada, in 1995 and 1996. Internet colleagues of Ravotas have also supplied documents. Any identifying names or details of both the written texts and the interviews have been removed to maintain confidentiality for the clients and the therapists involved.

The impetus for the larger study was Ravotas's concern (arising from her clinical practice) with her own discursive struggles in transforming material from the oral interviews with clients into a written report culminating in a billable diagnosis. We sought to determine the function of the DSM-IV in this task by examining the historical development of diagnostic nosology in psychiatry (see Berkenkotter and Ravotas, 1997), and we triangulated our analysis of therapists' texts with an analysis of the terms and concepts therapists used in our interviews to describe their goals as therapists and their production of written texts.

▪ ▪ Introduction to the Texts

The texts that were selected for this project were the psychosocial assessment texts produced in the process of therapy. The basic purpose of this document is to build a case for, or depiction of, the client's problems which will guide treatment and provide evidence showing that the client needs therapy. As most third-party payers require a diagnosis for payment, this "case for therapy" is also a "case" for the diagnostic formulation of the problem. These texts are typically read by the therapist, his or her supervisor, a psychiatrist or physician (if a referral is made for medication), and possibly a judge, a new therapist, or an insurance company reviewer. Although clients legally have a right to review their records, they rarely request—and therapists do not generally promote—this option. Therefore, the client is seldom seen as a potential audience.

Because of the confidential nature of therapy practice, therapists' competence and credibility are often based on the narratives they produce about their work either in written texts or in conferences with other professionals (Soyland, 1994; Barrett, 1988). Many of the therapists we interviewed reported that they use professional terminology in these accounts to communicate with their peers and also to indicate their competence as psychotherapists. Therefore, the texts are primarily written in this professional register, the therapist employing the descriptive language that can be traced to the DSM-IV (or ICD-10) classificatory categories. Interestingly, a commonly used expression among therapists, "clinical picture," is a rather revealing description of this practice. Clinicians' use of the diagnostic lingua franca, by establishing "categories of relevance" (Goodwin, 1996, p. 610; cf. Bowker and Starr, 1999, pp. 62–66), provides a shared way of *seeing* which foregrounds some features in a complex interdiscursive and intertexual field while backgrounding others.

In contrast, the work in which many therapists and clients engage is a joint production of solutions to a given problem (Ferrara, 1994). Some of the most recent theories of therapy contend that therapy, as an activity, should function to separate out the client from her or his problems and to foreground the client's strengths. Many therapists recognize the power and the influence of the joint production process, and they assume that assessment itself *is* an intervention. Yet, in their written psychosocial assessments, there is very little to indicate that these accounts are a description of the interactive process occurring within the session. Rather, the impression given to the reader is of a snapshot of the pathology located within the person, a concrete instantiation of the "psychiatric gaze" (Barrett, 1988, pp. 289–90).

▪ ▪ Contrasts between the Therapists' and Clients' Use of Membership Categories and Categorization Devices

The recontextualization of oral material into the first session's record is accomplished through the therapist's lexical choices and grammatical constructions, especially through the use of nominalizations. Nominalizations are often paraphrases of a client's statements cast in the categorizations and category-bound activities of psychiatric nomenclature. Excerpts #1 and #2 appear in two successive psychosocial evaluations of the same client. The first is a Screening Summary, typically written by the therapist on duty at a mental health clinic seeing walk-in clients; the second, the Extended Intake Summary, is made by the therapist subsequently assigned to the client. The language of these two assessments illustrates the differences between those membership categories drawn from the client's "lifeworld" (Mishler, 1984) and those from the psychiatric discourse community. The therapist has preserved the convention of using quotation marks for the client's words.

(1)   From Screening Summary (p. 1; italics added to direct quotations, nominalizations in bold for emphasis):

Presenting Concern: (Precipitating even duration, developmental history, how problems disrupts [*sic*] functioning): . . . "*I just seem to be falling apart lately.*" Ct. reports that ever since she and her current SO [significant other] began having problems in early June, she has been feeling progressively worse. She reports she was able to "*hold it together*" during the summer, but is finding it increasingly difficult do so now that school has started. On a day-day basis, client finds she is preoccupied with her relationship problems. She worries she has "*screwed up yet another relationship with (her) neediness*" and berates herself for not being able to control this. As a result she is having trouble concentrating on academic tasks, has a **predominantly dysphoric mood,** has withdrawn from socializing with friends, experiences **initial insomnia,** and complains of "*crying jags.*" She reports **occasional, passing thoughts of suicide,** but adds: "*would never do that.*" The ct. reports that she has "*never had a good relationship.*" She believes she has been "*screwed up*" by "*trying to get (her) dad's attention.*" . . .

(2)   From Extended Intake Summary (p. 1; nominalizations boldfaced for emphasis):

Summary of Initial Concerns: Ct. presents **with initial complaints of problems in an intimate relationship.** She reports she has been having problems in her current relationship since early June. At that time she reported noticing that she and SO began having increased arguments, and she seemed increasingly distant. . . . She has primarily reacted **with a series of depressive sx** [symptoms]. These include: **predominant dysphoric mood, difficulty concentrating, social withdrawal, loss of interest in usual activities, initial insomnia,** and **frequent crying spells.** Denies **anergia, changes in appetite or eating habits,** and feel-

ings of worthlessness. There are **no psychomotor abnormalities.** There are **occasional transitory thoughts of suicide without rumination, plan or intent.**

In the Screening Summary excerpt, the Presenting Concern is stated from the client's point of view represented through the therapist's use of direct and indirect quotations (Hickmann, 1993; see Ravotas and Berkenkotter, 1998, for a discussion of the various devices the therapists used for representing clients' speech). More important, this initial account of personal trouble is cast in the context of the client's interpersonal experience. That the topic and focus of the passage are from the client's lifeworld is foregrounded by the therapist's use of quotation marks. The use of direct quotations to show that the client's comments are reported verbatim (but see Tannen,1989; Clark and Gerrig, 1990) lends verisimilitude to the account. The salient categorizations of family and male/female relationships as well as the category-bound activities, "falling apart" and "screwed up" (in relationships, in the family), are, as well, foregrounded by the therapist's use of quotation marks.

In contrast, in the second excerpt , the Summary of Initial Concerns, which also putatively refers to the client's (oral) self-report, the writer reframes the contextual, experiential "raw material" provided by the client into the DSM-IV-based membership categorization device (MCD) "mental status," with its constitutive categories, "sx" (symptoms), including "predominant dysphoric mood," "difficulty concentrating," "social withdrawal," "loss of interest in usual activities," "initial insomnia," and "frequent crying spells." The therapist's use of these nominalized constructions emphasizes the distinction between the client's local, contextual, lifeworld categorization and the therapist's "expert" categorizations, the latter cast in the terminology of the professional register. Here a number of questions arise: What is the *rhetorical purpose* of such a contrast? What do these salient differences between client and therapist categorizations accomplish, given that this text is a psychosocial assessment? What is the significance of this dissonance between the client's and therapist's utterances, given that *both* are the therapists' representation?

In order to make the contrast between the therapist's lexical choices (in representing the client's speech) and her use of a professional nomenclature even sharper, we have placed the two kinds of description in two columns in table 17.1. The client's reported comments, which can be seen to express category-bound activities (CBAs), as seen through her use (for the most part) of active verbs, are in the left column of the table. (One no-

TABLE 17.1 **Contrasts between Therapist's and Client's Membership Categorization Devices (MCDs)**

CLIENT'S MCDS EXPRESSED AS CATEGORY-BOUND ACTIVITIES*	THERAPIST'S MCDS EXPRESSED AS NOMINALIZATIONS (ITALIC)
I just seem to be falling apart lately*	a *predominantly dysphoric mood*
I screwed up yet another relationship with my neediness*	a *previous relationship breakup*
	– symptoms of *depression . . . primarily reactive to a problematic relationship*
I never had a good relationship*	*Probable Adjustment Disorder*
I've been screwed up* [by] trying to get dad's attention*	client presents *w/predominant dysphoric mood** – *social withdrawal* – *initial insomnia*
She gave me a chance to vent*	
Counselor would have a different light on things	no *psychomotor abnormalities*
I caused our problems by being too needy*	*Adjustment Disorder w/Depressed Mood*
I always had similar problems in a relationship*	[sister also] experienced *relationship problems* and depression – *no suicidal ideation*
He needed me as much as I needed him*	
We just grew apart	Minimal Continued Dysphoric Mood
Parents cold and tense, brother moody	Minimal Continued Dysphoric Mood
I am a caring person	*establish predominant euthymic mood**

*Category-bound activities

table exception is the passive "I've been screwed up by trying to get dad's attention," which we shall discuss shortly.) The therapist's categories, which most frequently appear as nominalizations, are in the right column. In a few instances these nominalizations appear to be paraphrases (in professional nomenclature) of the CBA in the client's statement appearing across from it in the left column. For example, "a predominantly dysphoric mood" is a paraphrase that recontextualizes the client's "I just seem to be falling apart lately." Similarly, "a previous relationship breakup," is a paraphrase of "I screwed up yet another relationship with my neediness." Most of the other descriptions appearing in the two columns, however, are not parallel. Rather, we are suggesting with the visual contrast of client's and therapist's descriptors in the two columns that there is an interplay between these two "voices" (Mishler, 1984, 1986) as reported by the therapist: the dominant *voice of medical practice* as instantiated in the lexicon the therapist uses, and the *voice of the client* reflecting her lifeworld, that is, "that individual's contextual understanding of her problems in her own terms" (Mishler, 1986, pp. 142–43; but cf. Atkinson, 1995; Engeström, 1993; Engeström, 1995; Silverman, 1987). One does need to keep in mind, however, that the material in the left column is the therapist's *reconstruction* (usually from notes taken in session) of what the client said; thus, there may not be verbatim accuracy in the client's comments.

The client describes her troubles using lay categories of a sort that we might call *emic* in that they are densely contextual. Her meanings are expressed by such phrasal constructions as "falling apart," "hold it together," "never had a good relationship," "caused our problems by being too needy," and "always had similar problems in a relationship"—all CBAs. As previously mentioned, the client's predominant categorizations (MCDs) are family and relationships (familial, male/female), which are also implied by her use of the verb + participle, "screwed up" (a CBA). Such constructions are the raw materials of a narrative account, suggesting that the client perceives "the problem" as existing in her and sedimented from her early family interactions. For example, she describes the cause of her current dilemma using the passive construction "I've been screwed up," followed by the prepositional phrase "[by] trying to get dad's attention." The syntactical construction here makes the argument that it is the client's own actions ("trying to get dad's attention") that have made her the agent of her current problems. This construction is particularly interesting because of what it shows at the grammatical level of the client's inferencing process, that is, the client is responsible for her current inability to have a lasting relationship (i.e., "screwed up yet another relationship") because an earlier neediness ("trying to get dad's attention") has "screwed her up" in her adult relationships with men.

The client's choice of descriptive categories/categorizations, as can be seen in her grammatical and lexical choices and her syntax, instantiates her perception of a history of failed relationships. We can recognize in this account a common popular cultural narrative of women who are unsuccessful in maintaining relationships as adults because of their inability to have a healthy relationship with the male parent. In this sense the client constructs herself and her current problems within *a core narrative*, a culturally sanctioned story pattern, built from the categorizations (and the norms embedded therein) of "family" and "relationships." In this respect her use of the verb + participle "screwed up," in the context of her narrative, is particularly telling: "I screwed up in the family (with my father) and I'm screwing up now because of that history" (cf. Capps and Ochs, 1995).

In contrast to the contextually grounded, lifeworld categorizations appearing in the client's account, the therapist's use of MCDs is decontextualized and *etic*. That is, the categories the therapist uses are drawn from a classification system, the DSM-IV's classifications of psychopathology. For example, the therapist indexes a diagnostic categorization ("Adjustment Disorder with Depressed Mood") by using such nominalizations as "predominantly dysphoric mood," "social withdrawal," and "initial insomnia." The use of such phrases is especially important in the therapist's account because they operate to translate the client's emic categories into the professional psychiatric (etic) categorizations. The influence of the DSM-IV is particularly salient here, as descriptors such as "social withdrawal" and "initial insomnia" are those appearing on the symptom list of the DSM-IV's classification of "Major Depressive Episode" (although this diagnosis is ruled out in favor of "Adjustment Disorder w/ Depressed Mood"). "Predominant Dysphoric Mood," on the other hand, is a commonly used nominalization in the psychiatric register, one that is synonymous with "depressed mood." Through the use of such nominalizations, the therapist constructs the "clinical picture," built up from inference-rich membership categories, in this case those associated with the categorization of "Adjustment Disorder w/ Depressed Mood."

▪ ▪ Other Discursive Practices Indicating Recontextualization

One of the major problems arising from the therapist's use of etic categories is that the client's rich lifeworld account is lost in the therapist's account, with only vague temporal and location references appearing in subsequent assessments. With the context elided, actions, moments, and individuals significant *to the client* are missing from the written record. Over a period of time material in the Psychosocial Assessment may again be recontextualized (perhaps numerous times) by a number of other therapists, physicians, or other treatment providers reading the records to write background histories in further patient assessments. Consider, for example, the following excerpt from a Psychosocial Assessment of a man who has been in treatment for many of his thirty-six years.

(3) From Psychosocial Assessment (p.1; italics added to foreground writer's temporal references):

Mr. D. presented with mental illness symptoms *at age 17* ranging from thought disorder areas through delusions/hallucinations to manic behaviors. Denial and lack of expression of insight has been *long term historical.* Somatic ideation and perseveration qualities have also *historically influenced* expressed thought and behaviors.

The very general nature of this statement suggests that the therapist-writer most likely reviewed the client's previous records in order to write the case history. In this kind of brief narrative, the client's initial descriptive account, including his references to time and place (e.g., "For the last two weeks, I have been hearing the voice of my dead father when I go to bed at night"), is noticeably absent. The temporal indicators used ("presented at age 17," "long term historical," and "historically influenced") imply *ongoing, continuous* symptoms. The absence of specific temporal or locational references reinforces the presentation of the symptom as an enduring quality located within the person.

Another common technique for recontextualizing information the client provides is that of using *framing clauses* for reporting speech (Hickmann, 1993) which contain a *"verb of saying"* that implies a direct quotation will follow (e.g., "He stated . . ." "She reports . . ." "She verbalized . . ."). Occasionally direct quotations of what the client putatively said in the initial interview immediately follow the use of such framing clauses; however, more often, as can be seen in the example below, the therapist chooses to follow the verb of saying with a paraphrase in the professional register.

(4) From Psychosocial Assessment (p. 1; subject + "verb of saying" in bold):

She states he was abusive toward her and she finally left him when her daughter was eight.

In some cases the therapists in the study used a framing clause followed by an indirect quotation to recontextualize the client's utterances into nominalizations that can be attributed to a particular category of disorder belonging to the MCD "mental status." For example,

(5)   From Psychosocial Assessment (p. 2; subject + "verb of saying" in bold; italics added to highlight therapists' use of nominalizations):

He reported a *28 pound weight loss.* . . . **He also acknowledged** loss of *libido, impaired concentration, loss of interest, and feelings of helplessness.* . . . **He denied** any current *suicidal/homicidal ideation.*

In this excerpt the writer's use of framing clauses creates the impression that the client is directly reporting the nominalized material, that is, reporting some symptoms while denying others. Although readers are not directly aware of the therapist-writer's use of framing clauses plus nominalized paraphrases in professional nomenclature, the readers are predisposed to "allow the narrator's perspective to intrude upon the original utterances" (Hickmann, 1993, p. 65). At the microlevel, then, the use of such discursive techniques as those seen above also enables readers to infer the symptomatic diagnosis. In this manner the therapist-writer provides the elements of a clinical narrative that will culminate in a diagnosis. In effect, the client becomes the sum of his or her symptoms.

From a microlevel perspective, the recontextualization of oral material from the first session into the written record is accomplished through the therapist's lexical choices and grammatical constructions, especially through his or her use of nominalizations. These nominalizations may be translated (further reified) into numeric codes for use in another genre, the billing statement. We have tried to demonstrate through the above analysis the way in which therapists' lexical choices and syntactical constructions contribute to pathologizing the client. It is important to keep in mind that the therapist's objective, professional accounting (credibility, "billability") is carried out through the categories and categorizations she or he deploys in the written record. Significant in this process is the loss of context (and perspective) that is provided in the client's oral account. In this respect, the written record functions to both decontextualize and recontextualize the client's raw, experiential material (Hak, 1992;

see also Dreier, 1993; Mehan, 1993; McDermott, 1993) into an orthodox narrative.

▪ ▪ Conclusion

The practice of psychotherapy involves both the activities of talking to clients and transforming the raw material from the oral interaction into recognizable written forms—case notes, reports, and other genres. Our analysis suggests that somewhere along the way the client's richly descriptive narrative is lost, the result of the therapist's use of rhetorical and linguistic strategies that lend credence to his or her diagnosis, the primary practice for which he or she is billable. In this respect diagnosis is the all-important measure of the need for treatment, and the accompanying written material needs to support the diagnosis.

It is important to keep in mind that the microlevel linguistic practices that we describe above occur within the context of the many discursive activities (oral and written) of many actors and texts operating within multiple systems: mental health, actuarial, legal, inter- and intraprofessional, to name a few. It is also the case that the therapist engaged in her work is not aware of the historical practices and genres in which she participates (see Berkenkotter and Ravotas, 1997). Perhaps she experiences a "felt difficulty" with her writing practices, as was the case with Doris Ravotas, which led to the research we are reporting here. This feeling of dissonance (which many of our therapist-informants also expressed), we contend, is symptomatic of what Engeström called the "inner contradictions" within an organization reflecting changes in socioeconomic formation (1993, p. 72). Specifically, the therapist feels the tension between her role as healer-practitioner on the one hand and as cost-efficient producer and social accountant on the other. In a similar manner, the knowledge produced in the course of therapy reflects the tension between what Engeström refers to as its "use value" and its "exchange value" (p. 72), the client reaping the benefits of the former, the mental health clinic accruing the benefits of the latter.

There is, we believe, yet a third dimension to the knowledge, or learning, produced in therapy sessions. In one sense, it is local knowledge that is responsive to the context, roles, and interactions out of which it is produced. Yet the knowledge produced in a therapy session is also *structurally constitutive* (Giddens, 1984), in the sense that, in their use of membership categorization devices, therapists both *constitute* social structure (at the microlevel) and *reproduce* the social structures of their respective professional and institutional affiliations (Mehan, 1993; cf. Berkenkotter and Huckin, 1995).

From a sociohistorical perspective, the therapist's use of the categorizations of psychiatry's medical model needs to be viewed in the context of the relatively recent developments in the mental health field, in particular the "medicalization of psychiatry" in the 1970s, marked by the 1980 publication of the DSM-III. The effect of the DSM-III, and its revisions, the DSM-III-R and IV, was to *codify* the classifications of psychopathology and to mandate therapists' use of a nomothetic nomenclature, despite many therapists' insistence on the idiographic and interpersonal nature of their client's problems. Changes in the mental health system in the United States brought about by the requirements of Medicaid and other third-party payers made practitioners' use of a standardized nomenclature and a universal classification system even more necessary for reimbursement.

Notes

1. *Pathologizing*, a term used by narrative therapists, refers to the process through which therapists, who internalize concepts from the medical model of psychopathology in diagnosing their clients, come to perceive the client's problems as endogenous. This construction of identity makes it difficult for clients to access the personal resources they need to address their problems (S. Madigan, personal conversations, Conference on Narrative Ideas and Therapeutic Communication Practice: 4th Annual International Conference, Vancouver, BC, Canada, February 1996). For an understanding of the core concepts and goals of narrative therapy, see White and Epston (1990).

2. The authors are not implying that diagnosis is without value. Many individuals have benefited tremendously from careful diagnosis and treatment. It is our hope, however, that an understanding of the historical and discursive functions of diagnosis may be beneficial to therapists and other mental health care workers.

3. See Blashfield (1984) for an account of this period.

4. Psychotherapists, who make up the practitioner ranks in mental health agencies in the United States, are members of a professional community quite different in training and background from that of psychiatrists, the latter being educated as physicians before completing four additional years of training and residency in psychiatry. Although psychiatrists may practice psychotherapy, generally psychotherapists have Ph.D.'s in psychology or counseling or master's degrees in psychology, counseling, or social work. The clients whom therapists serve are most often to be found in an agency's outpatient facility or in private practice. These are persons with a wide spectrum of problems and difficulties, although generally not as disabling as those of chronically mentally ill individuals, who may turn up in outpatient facilities as well.

Part Five

. . . .

Visions for the Future

18

Clinical and Etiological Psychiatric Diagnoses: Do Causes Count?

KENNETH F. SCHAFFNER, M.D., PH.D.

IN THE PREFACE to the first edition of their classic book *Psychiatric Diagnosis* (1974), Goodwin and Guze wrote that

> there are few explanations in this book. This is because for most psychiatric conditions there *are* no explanations. "Etiology unknown" is the hallmark of psychiatry as well as its bane. Historically, once etiology is known, a disease stops being "psychiatric." Vitamins were discovered, whereupon vitamin-deficiency psychiatric disorders no longer were treated by psychiatrists. The spirochete was found, then penicillin, and neurosyphilis, once a major psychiatric disorder, became one more infection treated by non-psychiatrists. (1974, p. xiii)

In their most recent version (1996) of this book they reprinted that preface and did not appear to shift explicitly in favor of any etiological perspective. The 1996 edition does, however, cite a number of family studies that indicate partially genetic etiologies for psychiatric disorders such as schizophrenia and dementia. This increased use of genetic information is reconsidered later in this chapter.

This anti-etiological view of the role of initial causes in psychiatry is at odds with the rest of medicine—indeed, at odds with the health sciences in general. The tension between the Goodwin-Guze anti-etiological view and medical science was recognized by Kendell, who noted that "there is a longstanding and deeply rooted assumption in medicine that the most valid diagnoses are those whose etiology is known; and as a corollary that the most effective way of establishing the validity of a clinical syndrome is to elucidate its etiology" (1989, p. 46). Goodwin and Guze as well as Kendell ultimately found their positions on practical features of psychiatry and medicine. The reason that psychiatrists are concerned with diagnosis is so that they may make prognoses, both for those disorders that are treatable by interventions and for those that may at present not so be. Goodwin and Guze note that "classification in medicine is called diagnosis" and that "in choosing . . . [diagnostic] categories, the guiding rule was: *diagnosis is prognosis*" (1974, p. ix). For Kendell, an emphasis on etiology is justified on empirical grounds: "It is simply an empirical finding that the most aetiologically based classifications are more useful—because they embody a wider range of implications—than purely clinical classifications" (1989, p. 46).

The DSM-III, DSM-III-R, and DSM-IV also embodied a prima facie anti-etiological position,[1] although in the DSM-IV it was characterized more broadly as an "approach that attempted to be neutral with respect to theories of etiology" (American Psychiatric Association, 1994, p. xviii).[2] Again, like Goodwin and Guze's position (1996), a close reading of the specifics of some of the sections on disorders belies this neutral stance, particularly in the case of "Dementia of the Alzheimer's Type"—an example to which I return below.

Future DSMs will probably have to modify this general anti-etiological position, to reflect highly likely results emerging from advances in molecular genetics. In July 1995, the United Kingdom's National Health Service (NHS) released a report of a working group titled "The Genetics of Common Diseases."[3] At the beginning of that report it is stated that "a logical way to define diseases is based on aetiological factors and makes use of genetic information. *Diseases should where possible be classified on the basis of their pathophysiology rather than their phenotype*" (National Health Service, 1995, p. 5). The report adds:

> *Classification based on genetic susceptibility will have profound effects on the diagnosis and management of disease.* In many diseases little is likely to be achieved in explaining environmental risks or in refining therapeutic strategies until a clear aetiological classification is available. Modern molecular genetics now makes this feasible and is likely to prove fundamental in the study of many complex disorders such as schizophrenia, manic depressive psychosis, hypertension, stroke and ischaemic heart disease. A better understanding of how environmental factors interact with genes in the pathophysiology of disease

will be essential and although progress is being made it is unlikely that a full appreciation will be reached in the near future. (p. 6)[4]

In this chapter I examine the nature of possible etiological approaches to classifying psychiatric disorders within the context of the current molecular biological revolution. Although I do not ignore the importance of higher levels of analysis and aggregation, including organ, tissue, and cellular, the main focus is on biochemical and molecular etiological dimensions, in no small part because, as the NHS quotation indicates, it is at this level that finally some progress is hoped to be made in connection with psychiatric disorders such as schizophrenia (SZ) and bipolar disorder (BPD). This perspective requires that we address the concept of causation as it might be used in a reconfigured psychiatry. I also maintain that this concept of causation needs to be robust enough to reflect the complications of causal influences in as complex a subject as molecular biology and molecular genetics have become.

It might be useful before embarking on the details of the analysis to indicate the main theses that will emerge from this inquiry. These are eight in number:

1. The concept of cause can be analyzed in fairly simple terms at a high level of generalization using the counterfactual manipulation approach.

2. This concept of cause can be elaborated to include the nonspecific etiologies, a very powerful notion known as the INUS condition, and a probabilistic conception of causality, to be found in most psychiatric disorders.

3. Etiological approaches to disease may or may not offer special advantages, depending on alternative means of diagnosis and available interventions.

4. Phenotypic variability poses a dual problem in etiological approaches in psychiatry: a clinically based definition can make genetic investigations difficult, in terms of both identification and replication, and a clearer genetically related definition of a phenotype may not be as useful for clinical diagnosis.

5. Etiology in psychiatry, as in other domains, is only partially genetic and involves a complex network of interacting causes—causes that will remain probabilistic even as they are clarified at the molecular level.

6. The recent history of molecular and genetic inquiries into the Alzheimer diseases provides a good prototype for future psychiatric disorder characterization.

7. Research on the molecular aspects of behavior in simpler animal model organisms offers both discouragement and promise for etiological understanding of psychiatric disorders.
8. Conflicting values regarding the use of etiological markers will need to be addressed by future DSM working groups.

▪ ▪ Causes and Causes

As indicated in the previous section, because the concept of causation is central in the problem area sketched above, we need to have at least a preliminary notion of "cause" which can be robust enough to cover medicine, psychiatry, and molecular genetics. A review of the various approaches to causation which have been taken by philosophers over the past two millennia suggests that the concept of causation may not be unitary. In Aristotle we find four different senses of the term, and post-Humean analyses comprise such diverse approaches as regularity and conditional accounts, the activity or manipulability view, the (rationalist) logical entailment theory, a nonlogical entailment version, and the more recent possible world accounts (see Lewis, 1973; Brand, 1976; Earman, 1986).

In my view, several logical, epistemological, and metaphysical elements of these diverse approaches should be drawn on and intertwined to constitute an adequately robust analysis of causation for biology and medicine. I do not have an opportunity to do that here (I have done so elsewhere; see Schaffner, 1993b), but believe I can make my points well enough by referring to one such approach to causation which is widespread among research scientists in both the biological and the social sciences, including, possibly, scientists involved in clinical trials. This is the "manipulability" approach to causation. It can be found expressed very simply by Loehlin (1992) in his account of causal path analysis diagrams, in which we find letters representing variables connected by arrows (i.e., $C \rightarrow E$, where C is a cause and E is an effect; for an excellent example of path analysis in psychiatry see figure 1 from Kendler, Kessler, et al., 1993, "The Prediction of Major Depression," on the etiology of major depression, discussed in more detail below). Loehlin writes that "causes of various different kinds" can be represented in a path diagram and that the idea of cause is simply that "a change in the variable at the tail of an arrow will result in a change in the variable at the head of the arrow, all else being equal (i.e., with all the other variables in the diagram held constant)" (1992, p. 4). Loehlin also cites Mulaik's analysis of cause, which I read as being consistent with the views developed in this chapter.

In the second edition of the *Statistical Package for the Social Sciences,* or SPSS manual, we find an equivalent but more explicit definition as follows: "We propose the following 'operational' definition as an initial approximation to the idea of causation: X_1 is a cause of X_0 if and only if X_0 can be changed by *manipulating* X_1 and X_1 *alone.* We note first that the notion of causation implies prediction but prediction of a particular kind. It implies the notion of *possible* manipulation" (Nie et al., 1975, p. 384). In addition, the SPSS manual adds:

> The preceding definition of causation suggests both the criterion of
> causation and the means to measure causal effects. First to establish
> conclusively that X_1 is a cause of X_0, one must perform an "ideal" ex-
> periment in which all the other *relevant* variables are held constant
> while the causal variable is being manipulated. Second there should
> be some accompanying change in the dependent variable. We will
> use such validation as the ultimate criterion that X_1 is the cause of
> X_0. (p. 384)

This manipulation approach to causation, which is sometimes referred to as the "activity theory," can be found in the earlier work of Hart and Honoré (1985), as well as in the work of Collingwood (1940), Gasking (1955), and von Wright (1971); it is also stressed in Holland (1986) and Rubin (1978, 1986). It has been criticized as not being able to distinguish causality from mere correlation, but it fails on this ground only if the *counterfactual* interpretation of this approach is disallowed (also see Holland, 1986, and Glymour, 1986).[5] In counterfactual situations, we can conceptually hold other interfering factors constant and isolate causal contributions. In their recent book *Causation, Prediction, and Search,* Spirtes, Glymour, and Scheines (1993) also defend a manipulability approach, and one that explicitly permits counterfactuals. This counterfactual component is also contained in the earlier quote from the SPSS manual, in which the notion of a *possible* manipulation was explicitly appealed to.

That this approach may also be the sense of causation involved in clinical trials receives support from Howson and Urbach (1989), who point out, after describing a comparatively simple clinical trial with a control group, that "the reason for a control group is obvious. One is interested in the *causal effect* of the drug on the chance of recovery; so ideally one wants to compare how patients responded with the drug with how they *would have responded* without it" (pp. 251–52; my emphasis).

Again, it is important to note here that the idea of producing one thing by doing another has had a *counterfactual* aspect added to it. Other philosophers have made a similar point. For example, Mackie defends the following view: "The distinguishing feature of causal sequence is the conjunction of necessity-in-the-circumstances with causal priority." What this means is that "X is necessary in the circumstances for and causally prior to Y provided that *if x were kept out of the world* in the circumstances referred to and the world ran on from there, Y would not occur" (1974, p. 51).

I need to make it very clear at this point that the sense of cause introduced above is not committed to the notion of a specific etiology, even though it uses a notion of "necessity-in-the-circumstances" which looks like a necessary condition account, a condition that is a sine qua non. Such a notion is part of the concept of "specific etiology." This concept in relation to mental disorders was analyzed in depth by Meehl (1954) more than 20 years ago, and his definition is still valuable. Meehl characterized the notion in its strongest form as a disease that is present when the causal factor is present and absent when the causal factor is absent, that is, where the causal factor is a sine qua non. His example for this sense was Huntington disease, assuming complete penetrance. (Meehl provided more nuanced, weaker definitions of *specific etiology* as well [see Meehl, 1977, pp. 39–45], and he actually prefers his sense [3] [p. 39], which allows for the operation of additional variables, as well as a very high probability of occurrence, rather than only deterministic certainty.)

Meehl also adds, however, that an important conceptual analysis of *non*specific etiology must be mentioned for completeness, because of its ubiquity in biology and the social sciences as well as in medicine. Here he introduces another one of Mackie's analyses, known as the INUS condition. The notion of an INUS condition was developed by John Mackie on the basis of his reflections on John Stuart Mill's discussion of the plurality of causes problem. Mill recognized the complication of a plurality of causes by which several different assemblages of factors, say ABC as well as DGH and JKL, might each be sufficient to bring about an effect P. If (ABC *or* DGH *or* JKL) is both necessary and sufficient for P, how do we describe, for example, the A in such a generalization? Such an element, A (or any of the B . . . L factors, taken individually), is for Mackie an *i*nsufficient but *n*onredundant [alternatively = *n*ecessary] part of an *u*nnecessary but *s*ufficient condition—a complex expression for which Mackie uses the acronym INUS, on the basis of the first letters of the partially underlined words. Using this terminology, then, what is usually termed a cause is an INUS condition.

But our knowledge of causal regularities are seldom fully and completely characterized: we know some of the INUS conditions but rarely all the possible ones. Thus, causal regularities are, according to Mackie, "elliptical or gappy universal propositions" (1974, p. 66). One can represent this using Mackie's formalism after invoking *a causal field* of background conditions, F (a notion that Meehl also accepted in his accounts of specific etiology), which focuses our attention on some specific area or subject of inquiry, and noting that

In F, all $(A \ldots \bar{B} \ldots$ or $D \ldots \bar{H} \ldots$ or $\ldots)$ are followed by P and, in F, all P are preceded by $(A \ldots \bar{B} \ldots$ or $D \ldots \bar{H} \ldots$ or $\ldots)$.

The bar above B and H indicates that these types are functioning as negative causes in this generalization.

Finally, a cause in this sense can be described as either a qualitative (dichotomous) or a quantitative variable, and in the latter case an increase/decrease of the cause can have an increase/decrease (or decrease/increase) on the effect.

Although such an account of causal regularities looks on the surface quite abstract, good arguments can be provided that these notions of INUS conditions and incomplete generalizations can accurately capture our notions of causation in complex systems such as we encounter in psychiatry. The only additional emendation needed is to point out also that INUS conditions and gappy generalizations can also be found in *probabilistically* causal situations,[6] though here it may be required to modify Mackie's "elliptical or gappy universal propositions" to change "universal" to "general," so as to permit the use of statistical generalizations that may be excluded by connotations associated with the term *universal* (but see Mackie, 1974, chap. 9). We also need to stress that the generalizations that may be cited as potential explainers are likely to be of narrow scope and overlapping family character, a notion to which I return later, when I discuss the problem of phenotype definition. These complications such as INUS conditions and the use of gappy generalizations are all consistent with the general manipulability concept of causation—they represent elaborations of the manipulability notion which are required to accommodate real and complex systems.

I prefer this manipulability concept of causation because (bracketing some of the elaborations for a moment) it is in essence simple and easy to grasp yet it can handle causes at different levels of aggregation, including what is represented in path analytic diagrams as well as pathophysiology. Additional conditions can be added to it to sort out distinctions between causes that are (a) probabilistic, (b) populational, and (c) individual and deterministic (see Schaffner, 1993a, for additional details). It can also capture both the *etiological* sense of cause, and the important *pathogenetical* notion of causation, which is distinct, since we frequently know a considerable amount about the pathogenesis of disease states even when the initiating event (the etiology) is unknown. I also think that it is sufficiently flexible that, with the counterfactual aspects added, it can represent the complex types of causation we encounter in the networks of regulatory interactions in molecular genetics. The manipulability concept also admits of different ways of representing causation, from path analytic diagrams to the cartoons of molecular causation flow diagrams so widespread in molecular biology. However, even if the *concept* suffices as a robust representation, it will still be an empirical question whether a causal approach to psychiatric disorders is a useful one, with the notion of useful still to be unpacked further but including at least the dimensions of diagnosis, prognosis, and treatment of psychiatric illnesses.

▪ ▪ Cases in Which Biochemical/Molecular Causes Count

It would be wise to recall briefly some historical examples from nonpsychiatric domains before readdressing the nature of causality in psychiatric disorders. I do so because it is not entirely clear even where causal, and genetic, analysis have been accomplished that they are always of major use in medicine. Several cases will suffice to make these points clearer.

Diabetes Mellitus

Although diabetes mellitus had been long recognized as a disease, it was once clinically defined and in the past first confused with diabetes insipidus and known as the the "pissing evile" (Bliss, 1982, p. 20). Bliss recounts that the search for a cure "involved first finding the cause of the disease" (p. 25). Initially the organ at fault was thought to be the stomach, then the liver, and then, late in the nineteenth century, its origin was discovered to be due to the then unknown endocrinological function of the pancreas and to be attributed to the islets of Langerhans. In the 1920s, through a series of investigations carried out by Banting, Best, and others, the cause of diabetes mellitus was traced to a lack of insulin, and the exogenous administration of insulin was discovered to be what was touted at the time as a "cure" for the disease.

The importance of the cause is clear here—the lack of insulin depending on pancreatic pathology, though note that the etiology is *still* uncertain but thought to be autoimmune in nature. Insulin is also critically important for treatment in this disease. Further understanding of the pathophysiology has led to the distinction between juvenile insulin-dependent diabetes and adult-onset initially non-insulin-dependent forms of the disease. The distinct pathophysiological features that are part of the causal patterns in both forms of the disease are vital for prevention, diagnosis, and treatment.

HIV/AIDS-HIV

A similar success story even more specifically related to etiology can be found in detection, HIV life cycle, and pathology of AIDS. Initially defined as a syndrome in 1981, AIDS came to be understood as caused by a specific pathogen, the HIV virus. Preventing infection by the virus is of crucial importance in containing the disease. Understanding HIV's life cycle and its pathological effects on T4 lymphocytes led to rational drug design based on the life cycle, including AZT (zidovudine) and the protease inhibitors.

▪ ▪ Cases in Which Biochemical/Molecular Causes Don't Count (for Much)

Let us very briefly consider three cases in which causes don't count (for much—yet). Discovering the cause of sickle-cell anemia is a success story of molecular pathology and genetics. Linus Pauling termed sickle-cell anemia a "molecular disease" as long ago as 1947; a mutation at the β-6 position in the hemoglobin molecule causes a conformational change in the protein and the subsequent inability of the hemoglobin molecule to bind oxygen effectively.

But this molecular detail is not especially useful in diagnosis, which is made at the cellular level using a sickle-cell prep. In addition, hoped-for treatments based on the exquisitely detailed molecular pathology are still under development, after 50 years of having this knowledge.[7]

Similar stories could be told concerning cystic fibrosis (CF) and systemic lupus erythematosus (SLE), two other diseases about which a considerable amount is known regarding the molecular pathophysiology. These are contrast cases, however, in that the etiology of CF is known and attributed to a range of mutations (Walters and Palmer, 1997, pp. 29–30), whereas SLE has a well-defined pathogenesis but as yet no known etiology (Hahn, 1998). Efficacious treatments for both diseases are still in the process of development and constitute major research projects, but these are still unrealized, and treatments largely tend to be empirical.

The implication one can draw from these accounts of nonpsychiatric disease is that etiology may be useful in conceptually clarifying the nature of a disease but may also have a limited payoff in terms of diagnosis and treatment, even when the etiology is known down to the molecular level.

▪ ▪ Psychiatric Disorders and Diagnoses: The Problem of Incommensurable Validators and Criteria

In a perceptive article addressing how psychiatric nosology might become more "scientific," Kendler pointed out that many of the key issues in nosology in this area are "*fundamentally* nonempirical" (1990, p. 972). One of the issues Kendler identified was the potential nonagreement of different validators, such as clinical outcome, diagnostic stability, and familial aggregation. Kendler cited several studies of four subtypes of schizophrenia, comparing their relative advantages. Whereas the Tsuang-Winokur criteria gave the best results in terms of predicting outcome, ICD-9 criteria did better in terms of long-term stability and in detecting familial aggregation. Kendler added that "it may be that family studies provide a validator that is more closely related to etiologic factors" (1990, p. 971) but that this approach may not cohere well with the narrow standard DSM-III criteria for schizophrenia itself.

Kendell suggests that "the secrets of schizophrenia and bipolar disorder" are more likely to be uncovered "if the syndromes in question have been accurately identified to begin with" (1989, p. 46). In support of this view, he cites Noguchi's ability to attribute general paralysis to brain syphilis because "nineteenth century alienists had been able to discriminate fairly accurately between general paralysis and other forms of insanity" (p. 46). But this view assumes that psychiatric nosology is not likely to require significant regrouping as the molecular pathology is disclosed and that the phenotypes that we characterize clinically will be preserved in a smooth way as we "zoom down" to the molecular phenotype, etiology, and pathophysiology.

Anticipated by Kendler's (1990) concerns about the narrowness of the standard DSM-III (and DSM-III-R) criteria for schizophrenia, there is now additional, though still preliminary, evidence that research into the genetic components of schizophrenia (SZ) may require significant flexibility in the nosology of SZ to succeed. Whether this will necessitate finer subtyping, grosser amalgamation, or some reshuffling of existent diagnostic categories is as yet unclear. In the recent series of three papers and three letters, published in the November 1995 issue of *Nature Genetics,* four provided some fairly sound evidence for a schizophrenia vulnerability or susceptibility locus on the short arm of chromosome 6 (see Pelto-nen, 1995, for citations). But a major problem was encountered in the variable diagnostic definitions for schizophrenia used by the different research teams. Generally, each of the investigating teams used somewhat different diagnostic inclusion criteria, though several employed two or three different categories simultaneously seeking the strongest results (in terms of *lod* scores, a statistical estimate of significance used in identifying genetic effects). All utilized DSM-III-R (or roughly equivalent) diagnoses and related instruments. What most of the teams term a *narrow* definition of schizophrenia includes DSM-III-R schizophrenia and also schizoaffective disorder (Antonarakis et al., 1995, p. 236). An *intermediate* definition is typically more inclusive and adds to the narrow definition schizotypal personality disorder and also (in the case of Straub et al.) "all other nonaffective psychotic disorders (that is, schizophreniform disorder, delusional disorder, atypical psychosis and good-outcome SAD)" (1995, pp. 287–88). The *broad* category of Straub et al. *adds* to this intermediate category "mood incongruent and mood congruent psychotic affective illness, and paranoid, avoidant, and schizoid personality disorder" (1995, p. 288).

Straub et al. found their strongest links using this broad definition of the complex trait of "schizophrenia" and much weaker links using stricter criteria. Other research teams, however, utilized the narrow definition and obtained their positive linkage results with this stricter definition. One of these stricter groups noted critically that the broad diagnostic model "includes milder psychiatric disorders with *questionable genetic relatedness* to schizophrenia" (Schwab et al., 1995, p. 326; my emphasis). Interestingly, the Genetics Initiative of the National Institute of Mental Health (NIMH) has taken an agnostic approach to choosing between three different diagnostic models of schizophrenia of increasing inclusiveness, roughly approximating the three models discussed in the text, and it provides data (and DNA samples) on affected individuals and pedigrees listing the numbers of individuals identified satisfying each of the three diagnostic models (see National Institute of Mental Health, 1996).

This set of issues regarding the need possibly to alter psychiatric nosologies and possibly to redefine phenotypes as molecular genetics advances has been discussed by Tsuang et al. (1993) and Farmer, Williams, and Jones (1994). Given the pace and resources devoted to psychiatric genetics currently, additional analyses and competing proposals can be anticipated in the near future.

▪ ▪ Psychiatric Disorders and Diagnoses: The Complex Network of Etiological Factors

In the previous section, I stressed the *genetic* etiologic factor in psychiatric disease. But like all illnesses, etiology is only partially genetic, and in psychiatric disorders in particular, there will be not only environmental factors that play key roles but also complex interactions between the genetic and environmental factors extending over considerable periods of time.[8] Again I want to cite Kendler and his associates' work on etiology, but in this case in connection with his ongoing study of the etiology of major depression. In his model, a major depressive episode is traceable to a set of interacting causal factors, including genetic liability, childhood parental loss, and perceived parental warmth (Kendler, Kessler, et al., 1993). Additionally, social supports, a disposition to neuroticism, and recent stressful life events play the roles of intermediate causal variables. The complex interactions are depicted in his path analysis diagram. Follow-up studies by Kendler et al. (1995) have focused in on the interaction of genetics and stressful life events in women.[9]

A path analytic diagram such as Kendler's illustrates the partial, probabilistic, and still "gappy" features of causation discussed earlier. A second point is that these causes are best construed as INUS conditions. In addition, as those gaps are filled in, as other INUS conditions are identified, and as the underlying molecular etiology and pathophysiology are identified, we will *still* have a complex network of interacting causes. Further, the etiological determinants will almost certainly remain *probabilistic even at the molecular level,* perhaps with increasing sensitivity and specificity, but not deterministic, in their capacity to explain and predict major depression (see how this works in the Alzheimer disease example in the following section).[10] The issue as to *how* sensitive and specific etiological factors should be to become accepted as part of the criteria of a disorder is addressed through an example in the next section, and in connection with valuational issues at the end of this chapter.

▪ ▪ Alzheimer Disease(s) as a Potential Model for Other Psychiatric Disorders

The past half dozen years have seen significant progress in elucidating the genetic aspects of one long-recognized psychiatric disorder, Alzheimer disease. The upshot of this work, briefly reviewed in this section, has been to identify subtypes of AD which probably have a final common pathway but reasonably distinct etiologies. Allen Roses's group has made important contributions to AD genetics and has suggested that AD be considered as a prototype for common, complex trait disease (Roses, 1997). I would take this one step further and propose that AD (or ADs to emphasize the new understanding) be viewed as a model for other psychiatric diseases in connection with a causal understanding of the disease(s). Surprisingly perhaps, given its general anti-etiological stance, evidence of a genetic etiological and a laboratory dimension for AD is already present in the DSM-IV, a point to which I return below.

This AD model is not yet "ideal" as a prototype for an etiologically defined disease, because a clear picture of the etiology is still controversial (see Lendon et al., 1997). Nonetheless, enough information has become available to identify important components of the pathogenesis of AD that some general conclusions regarding etiology, nosology, and the role of molecular genetics can be tentatively extrapolated.

This information is largely of very recent origin. In an invited editorial in a 1991 issue of the *American Journal of Human Genetics,* Haines considered the conflicting data that then appeared to associate AD with a gene on chromosome 21, in contrast to chromosome 19 (Haines, 1991). This conflict was resolved if, as Haines noted, one distinguished *two* separate forms of AD, one early onset, associated with the APP gene on chromosome 21, and the other the more common form of AD, sometimes called "sporadic," that is, of late onset. In the intervening half dozen years, this distinction has been further confirmed, with *three* forms of *early* onset AD associated with the aforementioned APP gene, and two other genes, PS-1 and PS-2, known as presenilin genes, found on chromosomes 14 and 1, respectively. An excellent and current account of the genes and their possible roles in AD etiology and pathogenesis is developed in Lendon et al. (1997), where the provisional effects of the various AD predisposing genes are presented in a complex molecular pathophysiological account.

In his 1991 editorial, Haines also speculated that the then recent results obtained on genetic factors involved in AD might "serve as a paradigm for studies in other diseases of complex etiology" (p. 1021). Additional advances that have occurred since then provide confirming evidence for Haines' speculation. One of the 1991 investigations on which Haines commented in his editorial was a study by Pericak-Vance et al. (1991) of Allen Roses's group at Duke, which used one of the newer powerful methods of genetic analysis known as the affected pedigree method, a form of an allele sharing method, which was able to detect a linkage of AD to chromosome 19. Two years later, using another method of molecular genetics, association analysis, Saunders et al. (1993) in Roses's group identified the gene as APOE4, an allele of a gene coding for a lipoprotein that had been earlier implicated as a cardiovascular risk factor in the late 1970s.

The linkage of APOE4 to an increased susceptibility to AD was quite surprising and initially questioned by many investigators in AD genetics (see Lander and Shork, 1994, who say it was "dismissed"). Replications have almost uniformly confirmed the association, however, though some special populations do not appear to exhibit the association (Lendon, Ashall, and Goate, 1997). The main "bad actor" in this drama appears to be one of three variants of the APOE gene termed the e4 allele. The other two alleles are termed e2 and e3. Since individuals inherit two chromosomes, one from each parent, there are six possible genotypes. Individuals bearing the e2/e3 genotype appear to be at much less risk, whereas those with the e/4/e4 genotype are at the greatest for AD.

The APOE4 genotype can, moreover, play an important role as a diagnostic tool, if used in conjunction with other neuropsychiatric tests. For an individual with prior cognitive impairments and in the appropriate age range, with other causes excluded, APOE genotyping can increase the probability of a diagnosis of AD into the 94–98 percent probability range.[11] The instructions provided by the only firm licensed to market the APOE test (Athena Diagnostics Inc.) require that this neuropsychiatric workup be provided. It should be noted however, that the DSM-IV, since it was published in 1994, does not cite the APOE4 test. Goodwin and Guze (1996) do note that it is a risk factor. It will be interesting see if the APOE4 test will be included as a diagnostic component in the future editions of both texts.

It is important to note that the DSM-IV already cites under the heading of "Associated Laboratory Findings" in AD the classical senile plaques, neurofibrillary tangles, and so on found as part of the pathophysiology of this disease(s). In addition, some preliminary results regarding the genetics of the ADs are cited under the "Familial Pattern" rubric, though they do not appear in the diagnostic criteria per se.

It should also be stressed that the genetic successes with AD have been due in part to sustained efforts to refine and validate clinical and pathophysiological diagnostic criteria. In particular, the use of the CERAD criteria (Mirra et al., 1991) was of major assistance in clarifying the populations to be screened for genetic markers including APOE4.

▪ ▪ Lessons from "Simple" Organisms

An in-depth investigation by this author of the relation between genes and behaviors in comparative simple organisms, including the nematode, *C. elegans*, indicates that simple genetic etiologies for behavior *in general* are not to be expected (Schaffner, 1998). This is because the complexities involving tangled neural systems, and the roles of environmental influences on both development and function, generally make the likelihood of single genetic or oligogenetic effects quite small, if not undetectable. There are thus some important morals that follow from the inquiry into *C. elegans*—the simplest multicellular organism that exhibits rudimentary forms of behavior, possesses a nervous system, and in which we can trace the relations between genes and behavior. The principal take-home lesson there is that genes act in a complex interactive concert and *through* nervous systems, systems that are significantly influenced by development and exhibit short- and long-term learning that modifies behavior. The environment plays a critical role in development and also in which genes are expressed and when. Characterizing simple "genes for" behaviors is, accordingly, a drastic oversimplification of the connection between genes and behavior, even when we have the (virtually) complete molecular account.

But this is the story more for adaptive and more complex behaviors—and *C. elegans* does exhibit fairly complex forms of learning—than what we may encounter in some of the most significant psychiatric disorders. There, we might well expect to find one (rarely) or a few genes in more complex organisms, including *Homo sapiens*, which may have a strong effect on behavior. In my view, however, these strong effects will be more evident in the cases of *general derangements*—and perhaps including schizophrenia and manic-depressive (bipolar) disorder. This would be similar to the types of physical behavioral changes we encounter in neurotransmitter-based disorders such as Parkinson disease or in the pathology of neurodegeneration found in the ADs.[12] It may also be the case that normal personality genetic research may also discover some diffuse effects on behavior—much as Prozac and other neurotransmitter-affecting substances influence behaviors, including personality (in some cases)—but these are likely to be quite variable and not easy to classify nosologically.

This picture dovetails nicely with the AD story, since in the ADs we do encounter those simplifications in which we can rationally expect to detect strong genetic effects and a clearer etiology. In my view, there are two or three ways in which causal simplification may occur which may result in something close to a single-gene explanation of a portion of a behavior. One simplification, which can also perhaps provide points of potential intervention, occurs when a "common pathway" emerges. This is usually referred to as a "*final* common pathway" in medical and physiological etiology, in which many different parallel-acting weak causal factors (often termed "risk factors") can coalesce in a funneling toward a common set of outcomes. AD appears to represent just this type of disease, where multiple pathways can result in the well-known pathophysiological features including plaques, tangles, and neuronal loss (see Lendon, Ashall, and Goate, 1997). However, investigators probably need to be attentive to the possibility of common pathways emerging at any stage (early, intermediate, and final) in the temporal evolution of a complex network involving multiple causes and complex "crosstalk."[13] Determining the effects of factors in complex networks is methodologically difficult and typically requires complicated research designs with special attention to controls.[14] The existence of a common pathway, perhaps a specific neural circuit with a specific set of metabolites, might permit intervention by manipulation of the metabolites in such a common pathway.[15]

Another type of simplification which can emerge in a complex network of interactions is the appearance at any given stage of a *dominating* factor. Such a dominating factor exerts major effects downstream from it, even though the effects still may be weakly conditioned by other interacting factors.[16] I suspect that different neurotransmitters at different points in a complex system may be dominating factors, as may mutations that affect receptors or key cascades in intracellular signaling. (For evidence of this type of factor in *C. elegans,* see Sengupta, Colbert, and Bargmann, 1994.) Manipulation of such a dominating factor may thus have major effects on the future course of the complex system, though such effects can be quite specific and affect only a small number of event types. Such factors are major leverage points that can permit interventions, as well as simpler etiological explanations, which focus on such factors. Whether such dominating factors exist, as well as whether any common pathways exist, are empirical questions to be solved by laboratory investigation of specific systems.

This is, in fact, where the power of model organisms is likely to become most evident. Carrying out an investigation in an organism several orders more complex than *C. elegans* becomes considerably more difficult. One might hazard a guess that the difficulty may increase exponentially with the numbers of genes and neurons. Recognizing highly specific single gene and single neuron effects in complex organisms is likely to be accomplished only if highly homologous and strongly conserved genes can be identified in much simpler model organisms. Such identifications can give us powerfully directive hints where to look for such genes in more complex organisms and may help begin to characterize dominating factors or common pathways.[17] As in connection with the behaviors of even simple organisms such as *C. elegans* and *Drosophila*, however, the answer thus far appears to be that dominating factors and common pathways will be rare but extremely valuable both diagnostically and therapeutically when found.[18]

▪ ▪ The Unity of Causation, the Usefulness of Etiology, Triangulation, and Values Issues

I have argued above that a unitary notion of causation available in the philosophical literature can be applied to studies in psychiatry and holds all the way down to the molecular level. What we still need to consider is whether studies that identify various causal factors, especially those that are genetic and molecular, are of the most use in psychiatry. This requires that we consider the basic nature of psychiatry and its most fundamental goals.

Psychiatry, like medicine, is Janus faced. There are two aspects to psychiatry, as there are in all the healing disciplines. One is concerned with helping people with the care of their health—in this case mental health. The other is concerned with scientific goals—comprehensive explanations that are consistent with other well-entrenched scientific knowledge and which permit highly specific experimental predictions. The belief of most psychiatrists is that advancing the scientific aspect of psychiatry will provide the right tools for the helping function of psychiatry, and this view is strongly supported by the extraordinary success of biological-based psychiatry in addressing major mental illnesses with the aid of its armamentarium of drugs, lithium, the neuroleptics, and the serotonin reuptake inhibitors.

But the mesh between these two aspects may not always go well—there may be places where what seems clinically useful does not accord well with the biologically based perspective as indicated earlier using some citations from Kendler's work. I suspect that these gaps and potential clashes will be temporary ones when they occur and that in the long run a kind of triangulation—forcing Janus to look at the same entity, as it were—will succeed in providing the best kind of a unified psychiatry.

But in the shorter run, there will be some difficult choices to make, and much more research to conduct, regarding various scientifically convincing dimensions of mental disorders. The task forces that will be working on the DSM-V will have to balance what may occasionally be incommensurable goals of scientific and clinical validity. Consensus groups will have to work hard on identifying the sensitivity and specificity of various molecular and biological tests in various subpopulations that are certain to emerge in the next few years. In this endeavor, I would argue that they would be well advised to keep in mind the lessons that the AD prototype teaches, as well as be aware of the multifaceted etiological interactions that can be encountered in the thickets of the complex causation of mental illness.

▪ ▪ Conclusion: Considering Phenotype and Clinical Type

To summarize, the concept of cause can be analyzed in fairly simple terms at a high level of generalization using the counterfactual manipulation approach, and it can be elaborated to include the idea of nonspecific etiologies, in terms of a very powerful notion known as the INUS condition. I maintain that a probabilistic conception of causality, which is found in most psychiatric disorders, can be accommodated in this view. Etiological approaches to disease may or may not offer special advantages, depending on alternative means of diagnosis and available interventions. Phenotypic variability poses a problem in etiological approaches in psychiatry in two ways, in that a clinically based definition can make genetic investigations difficult, in terms of both identification and replication, and also that a clearer genetically related definition of a phenotype may not be as useful for clinical diagnosis. Etiology in psychiatry, as in other domains, is only partially genetic and involves a complex network of interacting causes—causes that will remain probabilistic even as they are clarified at the molecular level. Research on the molecular aspects of behavior in simpler animal model organisms offers both discouragement and promise for etiological understanding of psychiatric disorders. Finally, conflicting values regarding the use of etiological markers will need to be addressed by future DSM working groups.[19]

Notes

1. I use the term *prima facie* because many disorders from the DSM-III on have etiological terms in their names, for example, "Alcohol Intoxication" and "Posttraumatic Stress Disorder." I thank John Sadler for this point.

2. This sense of "anti-etiological" is probably designed to achieve the broadest possible consensus among psychiatrists and other users of the DSMs by bracketing possible competing theoretical etiologies. The text preceding this quotation cites the change from the DSM-I to the DSM-II which eliminated the widespread use in the DSM-I of the term *reaction,* based on Adolf Meyer's psychobiological theory (American Psychiatric Association, 1994, p. xvii). Also see Faust and Miner (1986) for a critique of the antitheoretical approach of the DSM-III.

3. I thank Dr. Eric Meslin, who was a member of the NHS Working Group, for providing me with a copy of this report.

4. The NHS recommendations envision the ultimate completion of the Human Genome Project (HGP), that at the end of what Walter Gilbert (1992) has termed the third phase of the HGP—which will probably require another hundred years of work—we will understand how all the genes work, in concert with their environments, to produce both normal and pathophysiological effects.

5. I stress the notion of counterfactuality, but it is not necessary to pursue this here. The need for counterfactuality is evident because causal statements go beyond the observed evidence and assert what would be the case if certain manipulations were done (which either were not done or have not yet been done). For a more detailed analysis of subjunctive and counterfactual conditions and their relation to causation, see Schaffner (1993b, pp. 299–302, and the references therein).

6. "Probabilistic causality," in which what is a cause increases the probability of its effect, has been treated extensively in the philosophical literature. See Schaffner (1993a) for references.

7. Note that in this section I indicate that the causal knowledge has not helped much yet. Come the end of Gilbert's third phase of the HGP, we may have much greater powers of intervention via genetic engineering in humans. I have suggested elsewhere, however, that genetic therapy is likely to be far more difficult than has yet been appreciated, even though some recent accounts of gene therapy have also begun to be less sanguine (see Andrews et al., 1994, and Walters and Palmer, 1997).

8. See Gottesman (1994) for some of these complexities in connection with SZ.

9. This is one of the best path analytic treatments in psychiatry related to depression. Moldin and Gottesman (1997) have urged that the next step to identify genetic and environmental contributions to SZ should be a large path analytic study of this disorder.

10. That there will be probabilistic or stochastic elements even at the molecular level is supported by recent work in molecular cancer genetics (see Schaffner and Wachbroit, 1994).

11. Bayes' theorem shows why this is the case. If the "prior" probability of AD is near 66 percent—that is, after an AD workup—the predictive value of a positive result (the e4/e4 genotype) for AD is in this mid to high 90s range (Roses, 1997).

12. The recently found effect on social behavior in mice of the Dishevelled (Dvi1) gene may be a good example (Lijam et al., 1997). This gene is found in *Drosophila,* where it was involved in early development. In the mouse, this gene has apparently duplicated (there are three probably overlapping Dv genes), and the Dvi1 mutation also affects sensorimotor gating.

13. The term *crosstalk* for complex regulatory interactions is used by Egan and Weinberg in their description of the *ras* signaling network (1993, p. 783).

14. See Schaffner (1992 and 1993b, esp. pp. 142–52) for a discussion of this type of problem.

15. It might be that focus *only* on common pathways could lead to an overly simplistic, reactive, and reductionistic approach to health care and to a downgrading of more complex "risk factor" types of influences. For cautionary comments along these lines, see Rose (1995).

16. It is possible that some of the work on temperament might reflect such a dominating factor/gene, or it may be that this is such a broad "phenotype" that generalizations in this area reflect many different factors. (See Kagan, 1994, for an account of this research area.)

17. A good example of the utility of model organisms is the discovery of the DNA repair gene in humans, termed hMSH2, which is strikingly similar to the MutS gene in *E. coli* and to the MSH2 gene in the eukaryotic yeast *S. cerevesiae* (see Schaffner and Wachbroit, 1994, for a discussion).

18. Bargmann takes a more optimistic view and believes not only that dominating factors will become evident as research proceeds but also that "dominant genes will be quite common in behavior once we succeed in breaking behavior down into small precisely defined components" (personal communication, August 1995).

19. The research leading to this article has been partially supported by the National Science Foundation's Studies in Science, Technology, and Society Program. I would like to thank Irv Gottesman, for suggesting numerous references for this chapter, and John Sadler, for reading and providing comments on an earlier draft.

19

. . . .

Defining Genetically Informed
Phenotypes for the DSM-V

IRVING I. GOTTESMAN, PH.D.

IT IS IRONIC THAT, as we complete the Decade of the Brain and begin to harvest the fruit from the heyday of the Human Genome Organization with a "decent" map in 2000 (Collins, 1999) and a complete gene map in 2001 (Collins, Guyer, and Chakravarti, 1997), no version of the DSM has a single criterion symptom for any mental disorder that involves a necessary and observable biological perturbation or a mutated gene (or gene region). Granting that the DSM-III-R and DSM-IV were not value-free guides to classification (Sadler, Hulgus, and Agich, 1994; Sadler, Wiggins, and Schwartz, 1994a, 1994b), an antineuroscience posture has not been among the complaints leveled against the convention-determining committees that formulated them. The explanation for our continuing reliance, 150 years after the founding of the Association of Medical Officers of Asylums and Hospitals for the Insane in the British Isles (Berrios and Freeman, 1991), on the workable phenomenological/descriptive approach, even though recently enhanced by structured interviews and criteria-mandating menu approaches, must mean that biologically or genetically informed rules are not yet ready for prime time. This chapter deals with some of the advances in the field of psychiatric genetics which guarantee that at least some of the criteria for classifying some of the mental disorders in the DSM-V will include population genetic and molecular genetic findings. Such findings will inform the nosology of mental disorders and be probabilistic indicators (Gottesman, 1997) rather than necessary or sufficient indicators, not unlike the rest of medicine.

■ ■ Genetic Heterogeneity

The same clinical phenotype may well have different genetic distal causes and, consequently, different courses and, in principle, different best treatments (Younkin, Tanzi, and Christen, 1998), as evidenced by dementia of the Alzheimer type (DAT). After coding *the* Alzheimer disease (AD) as if it were a unitary disease on Axis III (331.0), subtype coding on Axis I is required for DAT itself as a function of early versus late onset, with age 65 as the threshold, and as a function of one of four clinical presentations: uncomplicated, with delirium, with delusions, or with depression. For example, DAT with onset before age 65 with depression would be classified as 290.13. The future DSM-V will, at the least, have to take into account four or five different and relevant genotypes. The notation system used for them in *Online Mendelian Inheritance in Man* (OMIM) helps us to distinguish among them, and the latter can be accessed on the World Wide Web at www.ncbi.nlm.nih.gov/omim. Two to three dozen new entries per month have been recorded for the past twelve months, as have three hundred to sixteen hundred changes per month to previous entries. This resource is essential for those who would keep current with new discoveries both for the relatively simpler single major locus (SML) disorders, such as Huntington disease, and for the much more complex and common multifactorial disorders with genetic predisposing factors, for example, schizophrenia and the major affective disorders (Gershon and Cloninger, 1994; McGuffin et al., 1994; Kendler, 2000). For the former class of SML conditions, the identified gene is described as "causal," while for the latter class, the identified genes or gene regions are described as "associated with" or "contributing or predisposing to" susceptibility to the phenotype of interest.

Briefly, AD is heterogeneous in its genetic etiology, with three different rare forms now known to be transmitted in an autosomal dominant fashion: AD1 is found on chromosome (C) 21 [q21.3–q22.05], causing mutations in the amyloid precursor gene (APP); AD3 is found on C14 [q.24.3], causing a mutation in presenilin-1; and, AD4 is found on C1 [q.31–q42], causing a mutation in presenilin-2. AD2 is associated with yet another form of AD transmitted in a multifactorial manner implicating the APOE4 allele on C19 [cen-q13.2] as a susceptibility-increasing gene, a so-called QTL. A QTL, or quantitative trait locus, is a specific locus among the many that form the genetic component of complex traits. It is feasible, in humans, to detect a locus that contributes as little as 5 percent of the genetic variance, or heritability, of a disease or trait (Plomin, Owen, and McGuffin, 1994; Gottesman, 1997). Quite unlike the rare mutations above, each of us has two of the three alleles (e2, e3, e4) at the APOE locus, with e4 occurring in 15 percent of the general Caucasian population. This allele may have some kind of direct effect on AD processes as well as on general aging processes affecting cognitive functioning. An individual in the general population who is homozygous e4/e4 has about a 40 percent risk of developing AD by age 85, while such a homozygote from a family already selected by having an AD proband will have that risk augmented to 90 percent (McGuffin et al., 1994, pp. 204–6). By ignoring the rare SML forms of AD, it can be concluded that some 17 percent of the variance in the liability to developing AD in the general population is associated with the e4 allele, thus leaving 83 percent of the variance to unknown other distal and proximal contributors. In this context it is important to note that the e4 allele may provide useful information about the rate of cognitive decline in non-AD elderly (Feskens et al., 1994) and about the prognosis for the outcome of head injuries as a function of e4 genotype (Nicoll, Roberts, and Graham, 1996), as both are groups likely to be seen in liaison psychiatry. Newer gene regions, for example, on chromosomes 12 and 17, may also be implicated in AD but await confirmation (Marx, 1998; Roses, 1998a).

The rationale for the amount of detail above is to lay the foundation for the recommendation that a new axis, Axis VI, be implemented in planning for the DSM-V, one that will provide a location to record an individual's relevant genotype in respect to neuropsychiatric conditions that have a clinically relevant genetic component in our nosology of mental disorders (Gottesman et al., 1994). Axis III might be adapted for this purpose, but it would be burdened with somewhat different information; if, in the case of AD, it turns out that abnormal cerebrocortical amyloid deposition is an individualized final common pathway shared by all the dementias, such biological and phenotypic information (Gottesman and Shields, 1972; Singer and Reilly, 1996) could be recorded there. The suggestion about a new axis is made fully mindful of the hornet's nest of controversy that can be generated by yet another invasion of privacy and threat to insurability, not only for patients but for their unaffected relatives (Board of Directors of the American Society of Human Genetics, 1996; Pokorski, 1997; Rothstein, 1997). The risk-benefit issues will provide grist for the mills of bioethicists for many years to come. Such fundamental genotype information will require encryption with the keys only being made available to professionals needing to know for differential therapies, research, and genetic counseling.

▪ ▪ Genetic Pseudohomogeneity

Complacency about received wisdom, even for a neuropsychiatric disease as well known as Huntington disease (HD), can be shattered by the rapid pace of developing knowledge in psychiatric genetics. Not long after HD was clearly described in 1872 by the general practitioner George Sumner Huntington (1850–1916), it was clear to everyone that half the children and half the siblings of patients developed the disease if they lived long enough and were observed in the larger sibships of the day. HD is, or was, the prototype of a dominant gene disorder with apparently 100 percent penetrance, no gender difference, and an average age of onset in the mid-40s but with a very wide range from childhood into the 70s. Although the gene was finally mapped to the tip of the short arm of C4 in 1983, it took another ten years for the gene itself, IT15, or "huntingtin," to be localized to 4p16.3 and characterized as having abnormal expansions of the trinucleotide repeat CAG (Huntington's Disease Collaborative Research Group, 1993). All cases of HD studied worldwide have a repeat length in this very same gene which exceeds the ones seen in normal individuals. All HD patients were shown to have 36 or more repeats up to a maximum of 121; but Rubinsztein et al. (1996) were able to find a number of asymptomatic, but at-risk, and very elderly persons with repeat lengths of 36–39, thus proving that the HD gene was not necessarily fully penetrant as had been assumed up to now.

Furthermore, and here we return to nosology and the proposed Axis VI, Brinkman et al. (1997) found a very strong correlation between repeat length polymorphism and the age at onset of symptomatic HD with r square equal to 0.73. For example with CAG repeat sizes of 39 and 40, the median ages at onset were 66 and 59 respectively; at sizes 49 and 50, the ages of onset were 28 and 27 respectively; 90 percent of all HD cases were covered by the range 39–50. Recording the repeat size on Axis VI for both symptomatic and "asymptomatic" but at-risk relatives of probands who may be referred for prodromal cognitive or personality disorder traits or soft neurological signs of HD (Lyle and Gottesman, 1979) would be a logical consequence of the recommendations made here—with obvious value issues and bioethical alarms. The immediate practical gain would arise from the resolution of diagnostic ambiguities. Brinkman et al. (1997) point out the usefulness of such exquisite genotype information in the evaluation of clinical trials for new drug efficacy; the delay in expected onset age would provide indications of effectiveness in young persons with very large repeat sizes. Although this particular genetic mechanism of a dynamic mutation is associated with SML diseases, it is also being actively researched for multifactorial disorders such as schizophrenia and bipolar disorder (O'Donovan and Owen, 1996; Vincent et al., 1998), as it may characterize one of the numerous genes in an oligogenic system which could influence severity of disease or age of onset.

▪ ▪ From the Core to the Fringes of Lunacy

The naked and untrained eye can plainly see that kittens and puppies will develop into cats and dogs and be so classified. The naked and untrained eye will have great difficulty, however, classifying tadpoles as future frogs and caterpillars as future butterflies. Twin, family, and adoption strategies can inform the nosology of psychopathology by providing strong suggestions about which patently dissimilar disorders may be "spectrum" varieties of some core disorder and which disorders may be truly qualitatively different in the hope of minimizing category proliferation. Be forewarned that a "double standard" may be required wherein different rules should apply to classifying family members of a proband versus a random member of the general population, unrelated to a psychiatric case. For example, returning to HD and focusing only on phenotypic traits, we would *not* predict that fidgety children in the general population, given the very high base rate of such behavior, are at any significantly increased risk of developing HD; however, such children of HD parents would merit neurological surveillance. But a less common indicator, say a large discrepancy between the IQ test score of one at-risk child and all the other siblings (cf. Lyle and Gottesman, 1979) might be of use within such families, even if not useful in the general population.

An overview of six twin studies of schizophrenia conducted worldwide since 1963, comparing the concordance rates in the identical (MZ) and fraternal (DZ) co-twins for a DSM-like definition of schizophrenia, shows a median concordance rate contrast of 46 percent versus 14 percent , as contrasted with a population risk of 1 percent (McGuffin et al., 1994). The pattern was confirmed in a new study using ICD-10 criteria (Cardno et al., 1999). If there are nonstandard definitions of schizophrenia or schizophrenia-related disorders which can increase that MZ/DZ ratio over its current level of $46/14 = 3.3$, it should lead to a genetically informed nosology for this core class of disorders. We have found (Farmer, McGuffin, and Gottesman, 1987) that higher ratios go with higher heritabilities. Animal geneticists have found that (cf. Gottesman, 1997) complex traits with the highest heritabilities are the ones most amenable by dissection into quantitative trait loci (QTLs) using current techniques. Even more useful for research into the genetic aspects of mental disorders would be the heritability of each possible definition of schizophrenia—DSM, ICD, Research Diagnostic Criteria (RDC) , and so on—which would take into account the base rate of that particular definition in the general population (Spitzer, Endicott, and Robins, 1978). The heritabilities would then be calculated from twice the difference in the tetrachoric correlations in the liability to developing schizophrenia (Gottesman and Carey, 1983; Farmer, McGuffin, and Gottesman, 1987).[1]

Given the availability of detailed information on the Maudsley Twin Sample studied by Gottesman and Shields (1972), numerous studies have been conducted that vary the criteria and the definitions in the hope of improving nosology. In other words, how can we define the components of the schizophrenia spectrum in a scientific and refutable manner? In this study, initially, a panel of six experienced and blindfolded clinicians from Europe, the United States, and Japan with a diversity of perspectives about schizophrenia ranging from psychoanalytic to Schneiderian diagnosed the 114 MZ and DZ probands and co-twins. The ratio generated from the consensus diagnoses for "definite schizophrenia" was 4.1 but improved to 5.5 when the criteria were expanded to include a diagnosis of "probable schizophrenia" in the proband or the co-twin or both. For the judges as individuals, the ratios ranged from 1.5 to 7.6, and, most important, both too narrow (strict Schneiderian) and too broad (overly generous use of "schizotypal") attenuated the ratio.

The exercise then shifted to the use of operational criteria for different standard definitions of schizophrenia in the literature such as those made famous by Spitzer, Endicott, and Robins (1978) in the RDC, by Feighner et al. (1972) for the "St. Louis criteria," and by Carpenter et al. (1973) for "flexible criteria." The reliability of making the different diagnoses was promoted by the use of the OPCRIT checklist of symptoms and signs filled in from the case history information and verbatim interview material from a semistructured interview (McGuffin, Farmer, and Harvey, 1991). The top prizes here for a definition that would optimize finding any genes and thus have more "biological meaning" went to the RDC, either broad or narrow definitions, and to St. Louis criteria at the level of probable. The ratios generated were 5.2–5.5, and the heritabilities for these definitions were an impressive 0.83.

Given the results above, it might be anticipated that using the DSM-III would mirror the results obtained for such research-based criteria. Farmer, McGuffin, and Gottesman (1987), recycling the sample for this purpose, obtained a ratio of 5.0 and calculated a heritability for this definition of 0.85. We can infer that the DSM-III-R would yield virtually identical results based on the Norwegian twin study conducted by Onstad et al. (1991), who found MZ and DZ concordance rates of 48 percent and 4 percent. Considerations of sample size and power suggest a rather homogeneous picture.

At this juncture it is reasonable to inquire whether such approaches would support the classical Kraepelinian and DSM subtyping of schizophrenia into categories that vary across the dimension of severity but perhaps not taxonomically. Twin samples are not large enough to provide a definitive strategy once they have been subdivided into paranoid, hebephrenic, and catatonic proband groups, but the trends of twin and early family studies do not support qualitative subtyping as opposed to quantitative gene-plus-stressors dimensions (McGuffin, Farmer, and Gottesman, 1987). It was already apparent at the clinical level from longitudinal scrutiny of the Genain quadruplets (Rosenthal, 1963) that the members of this clone of four MZ individuals, all of whom developed schizophrenia, could each have any of the Kraepelinian subtypes over the course of their illnesses. Thus on any one day four "different" subtypes could be seen in this one genotype. The question was further explored by Farmer, McGuffin, and Gottesman (1984) using discriminant function analysis to posit two qualitatively different subtypes of schizophrenia, H (to remind of hebephrenia) and P (to remind of paranoid schizophrenia), in the Maudsley Twin Study. When twins were concordant for consensus-diagnosed schizophrenia, regardless of zygosity, fifteen out of nineteen pairs were both H or both P. However, such homotypia implying qualitative subtypes was diminished when examined with the usual twin perspective. The MZ concordance rate for H was 79 percent, while the MZ concordance rate for P was 33 percent with corresponding DZ rates, based on very few pairs, of 18 percent and 6 percent, respectively. Thus the pattern of results suggests that the two forms differ quantitatively on a multifactorial dimension of liability.

Newer family studies do not yet permit a resolution to this important question (Kendler et al., 1994; Kendler et al., 1997), thus leaving subtyping in limbo, awaiting advances in molecular genetics.

An equally important and unresolved question returns us to the nature of the schizophrenia spectrum (Shields, Heston, and Gottesman, 1975; Kendler, 1988; Kendler, McGuire, et al., 1993). Farmer et al. (1987) approached this problem head-on by observing the effect on the MZ/DZ concordance ratio, as one or more *other* diagnoses from Axis I and Axis II, observed in probands or co-twins, were added as evidence for concordance for an expanded definition of a schizophrenia spectrum. Recall that DSM-III schizophrenia yielded a ratio of only 5.01. Again, the suggestions can only be suggestions because of a lack of statistical power. Single additions of either affective disorder *with* incongruent delusions or schizotypal personality to the core diagnosis of DSM schizophrenia augmented the ratio of MZ to DZ concordance for schizophrenia to more than 6.0, while the addition of *any* DSM Axis I disorder (a continuum notion of psychosis antedating Kraepelin as favored by Crow [1998]) reduced the ratio to 2.39 and thereby reduced any enthusiasm for restoring pre-Kraepelinian preferences.

The addition of multiple diagnoses as putative indicators of the constituents of a schizophrenia spectrum provides new suggestions for nosological revisions. The most promising "compound" as indexed by a ratio of 7.68 arose from adding to schizophrenia itself the following: affective disorder with mood incongruent delusions, schizotypal personality, and atypical psychosis (psychosis, NOS). The addition of schizophreniform disorder left the ratio pretty much the same. Other additions, such as delusional disorder, nonpsychotic affective disorders, or other Axis I diagnoses, reduced the absolute size of the ratio, decreasing the likelihood of their being candidates for redefining a category of "schizophrenia spectrum disorder." The sample did not contain enough cases of schizoaffective psychosis or of schizoid personality to permit any conclusion about their utility, but both remain sentimental favorites in need of further testing.

The suggestions for a new definition from the Maudsley Twin Study could be idiosyncratic to the sample and the methods applied. Fortunately, the same rather specific results were obtained by Kendler et al. (1994, 1997) in their Irish, Danish, and Iowan schizophrenia family studies. Using three contrasting groups of probands with DSM-III-R diagnoses of schizophrenia, nonpsychotic affective illness, and normal controls together with large samples of their first-degree relatives, they found familial relationships between schizophrenia and schizotypal personality disorder, schizoaffective disorder, nonaffective psychotic disorders (schizophreniform, delusional, and atypical psychoses), and paranoid and schizoid personality disorders. The convergence toward a similar definition of schizophrenia spectrum disorder is encouraging and has already had an effect on what constitutes an affected individual in ongoing linkage and association studies of schizophrenia (Moldin and Gottesman, 1997).

Schizoaffective disorder has been nosologically problematic since it was introduced by Kasanin in 1933. The DSM-IV has coded it as 295.70 and placed firmly with the other variations on the schizophrenia theme. Many writers do not take this placement seriously and perpetuate a state of bafflement about what this disorder really is. A firm step toward clarity was already launched by Spitzer, Endicott, and Robins, (1978) with rules and specifications for variants in the RDC. A wealth of data on schizoaffective disorders exist which set the stage for further clarification when used in conjunction with twin, family, and adoption data and emerging genetic markers (Marneros and Tsuang, 1986; Bertelsen and Gottesman, 1995). The genetic strategies converge to support the hypothesis that schizoaffective disorder may well deserve separate nosological status as well as being, on the one hand, an atypical form of schizophrenia and, on the other, an atypical form of affective disorder; not a very neat state of affairs, but that is where empirical observations often lead us. We (Bertelsen and Gottesman, 1995; Gottesman and Bertelsen, 1989a, 1989b) have used the rare strategy of examining the adult offspring of couples in which one parent had schizophrenia and the other had a diagnosis of manic-depressive disorder, thus permitting the evaluation of the effects of the double predisposition to both schizophrenia and manic-depression. Our results, along with those from an updated early German study, show a distribution of offspring risks for schizophrenia and risks for manic-depression of the same magnitude as in children with one affected parent with either diagnosis, and a cluster of children with diagnoses of schizoaffective disorder per se; of course the total risk of psychosis to such offspring cumulates to very high levels. The findings are compatible with the idea of independent genetic transmission but not with the idea of a continuum of psychosis whereby the majority of offspring would have to have a diagnosis of schizoaffective disorder. The observed risks to offspring for schizoaffective disorder of 4–6 percent, against a background of schizophrenia risks of 4–14 percent and manic-depressive risks of 18–32 percent, from such dual-mating couples do not favor simple chance occurrence of the parental conditions. Although such clinical genetic information is far from definitive, it is illustrative of the kinds of strategies which can inform nosology.

▪ ▪ Toward a Genetically Informed DSM-V

The discussion so far using AD, HD, and schizophrenia as examples of the domains that have been influenced by genetic strategies leading to revisions of nosology can easily be extended to the mood and anxiety disorders (Carey, 1987; Kendler et al., 1992), ADHD (Faraone et al., 1998); autism (Le Couteur et al., 1996); and antisocial personality disorders (Lyons et al.,

1995; Gottesman, Goldsmith, and Carey, 1997). Often the powerful techniques of bivariate twin analyses have been used (Fulker and Cardon, 1993) to resolve the nagging classification problem of co-occurrence or comorbidity of diagnoses into shared genes, shared environments, or some combination of both.

The kinds of ideas and strategies emphasized in this chapter are not all new; observations near the turn of the century by Kraepelin and by E. Bleuler about the odd but not diagnosable symptoms in the visiting relatives of inpatients got them thinking along the lines presented here (Shields, Heston, and Gottesman, 1975). More recently, thoughtful discussions that would empower both clinical and molecular genetics as sources for values directed toward classification of mental disorders have added grist to the mills of nongeneticists (Kendler, 1990; Schaffner, Chap. 18 in this volume). Given the rapid pace of basic discoveries in the neurosciences, the DSM-V will be a very different guide to classification than its predecessors.

Note

1.   A simple formula for estimating heritability from correlations is $h^2 = 2 (MZ_R - DZ_R)$ where R = the observed correlation (tetrachoric or intraclass).

▶ ●

20

Values in Developing Psychiatric Classifications: A Proposal for the DSM-V

JOHN Z. SADLER, M.D.

IN THIS BOOK we have seen how values, at least in the sense in which I define them (as guides to action which are praiseworthy or blameworthy), can enter into a host of decisions about constructing a diagnostic classification, as well as be involved in the meaning of category descriptions, diagnostic criteria, and the like. We have considered arguments from those who would seek to eliminate values from a truly scientific classification as well as arguments from those who see value content in classification as a necessary part of (at least) certain kinds of human activity and who seek to resolve the associated value conflict in nosology through various means. In these deliberations, we have heard what I think is an important distinction regarding values in nosology, that is, that values may be involved in the *meaning of the nosological categories themselves* while, on the other hand, values may be *involved in the procedures and processes* involved in the development or construction of mental disorder classification. My presentation here is primarily concerned with the latter—the role of values in the *processes* of making a classification, namely, the recent DSMs.

My chapter is structured around three questions and their corollaries. I begin with, What kind of nosological processes are the DSM-III, DSM-III-R, and DSM-IV processes? The answer will be (in no particular priority) (1) scientific processes, (2) professional-interest or guild processes, (3) organizational-practical processes. But it is not the scientific, the professional, or the practical aspects of the DSM processes on which I place my main focus but instead how the *political* manifests itself in each of these.

The second part of the chapter considers, What role does the political take in the complex DSM process? The complete answer to this question would take considerably more time and space to answer, and Dr. Widiger's contribution to this volume (Chap. 3) has filled in some of the many gaps I have left here. Instead, I defend here a particular claim about the DSMs' politics—that is, there are growing *democratic elements* in the unfolding processes of the DSMs, particularly so in the DSM-III through DSM-IV. I will sketch some historical evidence that these democratic elements have grown in importance, which I will call simply the "democratizing" aspects of the DSMs.

If we accept the thesis that the recent-vintage DSMs have progressively democratized, one might wonder, democratized relative to what? My answer is: democratized relative to the popular images of knowledge-elitist, insular, and closed processes of scientific inquiry, and the knowledge-elitist, insular, and closed processes of the "medical establishment," for example, professional guild organizations such as the AMA and the APAs psychological and psychiatric. (Note that I say "popular images" because there are good reasons to doubt that these images are fair-minded or accurate.) The third question I want to address is, Do we want a democratized and democratizing DSM? My answer will be a resounding yes. Such a discussion will require the handling of a number of component issues: What values are involved, positive and negative, in such a democratized and democratizing DSM process? Why is such a direction a good one for the DSM-V and beyond? And if if it is, what directions should such further democratization take? The last presents the "proposal" part of the chapter. My extended thesis is that further democratization is not only desirable but pragmatically unavoidable, unless some controversial and autocratic (totalitarian might be an apt metaphor) action is taken by the American Psychiatric Association governance, a possibility I find most unlikely. Although I offer a number of specific suggestions about a further democratized DSM, they are offered not as a comprehensive "program" for a DSM-V process but rather as possibilities and options for what has been, and will be, an evolving, complex project involving the active participation of many people with many different points of view.

▪ ▪ The DSMs: What Kind of Nosological Process?

What does it take to put together a classification of mental disorders in the early twenty-first century? Perhaps foremost in many nosologists' minds is the need to secure credible and legitimate knowledge about mental disorders and to use such knowledge in categorization. One need only peruse superficially the literature surrounding the DSMs (beginning in the mid-1970s) to recognize the *scientific* investment in the DSMs' process, the aim being to create scientifically valid categories or diagnoses (see, for instance, the introductions to the DSMs III–IV [American Psychiatric Association 1980, 1987, 1994]; Frances, First, et al., 1991; Frances, Widiger, and Pincus, 1989; Kendler, 1990; Pfohl and Andreasen, 1978; Widiger et al., 1990). Indeed, Chapters 2 and 3 in this volume have emphasized the importance and value of an empirically based classification of mental disorders. Even the most strident of critics of the DSMs base many, if not most, of their criticisms on the DSMs' failure to be sufficiently scientific (see, for instance, Achenbach, 1980; Eysenck, 1986; Garfield, 1986; Grove, 1987; Jablensky, 1988; Klerman et al., 1984; Nathan and Langenbucher, 1999), which is still an endorsement of science-related values. From the perspective of the DSM authors, a DSM process should include, at bare minimum, scientific elements and procedures. I would not challenge this commitment.

But, as the DSM architects have considered, there are no simple relations between empirical research in psychopathology, clinical practice, and scientifically credible categories. What measures should be used in developing categories? Should categories be continuously varying dimensions or molar collections of related traits (syndromes)? What exactly are mental disorders, so we can choose their salient properties in describing our categories? How does the research construct relate to the clinical construct? Even if such complicated questions could be answered easily, there would remain the ripe potential for a classification of mental disorders to be completely unsuited for use by practicing clinicians. What if the most valid classification of disorders numbered them in the thousands, like that of Boissier de Sauvages's classification from the 1700s (Frances, First, and Pincus, 1995; Wallace, 1994)? Or quite the contrary, like Eysenck's minimalist, but empirically robust, classification of today (Eysenck, 1970, 1986), which grasps the psychopathologies by a handful? Such classifications could serve few of the practical interests of clinicians (at least under current practices) and likely do little to guide their treatments (Frances, First, and Pincus, 1995; Wallace, 1994, Frances, First, et al., 1991). So classification efforts must also serve another related set of values, those of instrumental efficacy and practical utility. The DSM architects have also wisely recognized this need, even elevating the value of clinical utility to the foremost value, as stated in the introduction to the DSM-IV (American Psychiatric Association, 1994) and in the *DSM-IV Guidebook* (Frances, First, and Pincus, 1995). But simply managing information and aiding treatment selection are not the only practical interests of the DSMs; indeed, there is a whole slew of them. First, the language of the manuals should not be too technical, so that a wide variety of users can understand the classification (Frances, First, et al., 1991). The classification should be compatible with the World Health Organization's classification of mental disorders, the ICD (Frances, Widiger, and Pincus, 1989; Kendell, 1991). The classified disorders should not deviate too far from those of prior manuals or traditional syndromes (Pincus et al., 1992). DSM diagnosis should be informed by (cross-) cultural beliefs and assumptions (Fabrega, 1992; Frances, First, et al., 1991; Kleinman, 1996; Lock, 1987; Lukoff, Lu, and Turner, 1992; Maser, Kaelber, and Weise, 1991; Mezzich, Fabrega, and Kleinman, 1992; Turner et al., 1995). New disorders should not proliferate too quickly so that the infrastructures of research and traditions of clinical practice are not destabilized or dismantled (Frances, First, and Pincus 1995, Pincus et al., 1992). These are only a few of these other practical interests. George Agich argued persuasively in this book and elsewhere that considering medical classification independently from actual clinical practice is a dire mistake, and I refer the reader to his discussions (Agich, 1994, 1997) for elaboration and defense of this claim. Agich supports, as the DSM authors and I do, that the manuals must grow out of the clinical encounter.

Not only must the classifications themselves meet practical needs, but the processes producing them have important practical constraints. For instance, each edition of the DSMs has involved a more complicated procedure in its construction, with progressively more people involved. Simply managing such a process requires still another brand of practical competencies, those of scheduling work group meetings, selecting committee members, dividing up workloads, setting work priorities, and ensuring communication among participants, to name only a few—hence my term for this aspect of the DSM processes as *practical-organizational.*

Moreover, processes of classification cannot overlook the central ethic of their entire activity, which is to aid individuals and families who suffer from mental disorders. Indeed, the very concept of *profession* includes, among other characteristics, a pledge to serve the interests of the client or patient, not to exploit them for personal gain, to secure expert knowledge to inform one's practice, and for professionals to regulate themselves in ethics and expertise toward these other objectives. (See Flexner, 1915; Metzger, 1975; and Pellegrino, 1979, 1990, for discussions of the ethics of the professions.) That these values are involved significantly in professional activities such as constructing diagnostic nosologies must be assumed, because to do otherwise is to impugn the professionalism of a very large group of practitioners, and widespread evidence is missing for the DSM processes pursuing purely or largely self-interested concerns.

But evidence of self-interest is not entirely missing from the DSM processes. Indeed, part of the ethics of profession involves pursuing some self-interested goals in order to advance other professional goals (e.g., the humane, service-oriented ones). One can use the turn-of-the-century advocacy of mental health professionals against the abuses of managed mental health care here as an example. As for the DSMs, their widespread sales success as well as that of their spinoff publications is well known, profits that benefit not just the American Psychiatric Press but the American Psychiatric Association as well (Sabshin, 1993). After examining the large range of APA-official DSM-IV publications, much less a DSM-IV trademark, only the most naive could deny that the pursuit of profit has not been a significant consideration in various phases of the DSM-IV project. I have already noted that every professional organization must serve its own interests in order to advance those of its patients or clients. However, where the purely professional organization's viability ends and the self-interested ambitions of the guild begin is precisely the dilemma that every profession and professional organization must contend with, and the DSM as a professional-organizational product is no exception. The point here is not to assess the role of guild interests in the DSMs but only to suggest that they play a role in determining the *kind* of process the DSM process is.

So we have three interrelated aspects of the DSM processes, that they are scientific, practical-organizational, and professional-guild type of processes. As we discuss the DSM processes further, we will see a few examples of how these aspects or interests of the DSM play out.

▪ ▪ What Role Does the Political Take in the DSM Processes?

Assuming my tripartite kinds of the DSM processes, we can perhaps place the politics of the DSMs among them. That is, we might look for examples of how the political manifests itself in the scientific, the practical-organizational, and the professional-guild interests of the overall process. More important, perhaps, we might look for the political in *how the balance between these kinds of interests* manifests itself. From my perspective as a relative outsider to the DSM processes, let me sketch some of the political interests as I have seen them reflected in the literatures surrounding the DSMs. Readers will note that I often use *politics, interests,* and *values* interchangeably here. This is not to suggest that these terms are always interchangeable. Rather, it is to admit that in the public sphere of developing a classification for mental disorders, a very diverse group of developers and users (e.g., mental health and related professionals) will make the politicization of values and interests hard to avoid.

The Political in the DSMs' Science

We tend to believe, and certainly wish to believe, that scientific processes reveal truths about the world independent of interests and values (see, for instance, Proctor, 1991, for a history of "value-free" science), much less frank politics. The idea that scientific knowledge is perspectival, incomplete, and infected with values and interests generates legitimate anxiety in all of us—for if we cannot anchor ourselves with scientific knowledge, on what basis can we rationally choose to act on the important problems that face us? But it is exactly this question—On what basis can we rationally choose to act?—that we must confront, scientist and layperson, patient and clinician. Scientists must choose as we all do: What are the important questions for research? Which methods will give us the most credible results? On what criteria shall we decide between conflicting theories and data? Whom should we admit as colleagues, and what should their qualifications be? It is in the particular answers to these questions that the politics of science emerges, and the DSMs' science is no exception.

Indeed, how did the science of the DSM processes answer these questions? Space permits only a selected example.

What were the important scientific questions for the DSMs? In the early days of forging the DSM-III, the "important" questions seemed to revolve around diagnostic reliability (again, see the introductions to the DSM-III [1980] and DSM-III-R [1987] ; Grove et al., 1981; Guze, 1992; Klerman et al, 1984; Millon 1983, 1986a, 1991): Can psychiatric diagnosis be reliable, so that different clinicians and different times for examinations result in the same diagnosis? How can we assure reliability? What diagnostic procedures should be used to improve reliability? As time went on, however, discussions from within and outside the DSM processes pushed for more validity, which was establishing that psychiatric diagnoses refer to distinctive and actual conditions in people, that they are not circular concepts, nominalistic constructions, or self-fulfilling prophecies. So in the DSM-IV era we find laborious efforts to review carefully the empirical literature on proposed categories (Widiger et al., 1990), not to introduce categories lacking sufficient empirical support (Blashfield, Sprock, and Fuller, 1990; Pincus et al., 1992), and to field-test the nosology more extensively

(Widiger et al., 1998). This change in defining the important question for the DSMs emerged from a value that is fundamental to all science, so fundamental that science cannot proceed without it—that value is *openness.* Openness in science means that every datum, theory, and assumption is open for review and question by anyone willing to make the effort (Grinnell, 1992). Without such openness the only epistemic recourse is domination/repression, or appeal to divine revelation or other authority. (That is, without the value of openness in science, the only way to settle disagreements about knowledge claims is to use power to suppress disagreement, or appeal to God to reveal the truth divinely.) Such openness was exhibited by the DSM processes in considerable measure—my evidence is the considerable published criticism both endured and assimilated by the DSM architects, criticism I draw on later. My point here about the political is that it is precisely this value of openness, so essential to scientific inquiry, which not only assures rigor and credible truth claims but also brings with it the valuational. The valuational becomes the political when the value-related decisions of scientific process are disclosed to, or discovered by, the public—the polity.

The Political in the Practical/Organizational DSM Interests

The political in the practical and organizational aspects of the DSM process is, in contrast to the scientific aspects, much easier to spot as well as easier to accept. After all, labors must be divided, committees appointed, work distributed, consensus reached, results approved (in our case, by the American Psychiatric Association).

The work must be done. But indeed, who should decide these matters, and by whose authority? In the case of the DSMs, the processes were initiated by the American Psychiatric Association's partially elected governance and were accountable to the same representatives within the APA (American Psychiatric Association 1980, 1987, 1994; Frances, First, and Pincus, 1995). But the criteria or principles used in the selection of groups, members, and leadership of the DSM effort are not so clear-cut; descriptions of the process in the DSM introductions and related literatures described a few general features: individuals were appointed to the DSM committees by nature of their research and clinical interests and diversity of viewpoints; moreover, effort was made to include people from other mental health professional groups and organizations so as to diminish provincialism. The practical requirement was that all such efforts ultimately had to exclude people if the overall effort was not to succumb to anarchy. This being the case, such exclusions did occur with the DSMs, ones that resurfaced in various literatures (see, for instance, Kirk and Kutchins, 1992, and Caplan, 1991a, 1991b, 1995).

Such selection criteria such as "interest in classification" and choosing people based on diversity of opinion do reveal particular political interests. For instance, choosing those "interested in classification" might well favor the expert's interests over those of the users (clinicians) as well as the patients. As another example, choosing "diversity" of representation might well foster a more conflictual but perhaps ultimately more amenable classification for the majority of users and "usees." In some cases, the practical-political is glaringly evident, as with the careful liaisons between the World Health Organization and the DSM processes, given each group's production of its own diagnostic manual for mental disorders (Frances, Widiger, and Pincus, 1989; Kendell, 1991; Sartorius, 1988). But these too are very brief yet, I hope, illustrative examples.

The Political in the Professional-Guild DSM Interests

Readers of professional psychology's and social work's responses to the various DSM endeavors will be quite familiar with the piquant exchanges over the DSM's singularity as the American diagnostic manual for mental health practice, one that happens to be produced by a particular "special-interest" group—psychiatry. (See, e.g., Cattell, 1983; Denton, 1989; Eysenck, 1986; Kirk and Kutchins, 1992; Kutchins, 1987; Larkin and Caplan, 1992; Schacht, 1985; Spitzer, 1985; Strong, 1993; Zubin, 1977.) Why should *psychiatrists*, as one group of mental health professionals, define mental health practices through their classifications? Why wasn't there more input from (fill in the blank) mental health professionals? What kind of professional hegemony is being perpetrated here? The most obvious answer to the last is, a hegemony based on a singularity, for example, psychologists and social workers have not produced a manual of their own, so the hegemony is by default.

However, the politics of the profession and guild run much deeper here than that of winning an unopposed "election." The politics of the DSMs for nonpsychiatrists concern the monopolizing not of classification (in which many clinicians have no formal interest at all) but of modes of professional practice, modes that may not fit with the professional practices assumed within the DSM approach to classification. That is, the DSMs shape not just diagnosis but reimbursement, case formulation, problem identification, everyday clinical language, and so on. (For more discussion of this point, see Berkenkotter and Ravotas [Chap. 17] and Schwartz and Wiggins [Chap. 13] in this book.) For instance, psychotherapists of various backgrounds and theoretical commitments have complained that the DSM's medical-model approach marginalizes their practice style (Chodoff, 1986; Dumont, 1987; Kovel, 1982; Kutchins, 1987; Radden, 1994), encourages them to label their clients in stigmatizing ways (Denton, 1989; Strong, 1993; Russell, 1994), and places a DSM diagnosis between the therapist and the client's interests (Denton, 1989; Kirk and Kutchins, 1992; Strong, 1993).

The aforementioned DSM profits, with their accompanying marketing efforts, have raised questions about proper role of the DSM's market "intentions"—Is this a profit-making enterprise? A public service that happens to make money for the American Psychiatric Association? A savvy effort to control the reimbursement of mental health care through market saturation? That the American Psychiatric Association profits from the DSMs is given; how one answers the questions about the proper role of profit making in a profession's diagnostic manual generate the politics.

The Political in the Balance between Science, Practice, and Professional Interests

This, in many ways, may be the area in which the politics are the most contentious. Politics live where the diverse interests of people play into the development of policy—social, legal, or professional, in our case. And as I have hoped to make clear in this brief discussion, there are many diverse interests at play in the DSM deliberations. To what degree should scientific interests and values prevail in influencing nosological decisions? What should be the criteria to reject or preserve diagnostic traditions? Should marketing considerations play a role in developing a diagnostic manual for mental disorders? What groups of individuals should participate in the manuals' development?

The DSM Response to Political Interests

The response of the DSM architects to politics must in some way reflect their values. In this section, I highlight some of the particularly *political* values revealed by the actions of the DSM leadership over the years. I address how aspects of the DSM process *function politically*. This should be distinguished from the *political intentions* of the DSM committees and leadership. I suspect, and this short thesis does not permit me to elaborate, that many of the aspects of the DSM process which I claim function politically were not intended for this purpose by the DSM powers that be. Rather, many of these aspects of the process were intended to meet other goals, some of which will be apparent from the discussion below.

In contrast to the DSM-I and DSM-II, Robert Spitzer's introduction to the DSM-III is remarkably detailed in its discussion of the sundry considerations in constructing the manual. Indeed, its opening paragraphs acknowledge and provide some explanation for the great interest in and controversy surrounding the document (American Psychiatric Association, 1980, p. 1). He explains the genesis of the DSM-III as a response to dissatisfactions not only with DSM-II but also with the ICD-8 with regard to clinical utility; moreover, the revision of the ICD-9 was imminent, requiring some action under the treaty agreement for compatibility which was briefly mentioned above. He describes the makeup and appointment of the DSM-III committees, the APA representatives and the processes related to their work, how the DSM-III process was to be accountable, the importance of involving other professional organizations, basic definition of concepts, and brief rationales for well-known controversial decisions (e.g., the marginalizing of the "neurosis" concept). This overall approach to orienting the user to the salient features of the process persists into the DSM-IV, in which even more details of the process, as well as handling of controversies, are addressed.

Given this marked change from the DSM-I and DSM-II manual, I think it is fair, even obvious, to conclude that the DSM-III moved in the direction of a much more open approach to the nosological process. This increased attention to the value of *openness* (at least informational openness) was accompanied by increasing weight to the value of *accountability.* That is, when DSM-relevant information is disseminated, the information is open to criticism and action by the public, and hence accountability is enhanced.

The openness value was furthered in the DSM-III-R and DSM-IV through soliciting more input from "outsiders," for instance, by distributing draft criteria and an "Options Book" (a draft DSM manuscript with various nosological options laid out, the committee's intention to get further input) and a proliferation of professional and lay articles with the primary objective of keeping the profession and public informed of the committees' deliberations and progress. So in addition to an *informational* openness in the DSM process, there was also some degree of *participatory* openness.

The "accountability" value also demonstrates evidence of growth. Not satisfied with simple appeals to scientific data, the committees through DSM-IV progressively systematized their scientific deliberations into formal and comprehensive literature reviews, even appealing to some theoretical sources for preserving "objectivity" in the literature reviews and their assimilation (see Widiger and Trull's [1993] careful discussion of the "consensus scholar"). Moreover, when member views suggested that the newly developed efforts to build the DSM-IV were premature or unnecessary, the APA responded by putting the matter to referendum vote (American Psychiatric Association, 1993b). So accountability means not only subject to criticism but also subject to political action—approval, curtailment, or revision.

"Respect for diversity" is a value that manifested itself early in the DSM-III days, through the concern for diverse membership in the committees, as well as soliciting participation from other mental health professional organizations. In the DSM-IV respect for diversity manifests as an explicit recognition of the culture ladenness of diagnostic concepts (Frances, First, et al., 1991; Lukoff, Lu, and Turner, 1992; Mezzich, Fabrega, and Kleinman, 1992; Turner et al., 1995) as well as a *theoretical* or *intellectual* diversity, as suggested by seeking diverse opinion on the matter of classification. Finally, the respect for diversity in the DSM manifested as a *professional* kind, whereby participation was sought by nonpsychiatrists as well as "outsider" input.

Encouragement of professional and public involvement, a value closely related to accountability, has subjected the DSM committees to significant scrutiny, criticism, and, indeed, hassles. Such investment in this value (noted through the aforementioned publications, professional meetings, debates, etc.) extracts a significant toll on committee members' energies: the tolerance of such "costs" reveals a deeply held commitment. Indeed, I believe it is reasonable to conclude that even this value has grown in importance, given the growth of committees, field trial efforts, extraprofessional input, and the like (Sadler 1996b).

There are a number of other important values reflected in the DSM process (most notably, scientific rigor, as I have noted above), but I have chosen to emphasize these particular values (openness, accountability, respect for diversity, encouragement of participation) because they and their opposites (political and informational opacity, tyranny, repression, exclusion) seemed most pertinent to the discussion of the DSM politics. It is no doubt clear by now that these positive values I have noted are explicitly *democratic* values; let me briefly expound on democratic values to set the stage for part three, which discusses furthering the implementation of democratic values in the DSM process.

Democracy, Democratic, and Democratizing

The political philosopher William Connolly cogently describes democratic values: "Democracy makes the state accountable to the people; it reduces unwarranted privilege; it protects the rights of citizens; it fosters allegiance to the public good by implicating its members in common projects; it encourages a healthy skepticism toward rules, authority, laws, experts, and regulations; it enables skeptical citizens to curtail governmental officials bent upon a destructive course" (1987, p. 3). Connolly is quick to note, however, that a democratic polity is not entirely benign and that the danger does not reside in simple threats to the democratic ideal. Rather, Connolly asserts, the dangers of democracy are intrinsic to the ideal itself.

Democracy is built upon the idea that an informed and involved public will perceive societal constraints, restrictions, and laws not as limits of freedom but as endorsed compromises—as Connolly puts it, expressions of citizenship. Rousseau (1978) believed that to seek freedom meant to seek the moral participation of the governed. But in seeking this participation, democracy must seek some balance between the often opposing poles of politics: the advancement and protection of individualism on the one hand and, on the other, the advancement and protection of the community. For instance, we have stop signs to protect the interests of the community; they do impose a constraint on my freedom, especially when I am in a hurry. But stop signs are also a constraint I endorse as a citizen because I recognize particular dangers (like being hit by another car) that are based on the limits and problems of wanton vehicular individualism (e.g., "auto"-anarchy, with pun apologies). Moreover, if my university attempted to constrain my presentation of this chapter for political reasons, I would oppose this undue constraint on my individual freedom and appeal to the university's policies regarding academic freedom. So the democratic polity can also constrain wanton communalism—for example, totalitarianism or tyranny.

One of the primary and intrinsic dangers for democracy, according to Connolly, is what he calls its tendency to "normalize" social institutions. Connolly's use of "normalizing" extends beyond the concept used in science or among students of psychopathology. "Normalizing" here refers to political movement toward a particular pole of the individualism-communalism continuum, movement favoring the pole of community interests. When community interests are overwrought, social forces are unleashed which tend to subvert or undermine individual rights, privileges, and expressions, ultimately homogenizing the society. For Connolly, the normalizing tendency in the democratic society manifests in multiple ways: in the development of increasingly complicated laws to regulate individuals at the margins of society (the criminal, the disabled, the mentally ill, the impoverished, etc.), the proliferation of governmental services to ensure just distribution of societal goods, the expanding development of science and technology to control nature and protect the polity from destabilizing perturbances, whether they be tornadoes, schizophrenias, or armed invasions. Normalizing consolidates the social/political around an increasingly powerful range of norms, norms that inevitably constrain individual liberties.

An analogy, I hope not too pretentious, might be of help here. As a wine-tasting hobbyist, I have on occasion read reviews in wine publications and then tasted on the basis of the reviews. Some of the wine publications use panels of tasters, which is more democratic, in a sense, compared with the methods of other publications, in which the reviews are governed by the taste of a single individual. Now what I find is that the committee-made reviews give good marks to wines that to my mind are very good but are lacking in personality, singularity, or distinctiveness. They all pretty much taste the same (good though), because the selection was made by a committee whose plurality selected out any perturbing idiosyncrasy in the wine's flavors. On the other hand, my solitary reviewer usually chooses wines with great personality and distinction, along with the occasional real clinker. (Once I found a single authority I trusted, I purchased according to his preferences, much like we would all prefer a benign despot, if there were any out there.) The preferences of the community, when they prevail, make for homogenized choices, a drift toward a "normalized" society, the society in which the individual, the unique, and the idiosyncratic are marginalized, like a unique wine in a tasting panel.

The point is that democratic processes, in which the citizenry participates but the majority rules, have an ontological peculiarity that tends to favor the interests of the *community,* a peculiarity (normalizing) that pushes the social world into increasingly sharper dichotomies: normal/abnormal; healthy/sick, functional/dysfunctional, rational/irrational, law abiding/criminal, stable/unstable. Connolly (along with numerous other social critics from Foucault to Nietzsche) claims that social institutions aimed at controlling, regulating, reforming, curing, and confining proliferate under democracy; and these institutions tend to normalize (bring into compliance with social norms) the criminal, the mentally ill, the illegal alien, the tax evader, the eccentric artist, and so on. Normalizing, it should be emphasized, is not necessarily an evil—rather, it is a condition of democratic process which must be accepted and contended with as a condition of democracy. Indeed, we can easily recognize the social value of normalizing institutions while also recognizing the need to modulate their undue constraints or excesses through the protection and celebration of the individual.

For Connolly the politics of normalization thrive on an assumed politics of concordance. Not having the space to elaborate Connolly's defense of this claim, I will simply note that the politics of concordance are built into particular notions of the democratic ideal. *Concordance* here means that participatory democracy permits a resolution of individual differences through negotiation, public discourse, legislation, and the like, so that the political disagreements as we know them can, in principle, dissipate. Readers of this book might wish, for instance, that a greater acknowledgment and sensitivity to values in classification would reduce conflict or facilitate "concordance." Connolly believes, as I do, that this is mistaken, not in that the possibilities for agreement are impossible, just in that the possibilities for democratic concordance are limited and a significant degree of discord is unavoidable in a democratic society (see Connolly, 1987, esp. chap. 1). The politics of concordance fuel normalization because discord is seen as, at best, a misunderstanding to be resolved and, at worst, an evil to be stamped out, rather than an ambivalent good inherent to the democratic process. That is, when the democratic ideal includes the assumption of complete or near complete conflict resolution, discord will be viewed as a problem for democracy rather than a condition woven into its fabric.

Now what of all this to the DSM process? I contend that the normalizing of psychiatric nosology is evident in the DSM product as well as in the kind of debate surrounding it. (We can see the tendencies for a DSM politics of concordance, for instance, in George Agich's claims in this book [Chap. 7].) I further contend that some of the particular varieties of normalizing in the DSM are directly related to a partial or incomplete commitment to a democratized DSM, the implication being that by furthering its democratization we diminish the destructive normalizing of the mental health field and enable a more productive discordance about the particulars of classification. In my concluding section, I develop and defend these claims.

▪ ▪ Democratization and a Future for the DSMs

Why the DSM Is Normalized and Normalizing

As I suggested above, normalization, in the democratic process, is the movement toward the pole of community interests rather than that of the individual. If we are to see how the DSM is normalized, we needn't look far. The evidence of normalization, presented below, is not given as a criticism of one or the other particular aspect of the DSMs; rather, the evidence presented illustrates the kind of product the DSMs are. Consider these points regarding the "normalized" status of the DSMs:

1. The manual is a committee product through and through. The broadest interests have been acknowledged and catered to. At once the manual seeks to serve the needs of clinical practice, research, administrative record keeping and coding, and third-party reimbursement (see the introductions in the DSM-III through DSM-IV, American Psychiatric Association 1980, 1987, 1994). Many criticisms of the DSMs have been leveled precisely at this all-things-to-all-people aspect (see, e.g., Kendell, 1991; Eysenck, 1986; Garfield, 1986).

2. The DSMs' standard-bearing status for clinical practice has led to themes of exclusion from critics. Exclusion from what? The idea here is that the DSMs' medical model of practice renders social or psychological approaches, indeed, even folk practices, which are not diagnosis dependent, difficult in terms of reimbursement for services, obtaining referrals, and the like (Chodoff, 1986; Denton, 1989; Rothblum, Solomon, and Albee, 1986; Strong, 1993, Schwartz and Wiggins, Chap. 13 in this volume).

   For specifics, consider the preference and importation (in the DSM-III through DSM-IV) of *en bloc* traditional-historical psychiatric diagnostic categories such as schizophrenia, manic-depressive (bipolar) disorder, depression, and personality disorders (Blashfield, 1984; Wallace, 1994; Wilson, 1993). These were preferred over novel "bootstrapped" quantitative taxa like those proposed by Meehl (1986), Corning (1986), Skinner (1986), and others (Blashfield, 1984). The DSMs embody an explicitly *medical* ethos and tradition of syndromatic, over construct-validated, diagnosis. This medical ethos contributes to a homogenized mental health field.

3. The thrust of science-based criticisms is that the DSM is too compromised a piece of science to warrant a meaningful claim for scientific status (Caplan, 1995; Kirk and Kutchins, 1992; Eysenck, 1986; Faust and Miner, 1986). The other practical (nonscientific) interests (user-friendliness, compatibility with the ICD, relevance to treatment selection, etc.) are too prominent to make the DSM a credible document (Schacht, 1985; Spitzer, 1985).

All these examples point to a relative imbalance of community over individual interests. As for evidence that they are "normaliz*ing*":

1. Most obvious to the claim that the DSMs are normaliz*ing* is their resounding success: other American classifications (e.g., RDC [Spitzer,

Endicott, and Robins, 1978]) find their way into research but not practice; the DSM is popular in countries and cultures whose official manual is the ICD (Frances et al., 1994; Jablensky, 1993; Hinton and Kleinman, 1993); and preferences for DSM categories and criteria prevail in
clinical psychiatric research. What room is there for alternative classifications (Schwartz and Wiggins, Chap. 13 in this volume)? It is the
DSMs' very success that has perpetrated an exclusive, and excluding,
control of the field.

2.   Several authors have noted that the DSMs are more suited to medical-
model practice styles than other mental health practice styles (Goodman, 1994; McKegney, 1982; Poland, Von Eckhardt, and Spaulding,
1994; Strong, 1993). Communication among clinicians often depends
on the DSM categories even though they may not reflect the approach
to mental health care embodied in the clinician's practice (see, e.g.,
Berkenkotter and Ravotas, Chap. 17 in this volume). The DSM language and concepts impose, in a sense, a consensus on the broad field
of mental health which doesn't really exist (Sadler, Hulgus, and Agich,
1994; Agich, Chap. 7 in this volume).

3.   Reimbursement often requires a DSM or ICD diagnosis, even if the diagnosis is not particularly relevant to the treatment plan, mode of
practice, or even the need for service (Sharfstein, 1987).

4.   The DSM, for better or for worse, is viewed by much of the public as a
normative document of mental health—for example, if you can be diagnosed with a DSM disorder, you have a mental disorder, with all the
social trappings and stigmata associated therein (Holden, 1986; Davis,
1997). Even minor conditions count as mental disorders (see, e.g.,
Davis, 1997) for some of the public. In the contrary case, conditions not
in the DSM can be disregarded as socially marginal mental health
problems, if mental health problems at all (see Shuman, Chap. 15 in this
volume).

5.   Several authors (Kirk and Kutchins, 1992; Rothblum, Solomon, and Albee, 1986; Kovel, 1982, Larkin and Caplan, 1992) view the DSM as an ex-
clusionary document aimed to further the economic and professional
interests of American psychiatry, a nosological imperialism, if you will.
In this view, the DSMs' purposes are to perpetuate a hegemony of mental health practice and to expand the boundaries of that practice, and
the policies and procedures of the DSM processes subserve these economic interests by excluding those with competing interests. Moreover, from these authors' point of view, the efforts to be inclusive, open,
and diverse in the DSM process (what I would call the "democratic" el-

ements) are instead merely rhetorical fodder purely intended to pacify the complainers at the margins of the DSM effort. This serves to permit the DSM's speedy approval by the American Psychiatric Association with the subsequent securing of professional turf. Again, the normalizing elements center around a DSM hegemony of diagnosis.

It is not my purpose here to answer these claims or even to assess their legitimacy; my purpose is to use them to exemplify particular kinds of political statements. Viewing them as political statements, I seek to fit them into a broader perspective, that of a democratic politics embedded in a professional/scientific debate. For my purposes here, I am not so much interested in the particulars about how these claims are supported or refuted or even if these views represent a small or large segment of opinion. Rather, I am interested in what these manifestations of the political mean to the DSM process.

And what do they mean? Particular value-related themes are noteworthy in this range of criticism, and the uniformity of these themes suggests to me that the democratization of the DSM process, while moving in the right direction, has not moved far enough. The most prominent of these themes is *exclusion:* the DSMs have taken over the mental health field (number 1 above), they marginalize "my" practice (number 2 above) and "my" models of mental health and illness (numbers 3 and 4 above), and, moreover, "I" haven't been included in the process (number 5 above). Other themes are notable, and the issue of *control* and *power* is prominent (the DSMs control or command mental health practice, etc.), but even these can be related to the issue of exclusion. Perhaps most notable in these critics' comments is an absence: an absence of a sense of full participation, of true political advocacy, of a fair hearing. These absences, in my view, could be addressed through a more complete commitment to a democratic DSM process—not to further a politics of concordance but rather to capture the full benefits of a democratic process that at present is suffering too many of the pitfalls of democracy (normalizing, discordance) without fully reaping its benefits (citizen participation, the potential to curtail governmental abuses, etc.). In some ways, the DSM process of the past promised more democracy than it delivered.

Furthering the Democratization of the DSM Process

In earlier papers of my own (Sadler 1996a, 1996b, 1997) and in collaboration with George Agich and Joe Hulgus (Sadler, Hulgus, and Agich, 1994), I have attempted to document and understand the "handling" of value issues in the DSMs. My general conclusions have been, and still are, that the DSMs' authors are profoundly ambivalent about the role of values in classification (readers will no doubt form their own opinions after reading this book). I wonder if the politics of concordance has been an assumed ideal in their deliberations; that concordance is the underlying political ideal for the DSM process. Perhaps concordance has been the DSM ideal of complete consensus and agreement instead of an ideal of a participatory democratic process. There is only indirect or circumstantial evidence favoring this hypothesis; most prominent is the often discussed desire for various kinds of "consensus" in the DSMs from DSM-III on. (See Sadler, Hulgus, and Agich, 1994, for more details about the "consensus" value in the DSM processes.) Various authors' (Gorenstein, 1992; Guze, 1992; Kendler, 1990; Schwartz and Wiggins, 1986) discussions around a positivistic scientific model for the DSMs indirectly support my conclusion: nosological science in positivist psychiatry should organize itself around objective data and procedure, seeking a single "truth" that can then unify the field.

The evidence for ambivalence about a "democratized" DSM process is easier to pin down. Earlier in this chapter I described various values embodied in the DSM processes which I considered explicitly democratic ones: openness, accountability, respect for diversity, and encouragement of participation or involvement. I said that although there was a clear commitment to these values, there was also a suggestion that the commitment was partial. Let me now specify why the "democratization" of the DSM is partial.

AMBIVALENCE OVER DEMOCRATIC VALUES

The DSM architects over the years have taken great pains to disclose their process through articles, books, meetings, and the like, but there are significant "closed" areas of the process. Moreover, even though there is evidence of a reaching out for diverse input and involving outsiders, there are significant gaps here, too. Let me mention a few examples :

1. The appointments to DSM task forces and work groups (the committees working on particular groups of disorders), as well as their leadership, were informal and nonpublic. There is no readily available public knowledge of why this or that individual was appointed over someone else; no knowledge of why these decisions were kept private; no open criteria for selection (only the very general ideas of interest and expertise already noted).

2. The DSM architects made considerable effort to invite "outsider" participation (e.g., draft criteria, the *Options Book,* inviting correspondence

with task force and work group members) yet provided no information how outsider suggestions, contributions, or input was to be assimilated by the individual work groups or the larger task force. That is, although outsider input was suggested, it was unclear how such input, or even *if* such input, would be considered or implemented. This was a source of indignation or frustration for some who endeavored to make contributions; the most vociferous of these would-be contributors were Paula Caplan and colleagues (Caplan, 1991a, 1991b, 1995; Larkin and Caplan, 1992), but similar echoes could be heard in the works of other DSM critics (e.g., several examples noted by Kirk and Kutchins, 1992). In my own (Sadler, 1996b) paper on the medication-induced movement disorders (MIMDs), I documented a discrepancy between task force guidelines or suggestions about incorporating new categories in the DSM-IV and the ways the inclusion of the MIMDs were actually justified in volume 1 of the *Sourcebook* (Widiger et al., 1994). While I did not interpret this inconsistency as evidence of pandering or extending gratuity to outsiders, I did note how such discrepancies could be construed as such.

3. The *Sourcebooks* in general provide little real justification for nosological decisions. They provide very good discussions of literature relevant to nosological considerations but often provide little insight into why one good, scientifically based option was favored over another good, scientifically based option. (In the abovementioned Sadler, 1996b, paper, I suggested that more explicit considerations of the values involved would clarify the rationales in the *Sourcebooks*. It would certainly be the case for the MIMDs.)

4. Perhaps the most important decisions about the DSMs concern the proper balance between scientific values, practical values, and the professional/guild values I have discussed earlier. Authors from within and outside the DSM matrix agree that the DSM-III through DSM-IV are bound to the interests of clinical practice as their primary value; but how exactly was this decision made? For instance, should we conclude that it was a purely politically expedient one (e.g., made to ensure approval of the DSM by the APA governance)? The point here is that the reasoning behind these centrally important decisions is almost completely opaque to the outsider. Such opacity clearly does not contribute to a sense of participation and ownership.

SHOULD THE DSM PROCESS BE MORE DEMOCRATIC?

I can understand some readers' chagrin at my suggestion that the DSM process should be more rigorously and thoroughly democratic, and I can anticipate their dread that such a move would bring an already too colossal, slow, and bureaucratic task to a complete standstill. There is cause for worry, but such a standstill needn't be the case.

Making the process more democratic only commits us to action around values such as openness, accountability, respect for diversity, and involvement of the polity. For instance, one could envision a DSM process, freely chosen, which limits the proliferation of committees, narrows objectives, and intends to satisfy a smaller audience rather than a larger one. The democracy of the United States government involves various approaches and divisions; each offers its tradeoffs in protecting democratic values. For example, the congressman may not be able to get done all he wants, but he also won't be much of a tyrant; the judge's opinion is quick and conclusive, but her judgment may trounce on someone's individual freedom. If we want a lean and mean DSM process, that can be democratically decided on as readily as one that has tremendous involvement by a large number of people. And how lean versus how comprehensive and diverse a DSM should be is precisely one of the questions for a democratic process, one that is analogously being bandied about our country at large, as we debate how much government is enough and how much is too much.

But what about science? Aren't we dragging down our scientific rigor by having to appeal to all kinds of nonscientific interests? Yes we are, and we are doing so under the status quo DSM process. But a democratic DSM process may elect to elevate scientific rigor as the prevailing value just as much as it elects to subject the process to nonscientific interests such as clinical traditions or compatibility with the ICD. Striking the proper balance between individual interests and collective interests is what the democratic process is about; if we had more citizen involvement, perhaps there would be more citizen identification with the product, as compromised (in the democratic sense) as it has been and will be. I believe the DSM should be seen as the expression of professional citizenship rather than the product of expert opinion and research, even under the condition of increased authority for expert opinion and research, if that is what the polity wants to do.

The normalizing tendency of democracy, the danger of the democratic ideal, is tempered by the continual flux of discord and discourse. In the context of a DSM process this means that open consideration of disagreement is valued because it continuously vitiates against a balance favoring community (normalizing) interests over individual interests. It ensures the vitality of a field that aims to liberate its patients from the constraints of mental illness, to aid patients in choosing their own lives, and not to fall to the temptations of domination or exploitation. It involves the mental health polity in a process in which it may be incompletely satisfied with the final product but "owns" the tradeoffs and compromises made.

VISIONS FOR FURTHERING A DEMOCRATIZED DSM PROCESS

Let me make some explicit suggestions about how future DSM processes might reduce the normalizing potential of the DSM process and product, increase public investment in the process, and foster a productive politics of discord for our fields. I am proposing these as a few of many options, many of which will contradict others in terms of the particulars of the resultant process and product. Quite frankly, before I would be willing to support or reject any of these options, a professional/public discourse is needed to elucidate the tradeoffs involved with any of them. Such a discourse would increase the sense of participation and enhance the sense of "ownership" of the DSM.

1. *Have the APA governance elect to support a process model of constructing a DSM:* Instead of subjecting the DSM manual (as product) to APA approval, subject a set of committees to approval. As long as such a task force and related committees follow some preset procedural requirements, the DSM product in whatever form would be approved at completion, irrespective of its form or content. This approach would in principle permit a direct discussion, perhaps even by referendum, of what kind of DSM the DSM should be, while giving an increased measure of freedom and efficiency to the nosological process and its architects. It would put to the democratic test what the APA membership (and perhaps other professional groups) really wants from a DSM. It could also up the ante regarding the participation of other mental health professional groups, which in turn could spur them to construct their own classifications. In these ways it could diminish normalization and stimulate diversification of mental disorder classification.

2. *Encourage the further development of DSMs cast toward particular practice groups:* The DSM-IV Primary Care (American Psychiatric Association, 1995b) would be only the beginning. This diversifying of the DSM product could denormalize it by diversifying its applicability and utility within and outside psychiatry. The downside is that this would diminish the cross-manual construct validity of the categories and makes a diagnosis more a practical construct rather than a scientific taxon. (This problem already exists, by the way, with the ICD and DSM.)

3. *Support the nosological efforts of competing groups:* I suspect a big chunk of the DSM's normalizing power resides in there being no alternative. Having a psychologists' classification of mental disorders (for instance) would permit the mental health consumer (whether patient, payer, or clinician) a clearer view of what kind of mental health care one is dealing with, as well as make explicit the differences in our plurality of theories, treatment approaches, and views on the proper balance of scientific, professional, and practical interests. Insurance companies may develop their own "styles" of handling mental health. Some practicable, viable alternatives to the DSMs would sharpen everyone.

4. *Make explicit the power hierarchies in the leadership and committees:* This in some ways is the most conservative of these suggestions. It assumes the preservation of the DSM-IV process much as it is and explicitly addresses some of the gaps in meeting the value of openness. There are a number of ways that openness and accountability could be enhanced. One might be to give explicit voting power to those groups that have direct or salient interests in the outcome of the manual, and I believe that includes representation by patients and their families. Another might be publicly specifying how DSM workers are appointed and by whom, how scientific evidence is weighed or judged as meritorious, how outsider input is to be considered (and not considered), how the balances between scientific, professional, and practical interests are to be struck, and so forth. A "Values Work Group" might serve to interpret and feed back values-related processes to the task force and work groups as the process unfolds. Such a group might aid in clarifying value considerations and priority setting before formal work begins on a DSM-V. Further, such a work group could articulate such considerations in the manual and its surrounding literatures.

The democratizing of the DSM began many years ago and has progressed steadily right up to the present. An irony of the history of the DSMs may be that as they became more political, they became more scientific! But this situation is only ironic if one accepts the premise that politics and science are necessarily opposed. In my view, furthering a democratic politics for a DSM will sharpen the scientific richness of the manual, its practical utility, its professional impact, and the constructive diversification of the mental health field. Perhaps most important, such rounding of the democratic DSM effort will enhance a sense of ownership in the result. Such personal investment in the DSM can only enhance our work and our care of patients.

21

Report to the Chair of the DSM-VI Task Force

from the Editors of *Philosophy, Psychiatry, and Psychology,*
"Contentious and Noncontentious Evaluative Language
in Psychiatric Diagnosis" (DATELINE 2010)

K. W. M. FULFORD, D.PHIL.

AUTHOR'S INTRODUCTION

This is a preview of a report commissioned in the year 2010 by the chair of the DSM-VI task force from the editors of *Philosophy, Psychiatry, and Psychology.* The report draws together in a practically useful form the remarkable advances in our understanding of the value structure of psychiatric classification and diagnosis in the sixteen years between the publication (in 1994) of the DSM-IV and the establishment (in 2010) of the DSM-VI task force. The importance of values in psychiatric classification had been widely accepted by the time the DSM-V was in preparation, but the detailed philosophical work and clinical field trials on which firm proposals could be based had not then been completed. This report reflects the results of this research. It covers: (1) sources of information; (2) the historical context within which the incorporation of values into the DSM should be understood; (3) a synopsis of the relevant philosophical theory, in particular on the relationship between factual and evaluative meaning; (4) a note on empirical research methods and the design of field trials in this area; (5) a case study suitable for inclusion in the DSM-VI case book (involving the differential diagnosis of spiritual experience and schizophrenia); (6) specific drafting proposals for selected parts of the DSM, in particular the introduction and the chapter on schizophrenia and other psychotic disorders; (7) materials for the DSM-VI Sourcebook; (8) notes on the implications of the proposals for psychiatric training and for the organization of services; (9) future research prospects; and (10) a glossary of key terms.

MEMORANDUM

University of Oxford
Department of Psychiatry

November 5, 2010

TO: The Chair,
        DSM-VI Task Force

FROM: The Editors,
        Philosophy, Psychiatry, and Psychology

RE: Report, "Contentious and Noncontentious Evaluative
        Language in Psychiatric Diagnosis"

Earlier this year you asked us to prepare a report for the DSM-VI
task force on the place of values in psychiatric classification and diagnosis.

Our brief was "to summarize and draw together in a practically
useful form the many advances in understanding of the value
structure of psychiatric classification and diagnosis which have
been made over the sixteen years since the publication of the DSM-
IV."

We have interpreted this brief as extending to concrete proposals
for redrafting relevant passages of the DSM. Thus Section 6 (on the
DSM-VI) and 7 (on the DSM-VI Sourcebook) include such passages. We should like to emphasize that our proposals for redrafting are not intended to be definitive. They are offered "for discussion" only. We have presented them in this concrete form in order
to indicate how readily values can be incorporated into the DSM in
a practically useful way without undermining the scientific validity
of the classification.

We respectfully submit our report for your consideration.

Report to the Chair of the DSM-VI Task Force

CONTENTIOUS AND NONCONTENTIOUS
EVALUATIVE LANGUAGE IN PSYCHIATRIC DIAGNOSIS

TABLE OF CONTENTS

Preface

Throughout most of the twentieth century psychiatry shared with the rest of medicine a model of science from which values were firmly excluded. According to what became known as the "medical" model, values were taken to be relevant only to the *application* of medical scientific knowledge in practice. Issues such as autonomy of treatment choice, therefore, or of the just distribution of resources figured large in the biomedical ethics of the day. But values were thought to have no place in the core scientific concepts on the basis of which medical knowledge of disease, and hence our systems of classification and diagnosis, were constructed.

Developments in the history and philosophy of science, however, over the last quarter of the twentieth century, showed the extent to which science itself is not value free. Many of the innovations described in this report represent the working out of the implications of these developments, mainly in the first decade of the present century, for psychiatry. The result, contrary to the expectations of the twentieth-century "medical" model, has been a psychiatry not at odds with the scientific paradigm but at the cutting edge of twenty-first-century medical science.

PART I—BACKGROUND

1.0   Sources

1.1 Much of the research on which this report is based has been published in the journal *Philosophy, Psychiatry, and Psychology* (PPP). Many relevant studies have been reported in other journals, however, and in a number of important books.

Notable among the latter are (1) the edited collection on conceptual issues in psychiatric diagnostic classification produced by John Sadler, Osborne Wiggins, and Michael Schwartz (1994b) to coincide with the publication of the DSM-IV, (2) the collection edited by John Sadler arising from the now legendary "Dallas Conference" in 1997 (Sadler, 2002),[1] (3) the series on philosophical psychopathology from MIT Press edited by Owen Flanagan and George Graham (the first book in this series, by Jennifer Radden [1996b], explored the ways in which values come into the definition and identification of dissociative disorders), and (4) Bill (K. W. M.) Fulford's *Moral Theory and Medical Practice* (1989), which set out the theoretical framework within which much of this work has taken place.

1.2 We have not attempted within the scope of this report to provide a comprehensive review of this now very large literature. It is covered in the review articles and Concurrent Contents sections of PPP (accessible online from 1998). Much of it is now available electronically, for example, in an annotated form in the University of Warwick's database of publications on the philosophy of psychiatry and in a database set up by Christian Perring at cperring@yahoo.com. Further references are given in Section 7 (which includes draft materials for the DSM-VI Sourcebook). Resources for training and research in this area are described in Sections 8 and 9, respectively, of this report.

2.0   The Historical Context

2.1 Among other salutary effects of the new millennium on psychiatry has been a greater recognition of the need to place new initiatives, whether in clinical work or research, in their historical context (Fulford, 2000a).

2.2 The history of twentieth-century psychiatry was a history of fashions—psychoanalysis, community care, a narrowly conceived "biological" psychiatry, all started as good ideas that, lacking the perspective of history, deteriorated into ideologies. The British empiricist philosopher and physician John Locke, writing in the seventeenth century, would have warned us against such "enthusiasms." But the history of psychiatry itself, as William Parry-Jones noted as early as 1972, shows the need for checks and balances, for diversity and pluralism, in this most difficult of subjects.

2.3 What are the lessons of history for our current enthusiasm for values in psychiatric classification and diagnosis?

2.4 A negative lesson is the danger of throwing out the scientific baby with the bath water of twentieth-century psychiatry's excessively narrow perception of its theoretical base. Many of the failings of psychiatry in the past century can be traced to its belief that the facts, mechanisms, and causes (psychological, social, or biological) by which it took science to be defined were the only "tools of the trade" it needed. There were distinguished dissenting voices—Karl Jaspers, no less, the founder of descriptive psychopathology, repeatedly emphasized the need for meaningful as well as causal explanations in psychiatry (see, e.g., Jaspers, 1913). Yet we should not lose sight of the fact that many of the *successes* of twentieth-century psychiatry, too, including the development of our present classifications, were achieved with just these scientific tools.

The danger, therefore, is that we will replace a twentieth-century enthusiasm (in John Locke's sense) for facts with a twenty-first-century enthusiasm for values. We recognize, now, that values are pervasive, not only in psychiatry but in medicine generally, and indeed throughout science as a whole. The *practical* importance of values, it is true, is more circumscribed. Even in psychiatry values are practically important in diagnosis and classification only where they are contentious (see below, Section 3, Philosophical Theory). But the lesson of history is that we need both, facts *and* values, science *and* philosophy, rather than either alone to the exclusion of the other.

2.5 A positive lesson of history is the importance of international cooperation. Most of the significant steps in the development of our current systems of psychiatric classification have been internationally based. The report to the World Health Organization, which resulted in the crucial shift from etiology-based to symptom-based categories in the ICD-8 and ICD-9, was produced by the British psychiatrist Erwin Stengel (Stengel, 1959); but it drew directly on the work of the American philosopher of science Carl Hempel (1961). Similarly, the International Pilot Study of Schizophrenia (World Health Organization, 1973) was successful precisely because it was a collaborative international study. More recently, the success of the DSM-V as a culturally decentered classification flowed directly from the earlier success of its predecessor, the DSM-IV, as a diagnostic system in countries other than America. The "Dallas Conference" built on this success by putting values on the research agenda of academic philosophy and psychiatry; and the "Florence 2000" meeting launched the wider international and multidisciplinary forum through which this agenda has been extended into clinical work and training in psychiatry and into the brain sciences.[2]

It is no accident that modern psychiatric classifications should have developed through international cooperation. For one thing, it is a plain matter of resources. Like the conquest of space and the Human Genome Project, there is too much for any one country to do. But it is also a matter of bringing together different perspectives and complementary skills. The journal PPP is a case in point. It was originally an initiative of the British Group, but it could not have survived through its early years in the 1990s without the unflagging commitment of its American partner; and its full flowering (intellectual and financial) has only recently been achieved through the support of our many new partners around the world.

3.0   Philosophical Theory

3.1 As a matter of philosophical theory, the debate about the place of values in our concepts of disorder is unresolved. Since the foundational work of the British sociologist Peter Sedgwick (1973), there have been those on both sides of the Atlantic who have argued that whatever their factual content, even such scientific concepts as disease and dysfunction are, really, evaluative concepts. Among the many distinguished early proponents of this view were Agich (1983), Engelhardt (1975), Fulford (1989, 2000b), Kopelman (1994), and Radden (1994).

Ranged against this "pro-value" team, though, has been an equally distinguished pro-fact team. Early members of the pro-fact team included the British chest physician John Scadding (1967), psychiatrists such as R. E. Kendell (1975) and Sir Martin Roth and Jerome Kroll (1986), antipsychiatrists such as Thomas Szasz (1960), social workers such as Jerome Wakefield (2000), and philosophers such as Christopher Boorse (1975, 1976). All of these authors argued, in one form or another, that the evaluative element in the meaning of the medical concepts could, in part at least, be excluded by redefining the concepts themselves in terms of value-free scientific norms of bodily and mental structure and functioning.

3.2 That this "values in *versus* values out" debate about the medical concepts remains unresolved comes as no surprise to us now that it has been recognized to be a *forme fruste* of an even longer-running debate in general ethical theory about the logical relationship (i.e., the relationship of meaning) between facts and values (or, more formally, between descriptive statements and judgments of value—see Fulford, 1989, chap. 3).

This so-called is-ought debate goes back at least as far as the eighteenth-century empiricist philosopher David Hume. Hume (1962) argued in effect that values were not reducible to facts ("no ought from an is" is the slogan by which this position is commonly summarized nowadays); and a number of philosophers in the twentieth century, notably the Oxford analytic philosopher R. M. Hare (1952 and 1981), took a similar pro-value line. Other philosophers, however, such as G. J. Warnock (1971), took an opposing pro-fact line. In ethical theory, Warnock's pro-fact position is called descriptivism (because it reduces evaluations to descriptions) in contrast to Hare's pro-value position, which is nondescriptivist (because it rejects the reduction of evaluations to descriptions. Hare's position was called prescriptivism because it emphasized the way value judgments prescribe actions. Prescriptivism is one form of nondescriptivist ethical theory).

3.3 Hare's pro-value nondescriptivism is a counterpart of the pro-value position in the debate about the medical concepts, while Warnock's pro-fact descriptivism is a counterpart of the pro-fact position in this debate. Like other debates in general philosophy, then, the importance of the debate, so understood, is not that it should come to a determinate conclusion. Rather, it is that it should deepen our understanding of the issues.

In the case of the debate about the medical concepts, understood as a form of the is-ought debate in ethical theory, the crucial deepening of understanding has been the recognition that the pro-value and pro-fact positions, although so radically opposed in principle, have similar (though not identical) practical implications for the place of values in psychiatric classification and diagnosis.

3.4 Nondescriptivism (the Hume/Hare position) shows the importance of values directly: if values cannot be reduced to facts, even in principle, they have to be taken seriously in their own right in practice. Descriptivism (the Warnock position) has the same practical consequence, but by way of a rather more involved route.

Thus, understood as a form of descriptivism, the pro-fact position in the debate about the medical concepts amounts, not to excluding values (as its proponents have generally supposed), but to reducing them to facts. Warnock (1971) persuasively argued that the reduction of values to facts was possible in certain circumstances. The relevant circumstances were, essentially, a high degree of agreement between people over the values in question. We can apply this to the medical concepts, then, for there is a high degree of agreement on values with respect to most experiences of physical illness—severe chest pain and collapse, for example, amount to a *bad* experience for nearly everyone. Hence, the concepts of disorder typically employed in physical medicine, although indeed evaluative concepts, may (if Warnock's theory is right) be reduced to the relevant descriptions.[3]

Descriptivism (reducing values to facts) offers a more self-consistent version of the pro-fact position than the value-excluding model standardly proposed in the debate about the medical concepts. In particular, it avoids the central logical objection to the value-excluding model, that even those most committed to a value-free definition of disease continue to use the concept with clear evaluative force (for example, see Fulford, 1989, chap. 3 and 7; Fulford, 2000b). Descriptivism avoids this internally contradictory feature of the value-excluding form of the pro-fact position. This is because the descriptions to which value terms are reduced in descriptivist ethical theory continue to operate as criteria for the value judgments in question—an excellent case of having one's cake and eating it!

In psychiatry, though, as opposed to physical medicine, Warnock's crucial condition for the reduction of values to facts is *not* satisfied. Psychiatry differs from physical medicine just in that *people differ widely over the relevant values*. Severe chest pain and collapse (in our earlier example; also nausea, dizziness, paralysis, and most other symptoms of physical illness) are indeed bad experiences for nearly everyone. Here, then, the values concerned are uncontentious, and they can thus be ignored for practical purposes when it comes to diagnosis. However, over such phenomena as motivation and emotion, sexuality, imagination and belief, the phenomena with which psychiatry is characteristically concerned, our values differ widely. This is not a matter of poor science, as some have suggested (Boorse, 1976, for example). Such variation in values is no more and no less than an important aspect of our very individuality as human beings. Hence, the descriptivist reduction of values to facts, even if possible in principle in physical medicine, would not be possible in psychiatry.[4]

The most self-consistent form of the pro-fact view (descriptivism), although diametrically opposed theoretically to the pro-value view, thus leads directly to the same conclusion as the pro-value view, that, in practice, values have to be taken seriously in psychiatric classification and diagnosis.

3.5 Which philosophical position one adopts, in the present state of development of philosophical theory, is partly a matter of professional identification. Descriptivism, as a philosophical interpretation of the pro-fact position, tends to be attractive to those who see the success of psychiatry as being measured by the extent to which it is able to follow in the wake of physical medicine. This is a "psychiatry second" view. Nondescriptivism, as an interpretation of the pro-value view, tends to appeal to those who see psychiatry as a trail-blazing discipline, developing at the cutting edge of medicine and establishing routes along which the older medical disciplines will eventually have to follow. This is a "psychiatry first" position (Fulford, 2000a, 2000b). It has a number of virtues: it is parsimonious (it offers a unified account of medical concepts rather than making psychiatry a special case); it protects human rights (descriptivism inevitably leads to a tendency to deny the variability of human values); it is theoretically fruitful (it connects psychiatry with important developments in the philosophy of mind and neuroscience; see Section 8); and, importantly, it is methodologically coherent with empirical research (Fulford, forthcoming).

4.0   Research Methodology and Field Trials

4.1 The philosophical work of Hare, Warnock, and others in the middle years of the twentieth century, which has proved so helpful to us in understanding the value structure of psychiatric classification and diagnosis, was not carried out originally with any direct practical payoff in mind.

That it should have turned out to be so useful practically is a direct reflection of the methodological congruence between philosophical work of this kind—it is called linguistic analytic philosophy—and empirical research (Fulford, forthcoming). Empirical research focuses on the way the world actually *is*; linguistic analytic philosophy focuses on the way language is actually *used*.

The idea behind the linguistic analytic method in philosophy is straightforward. We are on the whole better at using concepts than at defining them (try defining the concept of "time" if you doubt this). Hence, one way to become clearer about the meanings of the concepts employed in a particular area is to examine how these concepts are actually used. In medicine, this means looking at such sources as (1) the literature, including our existing classifications, but also (2) actual case histories and how they are described. (We come to a case history in Section 5.)

4.2 A different (although complementary) philosophical method, which has also been critically important in the development of twenty-first-century psychiatry, is phenomenology.

Phenomenology has contributed to our knowledge of (1) psychopathology, and hence to classification (see, e.g., the work of Bracken [forthcoming] on trauma and Philpott [1998] on dyslexia), and (2) the process of diagnosis (in particular, the role of tacit, or "craft," knowledge: this was highlighted, e.g., in foundational papers by Kraus (1994) in Germany and by Wiggins, Schwartz, and Northoff (1990) in America. Despite developments generally in what has become known as "naturalized phenomenology" (Petitot et al., 2000), phenomenology has not generally been concerned directly with the value structure of classification and diagnosis. Hence, in this section we will focus on the role of linguistic analytic philosophy.

4.3 Within the linguistic analytic tradition, nondescriptivist ethical theory, with its separation of descriptive and evaluative elements of meaning, has given us a particularly clear framework for the design both of primary research and of clinical field trials on specific areas of our classifications.

This framework distinguishes between three key expressions—*value term, value judgment,* and *descriptive criterion.* According to nondescriptivist ethical theory, a value *term* expresses a value *judgment* that is made on the basis of *descriptive criteria.*[5]

The descriptive criteria by which the categories of mental disorder in our classifications are defined, therefore, have two distinct roles: (1) they define a range of mental *conditions* descriptively (i.e., without introducing values), and (2) they operate as descriptive criteria for the value judgments involved in taking these mental *conditions* to be mental *disorders.*

4.4 In the traditional value-excluding medical-model conception of psychiatry, these two roles of descriptive diagnostic criteria, which we might call their descriptive and evaluative roles, were conflated. In a nondescriptivist value-including conception of psychiatry they are disentangled and hence can be studied separately. It is this separation that has proved to be so fruitful an approach in primary research and in clinical field trials on diagnosis and classification in psychiatry.

4.4.1 Primary Research. Building on the nondescriptivist separation of the two roles of the descriptive criteria for mental disorders, primary research in this area has had two correspondingly distinct objectives:

1. *descriptive*—to clarify further the descriptively defined characteristics of conditions with which psychiatrists are concerned, this being an extension of traditional descriptive psychopathology (as in the development of twentieth-century research instruments, such as the PSE [Wing, Cooper, and Sartorius, 1974], and, of course, the ICD and DSM classifications), though now informed by renewed interest in phenomenological methods; and

2. *evaluative*—to examine the extent to which these conditions, descriptively defined, are negatively evaluated by different groups and individuals and hence are, to this extent, correctly thought of as mental disorders. The latter research has yielded some surprising results. Notably, some conditions that traditionally had been thought to be uncontroversially pathological are now known to have nonpathological counterparts (e.g., schizophrenia and religious experience; see Sec. 5, Case Study, below).

4.4.2 Field Trials. Based as they have been on the results of this primary research, field trials in this area have also distinguished between these two objectives (descriptive and evaluative), though now in the form of two practically focused questions:

1. *descriptive*—are the descriptively defined conditions specified in our classifications reliably identifiable? and

2. *evaluative*—to what extent and in what ways is it clinically useful to make explicit the value judgments involved in deciding whether a given condition on a given occasion is properly thought of as a mental disorder?

Field trials around question 1 (descriptive) are an extension of twentieth-century research on the reliability of psychopathological and psychiatric nosological concepts. Field trials around question 2 (evaluative) have required new experimental paradigms. The latter, like their twentieth-century predecessors, have required the development of standardized interview schedules, training sessions for researchers, and so on, although in this case involving philosophers skilled in analytic methods as well as those (such as social scientists) with expertise in empirical methods (see also Training Methods, Sec. 8).

4.5 The design and implementation of this research has been mostly cross-disciplinary. There have been a number of studies by philosophers and practitioners working in isolation. But the most successful projects have been either collaborative or undertaken by the growing number of doubly qualified philosopher-psychiatrists. So far as field trials go, the work on models of disorder by Colombo and colleagues at Warwick and Oxford Universities and at the Institute of Psychiatry, and the series of papers from the Oxford-Southwestern Values Study Group, are cases in point.

In primary research, a remarkable range of empirical disciplines have been successfully paired with analytic philosophy in recent years. Besides wider developments in philosophy of mind, neuroscience, and schizophrenia (Hoerl, forthcoming), these include ethnography (in Robertson's [1996] study of the acquisition of professional values in medical training), linguistics (Van Staden's [1999] work on personal pronoun use and the process of change in psychotherapy), psychometrics (Sabat and Harré's [1997] study of Alzheimer sufferers), service planning (Marshall's [1994] need-for-care schedule), brain imaging (Spence's [1996] study of volition) and artificial intelligence (Wright, Sloman, and Beaudoin [1996] and Boden [1990] on connectionist architectures for the affective loading of cognitive processes in psychopathology).

Part II—Draft Materials for the DSM-VI

5.0   A Case Study

5.1 This section of our report offers a case study in the differential diagnosis of schizophrenia. There are many disorders in the DSM the diagnoses of which more obviously involve value judgments (e.g., conduct disorder—see below, Sec. 6.2). The diagnosis of schizophrenia, however, illustrates the way in which value judgments may be important in the diagnosis even of conditions that are not overtly value laden.

5.2 The case to be described, Simon, is based on a real person but with biographical and other identifying details changed to ensure confidentiality. Simon was one of a series of similar patients reported originally by the British psychologist Mike Jackson (1997). A detailed philosophical analysis of these cases appeared in an early issue of PPP (Jackson and Fulford, 1997).

5.3 Simon—Case History, Part 1

Simon, aged forty, was a senior, black American lawyer from a middle-class, Baptist family. Before the onset of his symptoms, he reported sporadic, relatively unremarkable psychic experiences. These had led him to seek the guidance of a professional "seer," with whom he occasionally consulted on major life events and decisions.

He gave the following history. Recently, his hitherto successful career had been threatened by legal action from a group of colleagues. Although he claimed to be innocent, mounting a defense would be expensive and hazardous. He had responded to this crisis by praying at a small altar that he had set up in his front room. After an emotional evening's "outpouring," he discovered that the candle wax had left a "seal" (or "sun") on several consecutive pages of his Bible, covering certain letters and words. He described his experiences thus. "I got up and I saw the seal that was on my father's Bible and I called x and I said, you know, 'something remarkable is going on over here.' I think the beauty of it was the specificity by which the sun burned through. It was . . . in my mind, a clever play on words." Although the marked words and letters had no explicit meaning, Simon interpreted this event as a direct communication from God, which signified that he had a special purpose or mission.

From this time on, over a period of some months, Simon received a complex series of "revelations" largely conveyed through the images left in melted candle wax. He carried photos of these, which left most observers unimpressed but were, for him, clearly representations of biblical symbols, particularly from the Book of Revelation (the bull, the twenty-four elders, the Ark of the Covenant, etc.). They signified that "I am the living son of David . . . and I'm also a relative of Ishmael, and . . . of Joseph." He was also the "captain of the guard of Israel." He found that this role carried awesome responsibilities: "Sometimes I'm saying—O my God, why did you choose me, and there's no answer to that." His special status had the effect of "increasing my own inward sense, wisdom, understanding, and endurance," which would "allow me to do whatever is required in terms of bringing whatever message it is that God wants me to bring."

He expressed these beliefs with full conviction. "The truths that are up in that room are the truths that have been spoken of for four thousand years." When confronted with skepticism, he commented: "I don't get upset, because I know within myself what I know."

He also described experiences of thoughts coming into his head: "If you're sitting and watching television, and then somebody turns on the vacuum cleaner, and the TV goes on the fritz, it's like that" . . . "the things that come are not the things I have been thinking about . . . , they kind of short circuit the brain, and bring their message."

5.4   Presented with this history in a study carried out toward the end of the twentieth century, most psychiatrists made a diagnosis of schizophrenia, with a differential diagnosis that included schizoaffective disorder, mania, organic disorder, and hysteria (Fulford, 1999). Their diagnostic reasoning was straightforward: Simon had at least one "characteristic symptom" (criterion A in the DSM IV—i.e., a delusional perception) and possibly a second (thought insertion). These experiences had been present for more than a month. Therefore, the likely diagnosis is schizophrenia or some related psychotic disorder.

This reasoning was fully consistent with traditional thinking about the diagnosis of schizophrenia and indeed with the then current ICD-10 (ICD-10's "symptoms . . . [of] . . . special importance to the diagnosis [of schizophrenia]" were broadly equivalent to the DSM's "characteristic symptoms"). Surprisingly, though, even at that time, the diagnosis could not have been made according to DSM-IV criteria without further information, for the DSM-IV (though not the ICD-10) added to the criterion of characteristic symptoms being present (criterion A) a further criterion (criterion B) of "social/occupational dysfunction" (American Psychiatric Association, pp. 285–86). What is surprising about this is that, although the DSM-IV had been available for three years at the time of the above study, few, if any, psychiatrists thought to ask whether Simon had shown a

reduced level of functioning "in such areas as work, interpersonal relations, or self care" as required by the DSM-IV's criterion B. We can get an
indication of whether criterion B was in fact satisfied from the way Simon's
story continued.

5.5 Simon—Case History, Part II

*Simon's experiences gave him the strength to take on and win the lawsuit that
was being mounted against him. This restored his self-confidence as a high-
achieving black attorney working in an area in which racism was still ram-
pant. His career flourished, and he used some of the large amount of money
he made to set up a new charitable foundation. Through all this, his revelations had continued, and he now saw that his purpose in life was to bring
about a reconciliation of Christianity and Islam.*

5.6 Clearly, then, by DSM-IV criteria, though not by the criteria in the
ICD-10, Simon did not have schizophrenia. His psychotic experiences, although conforming to the "characteristic symptoms" of schizophrenia,
were enabling rather than disabling. He was far from being ill: his experiences, although perhaps unusual, were religious or spiritual experiences
(other cases in the Jackson series had less flamboyant though still "psychotic" experiences). Why, then, was the correct differential diagnosis (of
normal religious experience) so consistently missed?

5.7 The reason, essentially, is that the correct diagnosis turns, crucially,
on a value judgment rather than on matters of fact. The relevant value
judgment, according to nondescriptivist ethical theory, was always implicit
in taking schizophrenia to be, not just a condition defined by characteristic symptoms, but a *negatively evaluated* condition (this being one of the
two key elements in the definition of a mental disorder—see below, Sec.
6.4.3). These value judgments were implicit in the ICD-10 and came close
to being explicit in the DSM-IV criterion B. But even here, the terminology used ("dysfunction") and the exclusive emphasis on science in the introduction of the DSM-IV suggested that criterion B was a matter simply
of further facts about the patient's condition, rather than of how that condition was evaluated.

5.8 The DSM-VI, building on the research described above (Sec. 4.0),
is now in a position to make the required value judgments fully explicit. It
could do this (1) by specifying that the required change in occupational/
social functioning must be "for the worse" and (2) by indicating the range
of value perspectives that must be taken into account in exercising clinical
judgment in this respect.

This is described further below, in particular in Section 6.5, on proposed changes to the DSM chapter "Schizophrenia and Other Psychotic Disorders," and in the diagnostic criteria proposed at the end of 6.5.2. Note that these sections of the report also cover proposals for incorporating into the DSM-VI certain refinements in our understanding of such terms as *clinical judgment, clinical significance,* and so on, together with revised definitions of key psychopathological concepts such as "delusion." A more extended treatment of Simon's case could be used in the DSM-VI Case Book to illustrate all of these. (A summary of the definitions proposed is given in Sec. 10, Glossary.)

6.0   Drafting Proposals for the DSM-VI

6.1 This section offers specific proposals for changes to the wording of the DSM. The proposals are put forward in this concrete way, not to preempt discussion and further changes, but in order to connect the theory on which they are based as closely as possible to the contingencies of day-to-day practice. One of the many strengths of the DSM has been its primarily *clinical* focus. The aim of the changes suggested in this report is to build on this strength rather than to dilute practical effectiveness with theoretical small print.

The texts to which the proposals relate are mainly from the DSM-IV rather than the DSM-V. This is because, although the importance of values in psychiatric classification had been recognized at the time the DSM-V was in preparation, the detailed philosophical work and clinical field trials on which firm proposals could be based had not then been completed.

In the following sections of our report, the location of proposed changes is identified by page and paragraph and/or line numbers (e.g., **p xv, para 1,** *l* 4). References are to the DSM-IV text unless otherwise specified. Proposed changes are indicated throughout by *italic font.* Original text is not italicized.

6.2 As indicated above (Sec. 3—Philosophical Theory), values are important practically in the diagnosis of many different kinds of mental disorder. Values are important practically for any mental disorder involving experience or behavior over which people's values differ to a significant degree. For such disorders, therefore, as described in Section 4 above, the value judgments relevant to diagnosis may be contentious. Hence, for any disorder of this kind, the required value judgments, and the procedures by which they are made, should be specified in sufficient detail to make fully explicit the evaluative, as well as the more familiar descriptive, diagnostic criteria for the disorder in question.

Rather than running through all the relevant disorders, however, which would be repetitious, we will illustrate the general approach to specifying values by reference to the diagnosis of psychotic disorders. These disorders are especially important in this respect because they are central (1) to the medical "disease" concept of mental disorder (it is in respect of psychotic disorders that the most significant advances in neuroscientific understanding have been made in the opening years of the millennium) and (2) to the special ethical status of mental disorders (it is psychotic disorders that continue to figure most prominently both in involuntary psychiatric treatment and in legal cases in which mental illness is offered as an excuse). However, (3) whereas values are overtly involved in the diagnosis of other less centrally placed disorders,[6] the value judgments involved in the diagnosis of psychotic disorders, although in fact diagnostically crucial (see the Case Study, Sec. 5), have not been widely recognized for what they are. (In this regard, see also Jerome Wakefield's chapter in Sadler, 2002). Hence, drawing these value judgments out and making them explicit provides a particularly effective illustration of the importance of values generally in psychiatric classification and diagnosis.

6.3 The particular focus of this section of our report is therefore the DSM chapter "Schizophrenia and Other Psychotic Disorders." First, however, in order to set our proposals in context, we will suggest possible changes to the introduction to the DSM.

6.4 The Introduction to the DSM. The introductory chapter to the DSM has traditionally provided important background information in particular on the ways in which each edition has built on its predecessors. The introduction to the DSM-VI should thus make explicit the precise role of *philosophy* in improving the practical utility of the classification. This will involve a number of changes, some small and others more extensive, to several sections of the introduction, in particular, (1) the opening paragraphs, (2) Historical Background, (3) The DSM-VI Revision Process, and (4) Definition of Mental Disorder. Further background to the proposed changes, particularly to the Definition of Mental Disorder section, is given in Section 7 of this report (draft materials for the DSM-VI Sourcebook).

6.4.1 The DSM-IV Opening Paragraphs. **p xv, para 1, *l* 2** "The utility and credibility of DSM-VI require that it focus on its clinical, research and educational purposes; *that it* be supported by an extensive empirical foundation; *and that its conceptual structure (including the values it embodies) be made as explicit as possible."*

p xv, para 1, *l* 5 "We hoped to make DSM-VI practical and useful for clinicians by striving for brevity of criteria sets, clarity of language, and explicit statements *both* of the constructs embodied in the diagnostic criteria, *and, where relevant, of the procedures by which judgments should be made as to whether the relevant criteria are satisfied in an individual case."*

p xv, para 1, *l* 7 *"The procedures specified in this Manual depend critically on good communication not only between clinicians but between patients and professionals and between different professionals in multidisciplinary teams. Hence, improving communication, as an essential prerequisite of validity in psychiatric diagnosis, was a central clinical objective of DSM-VI.* An additional goal was to facilitate research and improve communication *between* clinicians, *patients* and researchers."

p xv, para 2, *l* 3 "[DSM] is used by psychiatrists . . . , other health and mental health professionals, *and, increasingly, by patients and other users of services, by caregivers and by patient advocacy groups.* DSM-VI must be usable across settings . . . "

p xv, para 3, *l* 6 " . . . we selected Work Group members who represented a wide range of perspectives and experiences, *including in each case representatives of relevant advocacy groups.* Work Group members were instructed that they were to participate *primarily* as consensus scholars and not as advocates . . . "

p xv, para 4, *l* 7 "Conferences and workshops were held to provide conceptual and methodological guidance for the DSM-VI effort. *Philosophers from a number of disciplines made important contributions to these conferences, both as members of the Work Groups and Task Force and as external advisors. The conferences also* included . . . "

p xvi, para 3, *l* 4 "We received extensive correspondence from interested individuals who shared with us additional data and recommendations on the potential impact of the possible changes in DSM-VI on their clinical practice, teaching, research and administrative work *(in the case of mental health professionals), and on the extent to which the issues important to individual patients were properly identified (in the case of users, caregivers and advocacy groups).* This breadth of discussion helped us to anticipate . . . "

p xvi, para 4 "In arriving at final DSM-VI decisions, the Work Groups and Task Force reviewed all of the extensive empirical evidence, *analysis of concepts,* and correspondence that had been gathered. It is our belief that the major innovation of DSM-VI lies not in any of its specific content changes *(even the evaluative criteria now included were implicit in earlier* *classifications)* but rather in the systematic and explicit process by which it was constructed and documented. DSM-IV *was distinguished by the fact that it was* grounded in empirical evidence; *DSM-V took us an important step toward making explicit the framework of ideas (or concepts) by which this evidence is structured and given meaning; DSM-VI has completed this process by specifying the evaluative (as well as descriptive) criteria by which mental disorders are diagnosed."*

6.4.2   Historical Background. **p xvii, para 5** "In part because of the lack of widespread acceptance of the mental disorder taxonomy contained in ICD-6 and ICD-7, WHO sponsored a comprehensive review of diagnostic issues that was conducted by the British psychiatrist Stengel. His report, *which was directly influenced by the work of the American philosopher of science Carl Hempel,* can be credited with having inspired many of the recent advances in diagnostic methodology—most especially the need for explicit definitions as a means of promoting reliable clinical diagnosis. However, the next round of diagnostic revision, which led to DSM-II and ICD-8, did not follow Stengel's recommendations to any great degree. DSM-II was similar to DSM-I but eliminated the term 'reaction.' *It was only with ICD-9 and DSM-III that fully explicit descriptive criteria were finally adopted. History has repeated itself with DSM-IV, V and VI. Philosophical work, in this case from a number of other philosophical disciplines in addition to the philosophy of science, has helped to make explicit the evaluative elements in psychiatric diagnostic concepts; but it is only with DSM-VI (and ICD-12) that these elements have been fully incorporated into our classifications."*

p xvii, para 6 "DSM-III introduced *(and DSMs IV, V and VI have retained)* a number of important methodological innovations, including explicit diagnostic criteria, a multiaxial system, and an approach that, *consistent with the current state of the development of our knowledge of etiology is based mainly on the symptoms of mental disorder. In DSM-IV, this approach was called 'descriptive.' In DSM-VI, which makes explicit (where relevant) the evaluative as well as descriptive criteria for the diagnosis of mental disorder, it is called 'symptom-based.'"*

p xviii, para 2 " . . . corrections that led to the publication of DSM-III-R in 1987. *DSM-IV, which greatly extended the depth and sophistication of the empirical basis of the classification, followed in 1994. Dissatisfaction with a number of inconsistencies in the conceptual structure of DSM-IV resulted in philosophers being involved in the DSM-V Work Groups and Task Force. This was the first formal involvement of philosophers in the development of* *psychiatric classification since Carl Hempel's contribution to Stengel's report to the WHO. The shared understanding of working methods and objectives to which it led made possible the collaborative field trials on which the evaluative criteria incorporated in DSM-VI are based."*

6.4.3 The DSM-VI Revision Process. **p xviii, para 3, 16** "The Task Force on DSM-VI and its Work Groups conducted a three-stage empirical process that included (1) comprehensive and systematic reviews of the published literature, (2) reanalyses of already collected datasets, and (3) extensive issue-focused field trials. *DSM-V and DSM-VI have retained this systematic evidence-based approach. In addition, the inclusion of philosophers in the Task Force and Work Groups has allowed the epistemic values implicit in the review process to be made fully explicit (epistemic values determine the selection of data, criteria of significance, and so forth). The inclusion of users, caregivers and advocacy groups, has helped to make explicit the substantive values involved in the diagnosis and assessment of mental disorders."*

6.4.4 The DSM-V section "The Definition and Scope of Mental Disorder." (In DSM-IV this section was "Definition of Mental Disorder," pp. xxi–xxii.) Given the large number of small but important changes already introduced into this section in DSM-V, we have reproduced the relevant text in full. An expanded version of this section, providing additional details of the reasoning behind the changes to both DSM-V and DSM-VI, is given in Section 7 of this report, on the DSM-VI Sourcebook.

"*In earlier editions of DSM misgivings were expressed about the term 'mental disorder.' DSM-VI has followed its predecessors in retaining the term 'mental disorder' in its title. After extensive consultation and discussion, the Task Force concluded that, despite recent shifts in everyday usage, 'mental disorder' remains the term which most satisfactorily denotes the range of very diverse conditions with which psychiatrists are likely to be concerned professionally in their clinical work and research.*

"*Like all generic terms covering complex ideas, 'mental disorder' is open to misunderstanding. It does **not** imply that mind and body are wholly unconnected (importantly in psychiatry, mental disorders may have bodily causes and vice versa). It does **not** imply a sharp boundary between mental disorders and other conditions (any more than the existence of a distinct medical speciality of psychiatry implies a sharp boundary between psychiatrists and other doctors). It does **not** imply a determinate reference group, a well-defined set of conditions fixed for all time with which psychiatrists are properly concerned (the conditions with which any medical speciality is concerned vary with scientific advances and shifts of social convention). Finally, it does* *not* imply a unitary nosological principle (as in other areas of medicine, clas-sification in psychiatry is heterogeneous). This last point is especially impor-tant. Since DSM-III and ICD-9, psychiatric classification has benefitted from focusing on symptom-based categories of disorder. Most of the categories of disorder in DSM-VI remain similar in this respect to, say, migraine. But the categories of disorder appearing in subsequent editions of DSM are likely to become increasingly heterogeneous with future scientific advances.

"If it is clear what 'mental disorder' does not mean, it is much harder to say what it means. Again, this is characteristic of complex concepts. It is eas-ier to say what 'baroque' does not mean than to say what it means. The 'men-tal' part of 'mental disorder' is more straightforward than the 'disorder' part. 'Mental' denotes the 'higher' brain functions such as affect, thought, volition, desire, belief, intention and action. This is in contrast to the 'lower' functions, such as sensations (e.g. pain, nausea, dizziness) and movements (abnormal movements and paralysis), which, when disturbed, are characteristically 'physical' symptoms.

"The difficulty with the 'disorder' part of 'mental disorder,' although greater than the difficulty with the 'mental,' is not special to psychiatry. Med-icine as a whole lacks an adequate definition of the kinds of problems with which it is properly concerned. All the same, there is an important difference between psychiatry and more technological areas of medicine, namely that in psychiatry what we mean by mental disorder is practically as well as theoret-ically important (e.g. in involuntary civil commitment, in forensic cases, and so on). Hence the attempt in DSM-III (the first in a psychiatric classification) to make the way 'mental disorder' is understood explicit represented an im-portant advance. DSM-VI retains the changes to the definition of mental dis-order introduced in DSM-V. But it spells out, in addition, the points at which attributions of mental disorder depend on judgments of value.

"Thus, in DSM-VI, a disorder (bodily or mental) is defined as 'a syn-drome (or pattern) of behavior and/or experience which is either associated with or consists in clinically significant incapacity of the individual(s) con-cerned. A mental disorder is one in which the incapacity in question primar-ily involves one or more of emotion, thought, desire, volition, intention, belief and action.'

"Incapacity, as used in the above definition, includes but is broader than the notions of disability and dysfunction employed in earlier definitions (for example in DSM-IV). Incapacity implies a disturbance of normal agency; that is, a reduction (in one or more respects and to a greater or lesser degree) in the capacity to do or to experience the things the person concerned is ordi-narily able to do or to experience. Incapacity, so defined, may result from, re-

sult in, or even consist in, disturbances in one or more of the specific functional systems (biological, psychological or social) specified in earlier definitions. But incapacity may also involve loss of agency of a more global kind, defined by reference to the individual as a whole: certain disturbances of personal identity have to be understood in this way.

"Particular disorders (i.e., incapacities or patterns of incapacity) may be stipulated for particular purposes, e.g., legal, administrative, research or clinical. The set of disorders described in this manual are stipulative in this sense. Similarly, the procedures by which stipulatively defined incapacities are identified may be to a greater or lesser extent formalized.

"Stipulative definitions and formal procedures increase the reliability of judgments of incapacity, i.e., the degree of agreement on such judgments. Reliability, however, may be achieved at the expense of validity if its basis (in stipulative definitions and formal procedures designed for particular purposes) is forgotten. Hence, in particular, the inclusion in this manual of a particular category of mental disorder does not imply that the disorder meets legal or other nonmedical criteria for mental disease, mental disorder, or mental disability.

"Modern understanding of the concept of mental disorder, and hence of psychiatric diagnosis, thus extends the role of the psychiatrist as an expert. The psychiatrist is still required to be an expert to the facts. But the range of factual considerations to which he or she is required to be expert is considerably extended; and the basis of expert knowledge is now recognized to be tacit (acquired through experience) as well as explicit (including knowledge of conventional criteria).

"Thus, acting as an expert, the professional can offer clinical judgments of incapacity informed by knowledge and skills which go beyond (but are not thereby necessarily more important than) those of other professionals or of non-professionals (including 'consumers'). A diagnosis of mental disorder must therefore be based on, (1) identification of a relevant pattern or syndrome of experience and/or behavior (mostly but not exclusively those patterns defined stipulatively in current classifications—this is very much as in the twentieth-century medical model); (2) judgments of capacity against expert knowledge of the normal capacities of particular reference groups; and (3) judgments of value against, (a) expert knowledge of the values likely to be relevant (this includes those of the subject themselves, but also caregivers, other professionals, and the wider society), and (b) the values actually held by those directly concerned in the case in question as far as these can be ascertained by the clinician employing his or her skills as an expert. In addition, (4) the psychiatrist may have expert knowledge of causal factors, including brain mechanisms of experience and behavior.

6.5 The DSM-VI Chapter "Schizophrenia and Other Psychotic Disorders." In this section of our report we make specific proposals for changes to the chapter of the DSM concerned with disorders in which psychotic symptoms occur as a defining feature. Corresponding changes would be required for those disorders covered in other chapters of the DSM in which psychotic symptoms may occur but not as a defining feature (e.g., the subtype of Major Depressive Disorder with Psychotic Symptoms).

The following proposals are based on the philosophical theory and field trials summarized in Sections 3 and 4 of the report, respectively, and on the general principles just outlined in Section 6.4 (covering proposals for changes to the introduction to the DSM). As in earlier sections, the text is from the DSM-IV with proposed changes in italics.

6.5.1 Introductory Paragraphs to the DSM Chapter "Schizophrenia and Other Psychotic Disorders" (**p 273, paras 1–3**). "The disorders included in this section are all characterized by having psychotic symptoms as the defining feature. Other disorders *in which psychotic symptoms may occur* (but not as a defining feature) are included elsewhere in the manual (e.g., Major Depressive Disorder, With Psychotic Features, in the 'Mood Disorders' section).

"The term 'psychotic' has historically received a number of different definitions, none of which has achieved universal acceptance. *When the term is used of individual symptoms (as opposed to syndromes),* the narrowest definition of 'psychotic' restricts its use to delusion and to *true* hallucinations, i.e., *hallucinations that (prominent or not) are experienced as normal sensations and/or perceptions. The common phenomenological feature of delusions and true hallucinations is absence of insight. Hence, a slightly wider use of the term includes other experiences and behaviors in which insight is typically absent. These include in particular passivity phenomena, disturbances of agency in which experiences or behaviors normally under one's own control are attributed to some other agency (the symptoms most widely recognized as falling under this description include 'made' affect, movement and volition, and certain forms of thought disorder, such as 'thought insertion'). Note that 'insight' is a term that is used with a number of different meanings in psychiatry. Psychotic loss of insight means, specifically, that the subject believes (and persists in believing) to be real something that most other people are convinced is in the subject's imagination. (Phenomenologically, this is the counterpart of the idea that psychotic symptoms involve loss of ego boundaries.) Psychotic loss of insight is often a mark of pathology. It is particularly important to be aware, therefore, that psychosis is not necessar-*

ily pathological: psychotic experiences (as defined by lack of insight in this specific sense) are now recognized to occur, for example, in some forms of religious experience. Hence, this is one of the areas in which clinical judgment is crucial to the identification of clinically significant psychotic experiences and behavior.

"When the term 'psychotic' is used of syndromes (as distinct from individual symptoms), it means a condition in which clinically significant psychotic symptoms typically (though not necessarily invariably) occur. Psychotic symptoms may be a defining feature of mental disorder (as in this chapter of DSM) or an associated feature (as in other chapters in this manual). Particular psychotic disorders are differentiated by (1) characteristic psychotic symptoms (i.e., clinically significant psychotic experiences or behavior), (2) a variety of associated symptoms, and (3) other descriptive criteria (such as time course, causal factors, and, increasingly, differential sensitivity to antipsychotic drugs as measured by one or more of the biological markers now available).*

"In the case of schizophrenia, important associated symptoms include particular forms of (1) disorganized speech, (2) disorganized behavior, and (3) a variety of so-called negative symptoms. Hence, a diagnosis of schizophrenia may be made in a particular case in the absence of clinically significant psychotic symptoms if associated symptoms are clearly present (conventionally, at least two associated symptoms are generally required . . .*

"The different disorders in this section *thus* emphasize different aspects of the various *meanings* of 'psychotic.' *This is fully consistent with the heterogeneity of medical classifications, especially at times of rapid growth in understanding. In schizophrenia, schizophreniform . . .*" [*Note:* The particular disorders included here will depend on the recommendations of the DSM-VI Work Group on Psychotic Disorders and the DSM-VI Task Force.]

6.5.2 The DSM-IV section on Schizophrenia (**pp. 274 ff.** of DSM-IV). **para 1** "The essential features of schizophrenia are a mixture of characteristic signs and symptoms (both positive and negative) that have been present for a *clinically* significant portion of time during a 1-month period (or for a shorter time if successfully treated), with some signs of the disorder persisting for at least six months (criteria A and C). These signs and symptoms are associated with *clinically significant* social or occupational dysfunction (criterion B). The disturbance is not . . . [here DSM-IV lists excluded conditions and then introduces the range of recognized schizophrenic symptoms. It continues . . .] No single symptom is pathognomonic of schizophrenia. '*Bizarre delusions (as defined below) or true hallucinations, in the form of either a voice keeping up a running commentary on the person's behavior or thoughts, or two or more voices conversing with each other, are sufficient for a diagnosis of schizophrenia (provided the other criteria, B–F, are also satisfied): but* the diagnosis *usually* involves the recognition of a constellation of signs and symptoms associated with *clinically significant* impairment of occupational or social functioning.'

[*Note:* Subsequent paragraphs in the introduction to the section on schizophrenia in the DSM-V included a large number of small drafting charges designed to reduce as far as possible inconsistencies in the uses of key terms that persisted in the DSM-IV. For instance, in para 2 of the DSM-IV version, "delusions" was used to mean "distortions or exaggerations of inferential thinking," whereas in para 3, they became "erroneous beliefs that usually involve a misinterpretation of perceptions or experiences." These definitions implied (unproven) theories of delusion formation and were replaced in the DSM-V with the operational "clinically significant irrational belief with psychotic loss of insight" ("psychotic" being further defined as above—see also Sec. 10 of this report, Glossary of Terms).]

para 4 "Although bizarre delusions are considered to be especially characteristic of schizophrenia, *the clinical judgment of* 'bizarreness' *may be difficult. Delusions are clinically significant irrational beliefs with psychotic loss of insight. Bizarre delusions are clinically significant beliefs with psychotic loss of insight which are judged to be **very** irrational. The diagnosis of* 'bizarre delusion' *is thus a three-step process (although not normally carried out in distinct steps, except in contentious cases): <u>step 1</u> is to establish that there is psychotic loss of insight—this requires a descriptive or (factual) judgment that what the patient believes to be real is believed by most other people to be in his or her imagination; <u>step 2</u> is to establish that the belief is irrational—this is a mixed factual and evaluative judgment, involving such considerations as (a) the extent to which the subject's beliefs, if about matters of fact, are true or false or, (b) if involving value judgments, are consistent or inconsistent with his or her other and previous values; and in either case, (c) the extent to which the subject's beliefs are consistent with the actions (including failures to act) based on them; <u>step 3</u> is to establish that the belief is **very** irrational—this extends step 2 in one or more of its three main components: a belief that is **wholly** implausible as to matters of fact, and/or which expresses values that are **impossible** to understand, and/or which bear no relation to the intentional structure of the subject's actions, would be bizarre in this sense. Given the general criteria for clinical significance* (as above), *a bizarre delusion is necessarily clinically significant. An example of a bizarre* (*factual*) delusion is a person's belief that a stranger has removed his or her internal organs and has replaced them with someone else's organs without leaving any wounds or scars. An example of a nonbizarre (*factual*) delusion is a person's false belief that he or she is under surveillance by the police. *Delusional perceptions (as included in Schneider's list of 'first rank' symptoms) are not necessarily bizarre, although the notion of a 'primary delusion' (i.e., one arising apparently without pathological antecedents) does incorporate some elements of bizarreness in the sense used here (in particular, such delusions are discontinuous with the intentional structure of the subject's thinking). On the other hand, delusional interpretations of passivity experiences* of loss of control over mind or body *(though not the experiences themselves, which may occur in nonpsychotic forms), are generally considered to be bizarre; these experiences include a number of Schneiderian 'first rank' symptoms,* such as a person's belief that his or her thoughts have been taken away by some outside force ('thought withdrawal'), that alien thoughts have been put into his or her mind ('thought insertion'), or that his or her body or actions are being acted on or manipulated by some outside force ('delusions of control'). If the delusions are judged to be bizarre, only this single symptom is needed to satisfy criterion A for schizophrenia."

6.53 The DSM-VI Diagnostic Criteria for Schizophrenia
[Included in Summary Box, pp 285–86, DSM-IV]

Diagnostic Criteria for Schizophrenia

A.   **Characteristic Symptoms**: Two (or more) of the following, each present for a *clinically* significant portion of time during a 1-month period (or less if successfully treated):

(1)   delusions

(2)   *true* hallucinations

(3)   disorganized speech (with specific features, e.g., frequent derailment or incoherence)

(4)   disorganized behavior (*with specific features, e.g., catatonia; to be clinically significant, behavior must normally be grossly disorganized*)

(5)   negative symptoms, i.e., affective flattening, alogia or avolition

NOTE: Only one Criterion A symptom is required if delusions are bizarre or hallucinations consist of a voice keeping up a running commentary on the person's behavior or thought, or two or more voices conversing with each other.

B.   *Deterioration in* social/occupational function: For a *clini-cally* significant portion of the time since the onset of the *disorder,* one or more areas of functioning such as work, in-terpersonal relations, or self-care are markedly below the level achieved prior to the onset; or, when the onset is in childhood or adolescence, *there is marked* failure to achieve expected level(s) of interpersonal, academic, or occupa-tional *functioning. In either case the deterioration in social/ occupational functioning must be judged to be clinically sig-nificant.*

NOTE: *Clinical judgment is required to decide whether a change in (actual or anticipated) social or occupational functioning is clinically significant (i.e., pathological). A clinically significant change in social or occupational functioning is a change (1) for the worse, which (2) arises from or takes the form of incapacity. The values and capacities against which these two elements of clinical significance are respec-tively judged should normally (and always in contentious cases) be made explicit. The subject's own values and normal capacities should always be identified and should normally carry particular weight in the determination of this criterion. The subject's and the clinician's perspectives should be balanced by those of others, including, where appropriate, (1) relatives and caregivers, (2) other health profession-als in multidisciplinary teams, (3) nonclinical groups (e.g., lawyers, social workers, service user and/or advocacy groups, etc., in situations involving interagency cooperation).*

[criteria C–F unchanged]

7.0 Materials for the DSM-VI Sourcebook

In this section we give longer and more complete versions of the ma-terials included in the proposed changes to the introduction to the DSM (Sec. 6.4.4). This covers (1) The Term Mental Disorder, (2) What Mental Disorder Does Not Mean, (3) What Mental Disorder Means, (4) Incapac-ity, (5) Reliability and Validity, (6) Diagnosis, (7) The Role of the Expert, (8) Knowledge of Causes, (9) Culturally Competent Psychiatry, and (10) Individual Human Differences. In each case these materials can be read as drafts for sections of the DSM-VI Sourcebook.

[Note: In this section we have not differentiated between original DSM text and new or redrafted materials.]

7.1 (The Term Mental Disorder). "In earlier editions of DSM misgivings were expressed about the term 'mental disorder.' DSM-IV was openly apologetic about the continued use of this term in the title of the manual (the word 'unfortunately' occurs twice in the opening paragraph of the DSM-IV section on the definition of mental disorder).

"One particularly important result of involving philosophers in DSM-V was to give us a more realistic understanding of the properties of difficult concepts like 'mental disorder,' 'mental illness,' and so on. This led to a number of useful clarifications in the drafting of this section in DSM-V and to a correspondingly clearer approach in practice. Equally important, though, it produced a major shift in the self-image of psychiatry, from what has become known as the 'psychiatry second' mind-set of DSM-IV to the 'psychiatry first' mind-set of DSM-V. That is to say, instead of being apologetic about the difficulties presented by our key concepts, we have come to recognize that they make our discipline more *challenging* (clinically and in research as well as philosophically) than other conceptually-more-straightforward areas of medicine.

"DSM-VI has followed its predecessors in retaining the term 'mental disorder' in its title. After extensive consultation and discussion, the Task Force concluded that, despite recent shifts in everyday usage, 'mental disorder' remains the term which most satisfactorily denotes the range of very diverse conditions with which psychiatrists are likely to be concerned professionally in their clinical work and research."

7.2 (What Mental Disorder Does Not Mean). "Like all generic terms covering complex ideas, 'mental disorder' is open to misunderstanding. It does *not* imply that mind and body are wholly unconnected (importantly in psychiatry, mental disorders may have bodily causes and vice versa). It does *not* imply a sharp boundary between mental disorders and other conditions (any more than the existence of a distinct medical speciality of psychiatry implies a sharp boundary between psychiatrists and other doctors). It does *not* imply a determinate reference group, a well-defined set of conditions fixed for all time with which psychiatrists are properly concerned (the conditions with which any medical speciality is concerned vary with scientific advances and shifts of social convention). Finally, it does *not* imply a unitary nosological principle (as in other areas of medicine, classification in psychiatry is heterogeneous).

"This last point is especially important. Since DSM-III and ICD-9, psychiatric classification has benefitted from focusing on symptom-based categories of disorder. Most of the categories of disorder in DSM-VI remain similar in this respect to, say, migraine. As in physical medicine, however, other kinds of category are likely to become more prominent as we gain a firmer understanding of the causes of mental disorders (for example, categories based on structural pathology [e.g., ulcerative colitis], deviation from a physiological norm [e.g., hypertension], and external agents [e.g., pneumococcal pneumonia]). Medicine has always been opportunistic and pragmatic in the disorders it identifies. Psychiatry has the additional complication that clinically important causes of disorder are likely to be defined in terms of psychological and/or social processes (whatever their ultimate mediation through brain mechanisms). But what all this amounts to is that far from a unitary nosological principle, we should positively expect the categories of disorder appearing in our psychiatric classifications to become increasingly heterogeneous with future scientific advances."

7.3 (What Mental Disorder Means). "If it is clear what 'mental disorder' does *not* mean, it is much harder to say what it *means*. Again, this is characteristic of complex concepts. It is easier to say what 'baroque' does not mean than to say what it means.

"The 'mental' part of 'mental disorder' is more straightforward than the 'disorder' part, provided at least that we are careful to compare like with like, i.e., symptoms with symptoms, rather than conflating symptoms and causes. Understood in this way, then, 'mental' denotes the 'higher' functions such as affect, thought, volition, desire, belief, intention and action. This is in contrast to the 'lower' functions, such as sensations (e.g., pain, nausea, dizziness) and movements (abnormal movements and paralysis), which, when disturbed, are characteristically 'physical' symptoms. Paralysis is a helpful case in point: as a symptom of mental disorder paralysis is a disturbance of intentional action (as in dissociative states); as a symptom of bodily disorder it is a disturbance of movement. There are of course many intermediate and mixed cases.

"The difficulty with 'disorder' in 'mental disorder,' although greater than the difficulty with 'mental,' is not special to psychiatry. Medicine as a whole lacks an adequate definition of the kinds of problems with which it is properly concerned. Indeed much of the twentieth century debate about the meaning of 'mental illness' is now recognized to have been, really, a debate about the meaning of 'physical illness.' All the same, there is an important difference between psychiatry and the more technological areas of medicine, namely that in psychiatry what we mean by mental disorder is practically as well as theoretically important (e.g., in involuntary civil commitment, in "mad or bad" forensic cases, and so on). Hence the attempt in DSM-III (the first in a psychiatric classification) to make the way 'mental disorder' is understood explicit, represented an important advance; and the DSM-III definition was carried over essentially unchanged into DSM-IV. The DSM-III definition, however, depended on a number of elements of 'craft' or 'tacit' knowledge (e.g. in the concept of 'clinical significance'), which, under the influence of the philosophers of science in the DSM-V Task Force, have now been made explicit. The DSM-VI definition retains the changes introduced in DSM-V. But it spells out in addition the points at which attributions of mental disorder depend on judgments of value.

"Thus, in DSM-VI, a disorder (bodily or mental) is defined as 'a syndrome (or pattern) of behavior and/or experience which is either associated with or consists in clinically significant incapacity of the individual(s) concerned. A mental disorder is one in which the incapacity in question primarily involves one or more of emotion, thought, desire, volition, intention, belief and action.'"

7.4 (Incapacity). "This definition of disorder distinguishes between behaviors and/or experiences as such and the incapacity by which behaviors and/or experiences are marked out as pathological: even pain, although figuring prominently in earlier definitions, is only a symptom of disorder if it is associated with (either present or an increased risk of) incapacity. This distinction is especially important in psychiatry. As is now well recognized, even the traditional 'first rank' symptoms of schizophrenia, such as delusional perception, are not necessarily associated with incapacity and may indeed be strongly enabling.

"Incapacity, as used in the above definition of disorder, includes but is broader than the notions of disability and dysfunction employed in earlier definitions (for example in DSM-IV). *Agents* (paradigmatically, persons) have capacities; the *parts* of agents (livers, hearts, etc.) have functions (we speak of agents having functions only where they are parts of society, e.g. as doctors or parents). *In*capacity thus implies a *disturbance* of normal agency; that is, a reduction (in one or more respects and to a greater or lesser degree) in the capacity to do or to experience the things the person concerned is ordinarily able to do or to experience. Incapacity, so defined, may result from, result in, or even consist in, disturbances in one or more of the specific functional systems (biological, psychological or social) specified in earlier definitions. But incapacity may also involve loss of agency in a more global or holistic sense, defined by reference to the individual as a whole: certain disturbances of personal identity have to be understood in this way; and recent work in the philosophy of mind and artificial intelligence, suggest that delusion, a central symptom of mental disorder, is better understood in terms of disturbance of practical reasoning (i.e., of the rationality characteristic of an agent), rather than as a disturbance of cognitive functioning (i.e., as a disturbance in one or more of the specific cognitive systems on which practical reasoning partly depends)."

7.5 (Reliability and Validity). "Particular disorders (i.e., incapacities or patterns of incapacity) may be defined stipulatively for particular purposes, e.g. legal, administrative, research or clinical. The set of disorders described in this manual are stipulative in this sense. Similarly, the procedures by which stipulatively defined incapacities are identified may be to a greater or lesser extent formalized.

"Stipulative definitions and formal procedures increase the reliability of judgments of incapacity i.e. the degree of agreement on such judgments. Reliability, however, may be achieved at the expense of validity if it is forgotten that reliability depends on stipulative definitions and formal procedures designed for particular purposes. This is because judgments of capacity are made, not against absolute standards, but relative to norms defined for the relevant group (the 'reference group').

"Thus according to the medical model prevalent in the twentieth-century, capacities were objectively fixed, much as, say, the length of an object is fixed. Hence judgments of capacity were thought to be more complex than, but otherwise similar in principle to, the measurement of simple physical quantities. We now recognize that on the contrary, judgments of capacity are made relative to a background of, (1) expectations of normal capacities, and (2) a system of values defining good and bad departures from these normal capacities. Where the background is stable, reliability and validity go hand in hand. Both elements of the background, however, may vary widely, between cultures, at different historical times, and, in our heterogeneous society, even between individuals. As between different reference groups, therefore, the reliability of judgments of capacity can certainly be maintained by using stipulative definitions and formal procedures. But the very factors ensuring the reliability of diagnostic judgments in these circumstances will at the same time work to undermine their validity. This is why procedures which should be followed in making these judgments have been included, where relevant, in DSM-VI (for example, the range of value perspectives that should be identified in establishing whether there is clinically significant occupational/social dysfunction as in

Criterion B for schizophrenia—see e.g., Summary Box, at the end of Section 6 above)."

7.6 (Diagnosis). "The above considerations show that diagnosis is a considerably more complex process than had previously been recognized. In the twentieth-century medical model of disorder, doctors were taken to be experts in 'facts' with much the same properties as, say, facts about the length of an object. Modern understanding of the nature of mental disorder shows that this model was plausible only because the background against which the requisite judgments of capacity were made (at least in the dominant disciplines of acute 'high tech' hospital medicine) was relatively stable (in regard both to expectations of normal capacities and to values). In other words, although diagnosis is the same in *principle* in physical medicine as in psychiatry, physical medicine differs from psychiatry in operating (diagnostically) against a background which is largely stable. In physical medicine, therefore, the relativity of judgments of disorder can be ignored for *practical* purposes because the background is (largely) fixed rather than variable.

"This is an important aspect of the recent repolarization in medicine from a 'psychiatry second' mind-set to a mind-set of 'psychiatry first.' Diagnosis in psychiatry is more problematic than in physical medicine, not because psychiatry lacks a proper scientific basis, but because psychiatric diagnosis is a more complex procedure than diagnosis in physical medicine. The simplifications which allow diagnosis in physical medicine to *appear* to be equivalent to objective measures of simple physical properties, are simply not available to us in psychiatry."

7.7 (The Role of the Expert). "Modern understanding of the concept of mental disorder, and hence of psychiatric diagnosis, thus extends the role of the psychiatrist as an expert. In the twentieth-century medical model, the psychiatrist was an expert to the facts (there was much resistance to advising on questions of responsibility, for example). Modern understanding of mental disorder requires that the psychiatrist continues to be an expert to the facts. But the range of factual considerations to which the psychiatrist is required to be expert is considerably extended; and the basis of expert knowledge is now recognized to be tacit (acquired through experience) as well as explicit (including knowledge of conventional criteria). This means that judgments of incapacity are not exclusively a matter for 'experts' (in any field); but the expert, through professional training, gains a praxis-based knowledge of experiences and behaviors which are outside the range of normal. It is this which allows the psychiatrist (or in principle also anyone else with the relevant experience) to make judgments as an expert (in short, 'clinical judgments') of 'clinical significance.'

"Acting as an expert, the professional can offer *clinical* judgments of incapacity informed by knowledge and skills which go beyond (but do not thereby necessarily trump) those of other professionals or of non-professionals (including 'consumers'). A diagnosis of mental disorder should be based on, (1) identification of a relevant pattern or syndrome of experience and/or behavior (mostly but not exclusively those patterns defined stipulatively in current classifications—this is very much as in the twentieth-century medical model); (2) judgments of capacity against expert knowledge of the normal capacities of particular reference groups; and (3) judgments of value against, (a) expert knowledge of the values *likely* to be relevant (this includes those of the subject themselves, but also caregivers, other professionals, and the wider society), and (b) the values *actually* held by those directly concerned in the case in question as far as these can be ascertained by the clinician employing his or her skills as an expert. In addition, (4) the psychiatrist may have expert knowledge of causal factors, including brain mechanisms of experience and behavior."

7.8 (Knowledge of Causes). "Causal factors, like judgments of capacity, have to be handled more carefully in psychiatry than in physical medicine. In physical medicine, because the judgments involved in diagnosis approximate to objective measures of simple physical properties, knowledge of causal factors (often incorporated into disease concepts) has come to be thought of as equivalent to diagnostic judgments of pathology. In psychiatry, correspondingly, it is still sometimes assumed that once we have a more complete neuroscience, psychiatric diagnosis will come to look just like diagnosis in physical medicine, a matter of 'doing tests' on the brain rather as diagnosis in gastroenterology is a matter of 'doing tests' on the liver.

"The expectation, then, is that knowledge of brain science will one day remove the need for making judgments about the experiences of the person concerned. Explanation, on this model, will remove the need for understanding. But causal factors, in our twenty-first century understanding of mental disorder, are now recognized to be the 'dependent variable,' logically speaking—that is, they are defined *as* pathological by the pathological experiences and/or behaviors they cause, rather than vice versa. Hence, if an experience and/or behavior is uncontentiously an illness then its underlying causes will be uncontentiously pathological causes: many disease concepts in physical medicine are defined by such causes; and in these circumstances, diagnosing the disease may be equivalent to diagnosing the illness. But if (as is often the case in psychiatry) the experience and/or behavior of the person concerned is only *contentiously* an illness, then any causal factors, too, will be only *contentiously* pathological, and hence only *contentiously* diseases.

"All this was evident in principle even before recent advances in neuroscientific understanding of brain mechanisms. One unexpected result of these advances, however, has been to make it more, rather than less, important that psychiatrists should have expertise (based on both explicit and 'craft' knowledge) of experiences and behaviors which fall outside the range of most people's everyday experience. So long as the brain remained a 'black box,' there was little practical harm in the illusion that when we could look into the box, when we could explain the mechanisms of experience, the need for expert understanding of experience itself would gradually wither away. This illusion indeed, like many other illusions in the history of science, was a valuable heuristic. It motivated much fruitful research on the brain basis of abnormal experience, which, consistently with the twentieth-century medical model of disorder, was perceived as being on a par with research on the cardiac basis of angina. Conversely, though, it is precisely because we do now have a fairly detailed account of at least some of the brain mechanisms underlying experience, that it has become clear that knowledge of causes is independent of judgments of pathology.

"The first crack in the illusion came, of course, with the way neuroscience itself developed. So long as neuroscience was concerned with the mechanisms of (relatively) simple experiences (such as pain) it could take the nature of these experiences for granted (at least up to a point). Recent advances in our understanding of more complex experiences would not have been possible without the remarkable imaging techniques and AI models developed at the end of the twentieth-century. But as tools for exploring the mechanisms underlying more complex experiences, they remained largely blind until philosophers (notably from phenomenology and philosophy of mind) joined forces with neuroscientists and clinicians to give us sharper conceptual tools for understanding the structures of the experiences themselves.

"Even ten years ago philosophers, neuroscientists and clinicians were still somewhat taken aback to find themselves working together on shared problems. Now, with the perspective of hindsight, we see ourselves as simply taking up where the philosopher-psychiatrist Karl Jaspers left off. Jaspers, the founder of modern descriptive psychopathology, working in the early years of the twentieth-century, repeatedly emphasized the need for meaningful as well as causal explanations of mental disorder. Much of twentieth-century psychiatry was taken up with establishing the pre-conditions for causal explanations. Important among these pre-conditions was the development of reliable symptom-based classifications of mental disorder. But now, in the early years of the twenty-first century, as the labors of twentieth-century psychiatry are at last beginning to pay off, we find that our long-sought causal explanations depend critically on the deeper understanding of meanings to which Jaspers himself pointed."

7.9 (A Culturally Competent Psychiatry). "If, however, the illusion that knowledge of causes is sufficient for judgments of disorder (and hence for diagnosis) was shaken by developments in neuroscience, it was finally shattered by the more humble contingencies of day-to-day practice. An important side effect of the move from institutional to community based mental health services in the closing years of the twentieth-century was a recognition for the first time that patient-centeredness in health care meant patients having a say not only in the treatments they were given (the traditional bioethical principle of autonomy) but also in how their problems were understood in the first place. This inevitably brought values into the diagnostic frame. And this in turn led to the recognition that many of the phenomena by which traditional psychopathology had been defined could occur in positively as well as negatively evaluated forms, and hence were not necessarily pathological at all.

"This was realized first in what was called then cross-cultural psychiatry (DSM-IV had a whole section on cross-cultural issues). But it was quickly recognized that the values in psychiatric diagnosis are endemic to the subject as a whole. This meant 'Western' psychiatry foregoing the favored vantage point which the value-free, exclusively scientific, twentieth-century model of mental disorder seemed to offer. Even in the twentieth-century it was acknowledged that psychiatry, however scientific its self-image, had to be 'culturally sensitive' in the way that it deployed its diagnostic concepts. But with the recognition of the value-relative nature of clinical judgments of mental disorder, the favored vantage point had to be given up altogether. Our twenty-first century model of mental disorder is, literally, culturally de-centered. Such a model, then, generates a psychiatry which, although no less scientific in its genuinely scientific aspects, is culturally competent rather than merely culturally sensitive.

7.10 (Individual Human Differences). "The independence of knowledge of causes and judgments of pathology is, of course, a *logical* independence (i.e., the one does not strictly, or necessarily, imply the other). Hence it remains true that, logically independent as they are, where the relevant diagnostic judgments are uncontentious, knowledge of causes may in practice be used as a short cut to diagnosis no less in psychiatry than in physical medicine. The requisite circumstances must apply, of course: i.e., the background factors against which judgments of capacity are made (expectations of normal capacities and values) must be more or less fixed rather than variable, this in turn making the relevant clinical judgments uncontentious, this in turn making the experience (and/or behavior) in question uncontentiously an illness, and this in turn making the underlying causes of that experience (and/or behavior) uncontentiously a disease.

"Such short cuts have the practical utility of taking us directly to the most effective strategies for treatment and to the best estimates of prognosis. Knowledge of brain mechanisms, similarly, has brought dramatic advances as we move into the new millennium, not only new treatments (more selective antidepressants, notably) but also powerful preventative gene therapies (still limited to monogenic disorders, such as Huntington's; though with encouraging early results for schizophrenia and some forms of Alzheimer's disease). But precisely because these diagnostic shortcuts are so useful, we must be aware of the dangers of *mis*-using them, of trying to take a short cut to diagnosis through knowledge of causation where the key condition for the short cut to be legitimate—that the experience (and/or behavior) in question is uncontentiously an illness—is not satisfied. This is where the short cut ceases to be clinically useful and becomes clinically abusive. For the central thrust of all the recent work on the value structure of medicine and psychiatry has been to show that the contentiousness of judgments of illness in psychiatry turns (in particular though not only) on the diversity of our values as individual human beings (in the areas of experience and/or behavior with which psychiatry is concerned).

"Hence it is only by abolishing a centrally important component of our individual human natures (i.e., value diversity) that developments in brain science, and with them more advanced knowledge of causes, could make diagnostic short cuts as readily available in psychiatry as they are in physical medicine. It would be a sad irony indeed if psychiatry, as the medical discipline above all concerned with people and with individual human differences, should be misled by its very humanitarian concerns into contributing to what the twentieth-century literary scholar, C. S. Lewis, called 'The Abolition of Man.'"

PART III—WIDER CONSIDERATIONS

8.0 Implications for Psychiatric Training and for the Organization of Psychiatric Services

8.1 Psychiatric Training. Recognition of the importance of the tacit or "craft" knowledge involved in clinical judgments, and of the central place of values particularly in *psychiatric* clinical judgments, has led to a number of changes of emphasis in psychiatric training. Familiarity with the descriptive criteria for psychiatric diagnoses remains crucial, this being the key to consistent, and hence reliable, practice. Validity of diagnostic judgments, though, depends on the skills of assessment of capacities and values. Like other clinical skills, these are acquired primarily by practice under expert supervision. Hence, in medical training generally but especially in psychiatry, there has been a much greater emphasis on "hands on" learning.

A departure from tradition, however, has been an extension of the scope of the notion of "expert supervision." Traditionally, this meant feedback from more senior colleagues. Such feedback is still essential. But there is now a greater recognition of the need for feedback also from other professionals and from consumers of services. The effect of this has been to develop a strong sense of interagency cooperation and understanding as the key to psychiatric assessments that are valid (notably from the patient's point of view) as well as reliable.

For those in a more academic stream, the appearance of a growing number of opportunities for trainees to take courses in relevant philosophical disciplines is also to be welcomed. In addition to the generic skills of clear thinking, consistent argument, and an alert eye for meaning, this has given psychiatrists the specific skills needed to work alongside philosophers as successfully as, in the past, they have worked alongside empirical scientists. This has proved to be crucial to the cutting edge work now emerging from the neurosciences. (Philosophers have benefited equally from this new interdisciplinary field.)

8.2 Organization of Psychiatric Services. The key change that we have seen in the organization of services in the early years of this millennium has been an increasingly close and substantive involvement of patients and patient advisory groups (or "consumers") in all aspects of the organization and delivery of mental health services.

This trend is bound to be strengthened as the value judgments involved in psychiatric diagnosis are made increasingly explicit with the publication of the DSM-VI. Thus far, the involvement of users has been an extension of the old medical ethical principle of autonomy. This emphasized that patients should normally be able to choose how they are treated. In psychiatry, in which treatment critically involves social intervention, the notion of autonomy has been extended to cover involvement of patients in the overall resourcing and administration of mental health care. With greater visibility of the relevant value judgments, however, autonomy will come to mean involvement of patients also in their diagnoses. As the British psychiatrist Dr. Allison-Bolger (personal communication), put it, patients will increasingly have a say in how their problems are understood as well as in how they are treated.

That diagnosis involves values, however, will not mean, as some pessimists have feared, diagnostic chaos. Human values, after all, are not chaotic. Indeed, there are encouraging signs that the more explicit recognition of values in psychiatric diagnosis, and hence our greater ability to make clinical judgments that are well balanced and appropriately geared to the needs of individual patients, are making psychiatric diagnosis considerably less chaotic than it used to be. Certainly, it is less often grossly abusive.

9.0   Future Prospects

The picture of science developed by historians and philosophers in the second half of the twentieth century has given us in the twenty-first century a perspective on psychiatry which is quite different from that of our twentieth-century colleagues (Fulford, 2000a, 2000b).

Throughout the twentieth century, psychiatrists perceived their discipline as growing up, evolving steadily out of prescientific mythology as it secured an increasingly secure basis in objective science. We now understand the psychiatry of most of the twentieth century quite differently, that is, as being in a period of what the historian and philosopher Thomas Kuhn (1962) called 'normal "science." At the start of the twentieth century psychiatric science was in a revolutionary period, a period of rapid development and change, in the course of which the work of Jaspers, Kraepelin, and others established a conceptual framework within which empirical research would proceed for most of the century. This research, though, by the end of the century, had issued in developments, notably in neuroscience, which stretched the Jaspers/Kraepelin framework to the point where it was beginning to break down. These are the circumstances in which revolutionary rather than normal science again takes over.

At the start of the twenty-first century, then, we are once more in a revolutionary period, a period of conceptual change driven in this case by technological advance. By its very nature, a period of revolution is a period of uncertainty. The revolution involved in making explicit the value judgments in psychiatric diagnosis is sufficiently radical that we are unlikely to be able to anticipate its full effects with any confidence. What seems certain, though, is that we are in for exciting times before we return to another period of normal science.

Glossary of Terms

A number of closely related terms are used in the DSM and in this report. The following definitions reflect the changes in our understanding of the meanings of these terms in recent years, in particular as they reflect a recognition of the importance of (a) tacit or "craft" knowledge and (b) value judgments in the exercise of clinical skills.

1. Hallucination—a perception in the absence of a normal causal stimulus
2. Delusion—an irrational belief with psychotic loss of insight (not all irrational beliefs involve loss of insight; e.g., obsessional and phobic beliefs)
3. True hallucination—a perception in the absence of a normal causal stimulus which is delusionally believed to be real
4. Psychotic loss of insight—the subject believes and persists in believing to be real something that most other people believe to be in the subject's imagination
5. Pathological loss of insight—clinically significant loss of insight. Note: this usually takes the form of the person concerned understanding his or her experiences, not as something mentally wrong with him or her, but either as something that he or she is doing/has done (e.g., delusions of guilt) or as something that is being done or is happening to him or her (e.g., delusions of persecution and hypochondriacal delusions, respectively).
6. Clinically significant—judged by someone exercising relevant expertise to be clinically significant
7. The exercise of relevant expertise—the actual exercise of clinical judgment by someone with the necessary skills and experience (note that this includes but is not limited to psychiatrists)
8. Clinical judgment of disorder—a judgment that an experience and/or behavior is clinically significant

9. A clinically significant experience and/or behavior—one that is incapacitating, that is, (a) involves *an alteration* of agency as defined by the
   expectations of normal capacities in the subject's reference group and
   (b) is *negatively evaluated* by the value norms of the subject's reference
   group
10. The subject's reference group—the group (defined by age, sex, culture,
    etc.) with which the subject would normally identify

Notes

1. "Values in Psychiatric Nosology," held in Dallas, Tex., December 4–6, 1977, under
   the auspices of the Department of Psychiatry, the University of Texas Southwestern Medical Center at Dallas. In this chapter only, references to the current volume
   are cited as "Sadler, 2002."
2. "Madness, Science and Society: Florence, Renaissance 2000," held in Florence,
   Italy, August 26–29, 2000, under the auspices of the Società Italiana di Psichiatria
   (Italian Society for Psychopathology) and the Royal College of Psychiatrists Philosophy Group. The network referred to is the International Network for Philosophy and Psychiatry.
3. Again, see Fulford (1989) for a fuller account of all these theoretical points, especially chaps. 3, 4, and 5.
4. Bill Fulford and Sidney Bloch (2000) described the differences between physical
   medicine and psychiatry in this respect in one of the first major new textbooks of
   psychiatry this century, *The New Oxford Textbook of Psychiatry*, as the difference
   between a constant and a variable. By analogy with these terms in science, the values involved in diagnosis in physical medicine are a constant, whereas those involved in diagnosis in psychiatry are a variable. This is why these values are by and
   large uncontentious in the former but contentious in the latter.
5. This oversimplifies the framework to the extent that a value term need not express
   a value judgment directly. The more accurate way of putting it is to say that a value
   term is a term the meaning of which includes an evaluative element. This evaluative element of meaning may be deeply hidden but remains operative in the way
   the term is used. *Disease* is an example of such a term. According to nondescriptivist ethical theory, disease carries overtly descriptive meaning; yet the way the
   term is actually used (not least by philosophers, like Boorse, 1975, espousing a
   value-free definition of the term) can only be explained on the basis that, although
   masked by its descriptive meaning, there is also an essential evaluative element in
   the meaning of the term. See Fulford (1989, chaps. 3 and 6); also Fulford (2000b,
   esp. pts. 2 and 3).
6. Criterion A for Conduct Disorder, for example, starts with "A repetitive and persistent pattern of behavior in which the basic *rights* of others or major age-appropriate societal *norms or rules* are violated" (American Psychiatric Association, 1994,
   p. 90; emphasis added).

References

Achenbach, Thomas M. 1980. DSM-III in light of empirical research on the classification of child psychopathology. *Journal of the American Academy of Child Psychiatry* 19:395–412.

Agich, G. J. 1983. Disease and value: A rejection of the value neutrality thesis. *Theoretical Medicine* 4:27–41.

———. 1994. Evaluative judgment and personality disorder. In J. Z. Sadler, O. P. Wiggins, and M. A. Schwartz, eds., *Philosophical Perspectives on Psychiatric Diagnostic Classification*, pp. 233–45. Baltimore: Johns Hopkins University Press.

———. 1997. Toward a pragmatic theory of disease. In J. M. Humber and R. F. Almeder, eds., *What Is Disease?*, pp. 221–46. Totowa, NJ: Humana Press.

Ake v. Oklahoma, 470 US 68 (1985).

Allison-Bolger, V. Y. Personal communication.

American Psychiatric Association. 1952. *Diagnostic and Statistical Manual of Mental Disorders*. Washington, DC: American Psychiatric Association.

———. 1968. *Diagnostic and Statistical Manual of Mental Disorders*. 2d ed. Washington, DC: American Psychiatric Association.

———. 1980. *Diagnostic and Statistical Manual of Mental Disorders*. 3d ed. Washington, DC: American Psychiatric Association.

———. 1987. *Diagnostic and Statistical Manual of Mental Disorders*. 3d ed., rev. Washington, DC: American Psychiatric Association.

———. 1991. *DSM-IV Options Book—Work in Progress*. Washington, DC: American Psychiatric Association.

———. 1993a. *DSM-IV Draft Criteria*. Washington, DC: American Psychiatric Association.

———. 1993b. *Official Ballot for APA Officers, Amendments, and Referendum.* Washington, DC: American Psychiatric Association.

———. 1994. *Diagnostic and Statistical Manual of Mental Disorders.* 4th ed. Washington, DC: American Psychiatric Association.

———. 1995a. *Diagnostic and Statistical Manual of Mental Disorders.* 4th ed., International Version. Washington, DC: American Psychiatric Association.

———. 1995b. *Diagnostic and Statistical Manual of Mental Disorders.* 4th ed., Primary Care Version. Washington, DC: American Psychiatric Association.

Andrews, L., Fullarton, J., Holtzman, N., and Motulsky, A. 1994. *Assessing Genetic Risks.* Washington, DC: National Academy Press.

Antonorakis, S. E., Blouin, J.-L., Pulver, A. E., Wolyniec, P., Lasseter, V. K., Nestadt, G., Kasch, L., Babb, R., Kazazian, H. H., Dombroski, B., Kimberland, M., Ott, J., Housman, D., Karayiorgou, M., MacLean, C. J. 1995. Schizophrenia susceptibility and Chromosome 6p24-22. *Nature Genetics* 11:23–236.

Anzaldua, G. 1987. *Borderlands / La Frontera: The New Mestiza.* San Francisco: Aunt Lute.

Aristotle. 1941a. *Metaphysics.* In R. McKeon, ed., trans., *The Basic Works of Aristotle,* pp. 691, 953, 981. New York: Random House.

———. 1941b. *Nichomachean Ethics.* In R. McKeon, ed., trans., *The Basic Works of Aristotle,* pp. 1028–29. New York: Random House.

Atkinson, P. 1995. *Medical Talk and Medical Work: The Liturgy of the Clinic.* London: Sage.

Barefoot v. Estelle, 463 US 880 (1983).

Barrett, R. 1988. Clinical writing and the documentary construction of schizophrenia. *Culture, Medicine, and Psychiatry* 12:265–99.

Bartley, W. W. 1984. *The Retreat to Commitment,* 2d ed. New York: Knopf.

Bayer, R. 1981. *Homosexuality and American Psychiatry.* New York: Basic Books.

———. 1987. Politics, science, and the problem of psychiatric nomenclature: A case study of the American Psychiatric Association referendum on homosexuality. In H. T. Engelhardt Jr. and A. Caplan, eds., *Scientific Controversies: Case Studies in the Resolution and Closure of Dispute in Science and Technology,* pp. 381–100. Cambridge: Cambridge University Press.

Bayer, R., and Spitzer, R. L. 1982. Edited correspondence on the status of homosexuality in DSM-III. *Journal of the History of the Behavioral Sciences* 18:32–52.

———. 1985. Neurosis, psychodynamics, and DSM-III: A history of the controversy. *Archives of General Psychiatry* 42:187–95.

Bazerman, C. 1995. Influencing and being influenced: Local acts across large distances. *Social Epistemology* 2:189–99.

Benjamin, L. 1993. *Interpersonal Diagnosis and Treatment of Personality Disorders.* New York: Guilford Press.

Beresford, E. 1996. Can phronesis save the life of medical ethics? *Theoretical Medicine* 17: 209–23.

Bergner, R. M. 1997. What is psychopathology? And so what? *Clinical Psychology: Science and Practice* 4:235–48.

Berkenkotter, C., and Huckin, T. N. 1995. *Genre Knowledge in Disciplinary Communication: Cognition/Culture/Power.* Hillsdale, NJ: Erlbaum.

Berkenkotter, C., and Ravotas, D. 1997. The function of genre in the transmission of practice over time and across professional boundaries. *Mind, Culture, and Activity* 4 (4): 256–74.

Berner, P., Katschnig, H., and Lenz, G. 1986. The polydiagnostic approach in research on schizophrenia. In A. M. Freedman, R. Brotman, I. Silverman, and D. Hutson, eds., *Issues in Psychiatric Classification: Science, Practice, and Social Policy,* pp. 70–91. New York: Human Sciences Press.

Berofsky, B. 1995. *Liberation from Self: A Theory of Personal Autonomy.* Cambridge: Cambridge University Press.

Berrios, G. E. 1996. *The History of Mental Symptoms: Psychopathology since the Nineteenth Century.* Cambridge: Cambridge University Press.

Berrios, G. E., and Freeman, H., eds. 1991. *150 Years of British Psychiatry, 1841–1991.* London: Gaskell.

Berrios, G. E., and Porter, P. 1995. *A History of Clinical Psychiatry: The Origin and History of Psychiatric Disorders.* London: Athlone Press.

Bertelsen, A., and Gottesman, I. I. 1995. Schizoaffective psychoses—genetical clues to classification. *American Journal of Medical Genetics* 60: 7–11.

Bickman, L., Guthrie, P. R., Foster, E. M., Lambert, E. W., Summerfelt, W. T., Breda, C. S., and Heflinger, C. A. 1995. *Evaluating Managed Mental Health Services: The Fort Bragg Experiment.* New York: Plenum Press.

Bijker, W., Hughes, T., and Pinch, T., eds. 1984. *The Social Construction of Technological Systems: New Directions in the Sociology and History of Technology.* Cambridge: MIT Press.

Black, D. W., and Andreasen, N. C. 1994. Schizophrenia, schizophreniform disorder, and delusional (paranoid) disorder. In R. E. Hales, S. C. Yudofsky, and J. A. Talbott, eds., *Textbook of Psychiatry,* 2d ed., pp. 411–63. Washington, DC: American Psychiatric Press.

Blashfield, R. K. 1982. Invisible colleges and the Matthew Effect. *Schizophrenia Bulletin* 8:1–6.

———. 1984. *The Classification of Psychopathology: Neo-Kraepelinian and Quantitative Approaches.* New York: Plenum Press.

Blashfield, R. K., Blum, N., and Pfohl, B. 1992. The effects of changing Axis II diagnostic criteria. *Comprehensive Psychiatry* 33:245–52.

Blashfield, R. K., and Livesley, W. J. 1991. Metaphorical analysis of psychiatric classification as a psychological test. *Journal of Abnormal Psychology* 100: 262–70.

Blashfield, R. K., Sprock, J., and Fuller, A. K. 1990. Suggested guidelines for including/excluding categories in the DSM-IV. *Comprehensive Psychiatry* 31:15–19.

Blashfield, R. K., Sprock, J., Haymaker, D., and Hodgin, J. 1989. The family resemblance hypothesis applied to psychiatric classification. *Journal of Nervous and Mental Disease* 177:492–97.

Bliss, M. 1982. *The Discovery of Insulin.* Chicago: University of Chicago Press.

Board of Directors of the American Society of Human Genetics. 1996. ASHG report: Statement on informed consent for genetic research. *American Journal of Human Genetics* 59:471–74.

Boden, M. A. 1990. *The Creative Mind: Myths and Mechanisms.* London: Butler and Tanner.

Boorse, C. 1975. On the distinction between illness and disease. *Philosophy and Public Affairs* 5 (Fall): 49–68.

———. 1976. What a theory of mental health should be. *Journal of Theory of Social Behavior* 6:61–84.

———. 1982. What a theory of mental health should be. In R. B. Edwards, ed., *Psychiatry and Ethics,* pp.29–49. Buffalo: Prometheus Books.

———. 1987. Concepts of health. In D. Van De Ver and T. Regan, eds., *Health Care Ethics: An Introduction,* pp. 359–93. Philadelphia: Temple University Press.

Bornstein, R. F. 1997. Dependent personality disorder in the DSM-IV and beyond. *Clinical Psychology: Science and Practice* 4:175–87.

Bowker, G. C., and Star, S. L. 1999. *Sorting Things Out: Classification and Its Consequences.* Cambridge: MIT Press.

Bracken, P. Forthcoming. *Meaning and Trauma in the Post-Modern Age: Heidegger and a New Direction for Psychiatry.* London: Whurr Books.

Brand, M. 1976. *The Nature of Causation.* Urbana: University of Illinois Press.

Braude, S. 1991. *First Person Plural: Multiple Personality and the Philosophy of Mind.* London: Routledge.

Brinkman, R. R., Mezei, M. M., Theilmann, J., Almqvist, E., and Hayden, M. R. 1997. The likelihood of being affected with Huntington-disease by a particular age, for a specific CAG size. *American Journal of Human Genetics* 60:1202–10.

Brown, P. 1990. The name game: Toward a sociology of diagosis. *Journal of Mind and Behavior* 11 (3, 4): 385–407.

"Call for Papers: Values in Psychiatric Nosology: A Conference for Philosophers and Mental Health Clinicians." 1997. Department of Psychiatry, the University of Texas Southwestern Medical Center.

Cantor, N. 1990. From thought to behavior: "Having" and "doing" in the study of personality and cognition. *American Psychologist* 45:735–50.

Caplan, P. J. 1991a. How *do* they decide who is normal? The bizarre, but true, tale of the *DSM* process. *Canadian Psychology / Psychologie Canadienne* 32:162–70.

———. 1991b. Response to the DSM wizard. *Canadian Psychology / Psychologie Canadienne* 32:174–75.

———. 1995. *They Say You're Crazy: How the World's Most Powerful Psychiatrists Decide Who's Normal.* Reading, MA: Addison-Wesley.

Caplan, P. J., McCurdy-Myers, J., and Gans, M. 1992. Should "premenstrual syndrome" be called a psychiatric abnormality? *Feminism and Psychology* 2:27–44.

Capps, L., and Ochs, E. 1995. *Constructing Panic: The Discourse of Agoraphobia.* Cambridge: Harvard University Press.

Cardno, A. G., Marshall, E. J., Macdonald, A. M., Coid, B., Ribchester, T. R., Davies, N. J., Venturi, P., Jones, L. A., Lewis, S. W., Sham, P. C., Gottesman, I. I., Farmer, A. E., McGuffin, P., Reveley, A. M., Murray, R. M. 1999. Heritability estimates for psychotic disorders: The Maudsley twin psychosis series. *Archives of General Psychiatry* 56:162–68.

Carey, G. 1987. Big genes, little genes, affective disorder, and anxiety: A commentary. *Archives of General Psychiatry* 44:486–91.

Carpenter, W. T., Strauss, J. S., and Bortko, J. J. 1973. Flexible system for the diagnosis of schizophrenia: Report from the World Health Organization International Pilot Study of Schizophrenia. *Science* 182:1275–78.

Carson, R. C. 1991. Dilemmas in the pathway of the DSM-IV. *Journal of Abnormal Psychology* 100:302–7.

———. 1996. Aristotle, Galileo, and the DSM taxonomy: The case of schizophrenia. *Journal of Consulting and Clinical Psychology* 64:1133–39.

Cattell, R. B. 1983. Let's end the duel. *American Psychologist* 38:769–76.

Cauwels, J. 1992. *Imbroglio: Rising to the Challenge of Borderline Personality Disorder.* New York: W. W. Norton.

Cawley, R. H. 1993. Psychiatry is more than a science. *British Journal of Psychiatry* 162:154- 60.

Chapin, J. B. 1880. Experts and expert testimony. *Albany Law Journal* 22:365–67.

Chessick, R. 1993. The outpatient psychotherapy of the borderline patient. *American Journal of Psychotherapy* 47: 206–27.

Chodoff, P. 1986. DSM-III and psychotherapy. (Editorial). *American Journal of Psychiatry* 143 (2): 201–3.

Clark, H., and Gerrig, R. J. 1990. Quotations as demonstrations. *Language* 66:764–805.

Clark, L. A., and Watson, D. 1996. Constructing validity: Basic issues in scale development. *Psychological Assessment* 7: 309–19.

Clark, L. A., Watson, D., and Reynolds, S. 1995. Diagnosis and classification of psychopathology: Challenges to the current system and future directions. *Annual Review of Psychology* 46:121–53.

Cloninger, R. C., Martin, R. L., Guze, S. R., and Clayton, P. J. 1986. Somatization in men and women: A prospective follow-up and family study. *American Journal of Psychiatry* 143:873–78.

Clouser, K. 1977. Clinical medicine as science. *Journal of Medicine and Philosophy* 2:1–7.

Collingwood, R. G. 1940. *An Essay on Metaphysics.* Oxford: Clarendon Press.

———. 1945. *The Idea of Nature.* Oxford: Clarendon Press.

Collins, F. S. 1999. Shattuck lecture: Medical and societal consequences of the human genome project. *New England Journal of Medicine* 341 (1): 28–37.

Collins, F. S., Guyer, M. S., and Chakravarti, A. 1997. Variations on a theme: Cataloging human DNA sequence variation. *Science* 278:1580–81.

Connolly, W. E. 1987. *Politics and Ambiguity.* Madison: University of Wisconsin Press.

Cooper, A. M., and Michels, R. 1988. Book review of DSM-III-R. *American Journal of Psychiatry* 145 (10): 1300–1301.

Cooper, H. M. 1984. *The Integrative Research Review.* Beverly Hills, CA: Sage.

Cooper, J. E. 1995. On the publication of the *Diagnostic and Statistical Manual of Mental Disorders:* Fourth Edition (DSM-IV). *British Journal of Psychiatry* 166:4–8.

Corning, W. C. 1986. Bootstrapping toward a classification system. In T. Millon and G. L. Klerman, eds., *Contemporary Directions in Psychopathology,* pp. 279–303. New York: Guilford Press.

Cosmides, L., and Tooby, J. 1999. Toward an evolutionary taxonomy of treatable conditions. *Journal of Abnormal Psychology* 108:453–64.

Cronbach, L. J., and Meehl, P. 1955. Construct validity in psychological tests. *Psychological Bulletin* 52:281–302. Also reprinted in Meehl, P. 1973. *Psychodiagnosis: Selected Papers,* pp. 3–31. Minneapolis: University of Minnesota Press.

Crow, T .J. 1998. From Kraepelin to Kretschmer leavened by Schneider: The transition from categories of psychosis to dimensions of variation intrinsic to Homo Sapiens. *Archives of General Psychiatry* 55:502–4.

Culver, C. M., and Gert, B. 1982. *Philosophy in Medicine: Conceptual and Ethical Issues in Medicine and Philosophy.* New York: Oxford University Press.

Cushman, P. 1995. *Constructing the Self.* New York: Addison-Wesley.

Damasio, A. R. 1994. *Descartes' Error: Emotion, Reason, and the Human Brain.* New York: G. P. Putnam's Sons.

Daubert v. Merrell Dow Pharmaceuticals, Inc., 113 S. Ct. 2786 (1993).

Davidson, D. 1984. *Inquiries into Truth and Interpretation.* Oxford: Oxford University Press.

Davis, L. J. 1997. The encyclopedia of insanity: A psychiatric handbook lists a madness for everyone. *Harper's Magazine* (February): 61–66.

Davis, W., Widiger, T. A., Frances, A. J., Pincus, H. A., Ross, R., and First, M. B. 1998. Introduction to final volume. In T. A. Widiger, A. J. Frances, H. A. Pincus, R. Ross, M. B. First, and M. Kline, eds., *DSM-IV Sourcebook,* 4:1–15. Washington, DC: American Psychiatric Association.

Dawes, R. M. 1994. *House of Cards: Psychology and Psychotherapy Built on Myth.* New York: Free Press.

Dawes, R. M., Faust, D., and Meehl, P. E. 1989. Clinical versus actuarial judgment. *Science* 243:1668-74.

Denton, W. H. 1989. DSM-III-R and the family therapist: Ethical considerations. *Journal of Marital and Family Therapy* 15 (4): 367–77.

Docherty, J. 1992. To know borderline personality disorder. In John F. Clarkin, Elsa Marziali, and Heather Munroe-Blum, eds., *Borderline Personality Disorder: Clinical and Empirical Perspectives*, pp. 329–38. New York: Guilford Press.

Dreier, O. 1993. Re-searching psychotherapeutic practice. In S. Chaiklin and J. Lave, eds., *Understanding Practice: Perspectives on Activity and Context*, pp. 104–24. Cambridge: Cambridge University Press.

Dumont, M. P. 1987. A diagnostic parable (first edition—unrevised). *Readings: A Journal of Reviews and Commentary in Mental Health* (December): 9–12.

Dunne, J. 1993. *Back to the Rough Ground: "Phronesis" and "Techne" in Modern Philosophy and in Aristotle*. Notre Dame: University of Notre Dame Press.

Earman, J. 1986. *A Primer on Determinism*. Dordrecht, the Netherlands: Kluwer.

Edwards, R. B. 1981. Mental health as rational autonomy. *Journal of Medicine and Philosophy* 6:309–22.

Egan, S. E., and Weinberg, R. A. 1993. The pathway to signal achievement. *Nature* 365:781–83.

Elliott, C. 1996. *The Rules of Insanity: Moral Responsibility and the Mentally Ill Offender*. Albany: SUNY Press.

Engelhardt, Jr., H. T. 1975. The concepts of health and disease. In H. T. Engelhardt Jr. and S. F. Spicker, eds., *Evaluation and Explanation in the Biomedical Sciences*, pp. 125–41. Dordrecht, the Netherlands: D. Reidel Publishing.

———. 1996. *The Foundations of Bioethics*, 2d ed. New York: Oxford University Press.

Engeström, R. 1995. Voice as communicative action. *Mind, Culture, and Activity* 2 (3): 192–215.

Engeström, Y. 1993. Developmental studies of work as a testbench of actvity theory: The case of primary care medical practice. In S. Chaiklin and J. Lave, eds., *Understanding Practice: Perspectives on Activity and Context*, pp. 63–104. Cambridge: Cambridge University Press.

Eysenck, H. J. 1970. A dimensional system of psychodiagnostics. In A. R. Mahrer, ed., *New Approaches to Personality Classification*, pp. 169–208. New York: Columbia University Press.

———. 1986. A critique of contemporary classification and diagnosis. In T. Millon and G. L. Klerman, eds., *Contemporary Directions in Psychopathology: Toward the DSM-IV*, pp. 73–98. New York: Guilford Press.

———. 1994. Normality-abnormality and the three-factor model of personality. In S. Strack and M. Lorr, eds., *Differentiating Normal and Abnormal Personality*, pp. 3–25. New York: Springer.

Eysenck, H. J., and Rachman, S. 1957. *The Causes and Cures of Neurosis*. San Diego, CA: Robert R. Knapp.

Faber, K. 1923. *Nosography in Modern Internal Medicine*. New York: Hoeber.

Fabrega, H., Jr. 1992. Diagnosis interminable: Toward a culturally sensitive DSM-IV. *Journal of Nervous and Mental Disease* 180 (1): 5–7.

Faigman, D. L., Porter, E., and Saks, M. J. 1994. Check your crystal ball at the courthouse door, please: Exploring the past, understanding the present, and worrying about the future of scientific evidence. *Cardozo Law Review* 15:1101–36.

Faraone, S. V., Biederman, J., Mennin, D., and Russell, R. 1998. Bipolar and antisocial disorders among relatives of ADHD children: Parsing familial subtypes of illness. *American Journal of Medical Genetics* 81:108–16.

Farber, S. 1993. *Madness, Heresy, and the Rumor of Angels.* New York: Open Court.

Farmer, A., McGuffin, P., and Gottesman, I. I. 1984. Searching for the split in schizophrenia. *Psychiatry Research* 13:109–18.

———. 1987. Twin concordance for DSM-III schizophrenia: Scrutinizing the validity of the definition. *Archives of General Psychiatry* 44:634–41.

Farmer, A. E., Williams, J., and Jones, I. 1994. Phenotypic definitions of psychotic illness for molecular genetic research. *American Journal of Medical Genetics (Neuropsychiatric Genetics)* 54: 365–371.

Faust, D., and Miner, R. A. 1986. The empiricist and his new clothes: *DSM-III* in perspective. *American Journal of Psychiatry* 143 (8): 962–67.

Fed. R. Evid. 702, 1974.

Feighner, J. P., Robins, E., Guze, S. B., Woodruff, R. A., Winokur, G., and Munoz, R. 1972. Diagnostic criteria for use in psychiatric research. *Archives of General Psychiatry* 26:57–63.

Feinstein, A. R. 1977. A critical overview of diagnosis in psychiatry. In V. M. Rakoff, H. C. Stancer, and H. B. Redward, eds., *Psychiatric Diagnosis,* pp. 189–206. New York: Brunner/Mazel.

Ferrara, K. W. 1994. *Therapeutic Ways with Words.* New York: Oxford University Press.

Feskens, E. J. M., Havekes, L. M., Kalmjin, S., de Knijff, P., Launer, L. J., and Kromhout, D. 1994. Apolipoprotein e4 allele and cognitive decline in elderly men. *British Medical Journal* 309:1202–7.

Feyerabend, P. 1978. *Against Method.* London: Verso.

———. 1988. *Against Method.* New York: Routledge, Chapman, & Hall.

———. 1991. Gods and atoms: Comments on the problem of reality. In D. Cicchetti and W. M. Grove, eds., *Thinking Clearly about Psychology,* 1:91–99. Minneapolis: University of Minnesota Press.

Fields, L. 1996. Psychopathology, other-regarding moral beliefs, and responsibility. *Philosophy, Psychiatry, and Psychology* 3 (4): 261–77.

Fiester, S. J. 1997. Nicotine use disorder. In A. Tasman, J. Kay, and J. A. Lieberman, eds., *Psychiatry,* 1:853–66. Philadelpha: W. B. Saunders.

Fingarette, H. 1988. *Heavy Drinking: The Myth of Alcoholism as a Disease.* Berkeley: University of California Press.

Flaum, M., Amador, X., Gorman, J., Bracha, H. S., Edell, W., McGlashan, T., Pandurangi, A., Kendler, K. S., Robinson, D., Lieberman, J., Ontiveros, A., Tohen, M., McGorry, P., Tyrrell, G., Arndt, S., and Andreasen, N. C. 1998. Field trial for schizophrenia and other psychotic disorders. In T. A. Widiger, A. J. Frances, H.

A. Pincus, R. Ross, M. B. First, W. Davis, and M. Kline, eds., *DSM-IV Source Book,* 4:687–713. Washington, DC: American Psychiatric Association.

Flexner, A. 1915. Is social work a profession? In *Proceedings of the National Conference of Charities and Correction, 42nd Annual Meeting,* Baltimore, May 12–19, 1915. Chicago: National Conference of Charities and Correction.

Follette, W. C., and Houts, A. C. 1996. Models of scientific progress and the role of theory in taxonomy development: A case study of the DSM. *Journal of Consulting and Clinical Psychology* 64:1120–32.

Forstrom, L. 1977. The scientific autonomy of clinical medicine. *Journal of Medicine and Philosophy* 2:8- 19.

Foucault, M. 1965. *Madness and Civilization.* Trans. R. Howard. New York: Random House.

———. 1970. *The Order of Things: An Archaeology of the Human Sciences.* New York: Vintage Books.

———. 1980. *Power/Knowledge.* Trans. C. Gordon. New York: Pantheon Books.

———. 1987. *Mental Illness and Psychology.* Trans. A. Sheridan. Berkeley: University of California Press.

———. 1990. *History of Sexuality.* Trans. R. Hurley. New York: Vintage Books.

Frances, A. J. 1982. Categorical and dimensional systems of personality diagnosis: A comparison. *Comprehensive Psychiatry* 23:516–27.

Frances, A. J., First, M. B., and Pincus, H. A. 1995. *DSM-IV Guidebook: The Essential Companion to the Diagnostic and Statistical Manual of Mental Disorders, Fourth Edition.* Washington, DC: American Psychiatric Press.

Frances, A. J., First, M. B., Widiger, T. A., Miele, G. M., Tilly, S. M., Davis, W. W., and Pincus, H. A. 1991. An A-Z guide to DSM-IV conundrums. *Journal of Abnormal Psychology* 100 (3): 407–12.

Frances, A. J., Pincus, H. A., Widiger, T. A., Davis, W. W., and First, M. B. 1990. DSM-IV: Work in progress. *American Journal of Psychiatry* 147:1439–48.

Frances, A. J. , Pincus, H. A., Widiger, T. A., First, M. B., Davis, W. W., Hall, W.,Mc Kinney, K., and Stayna, H. 1994. DSM-IV and international communication in psychiatric diagnosis. In J. E. Mezzich, Y. Honda, and M. C. Kastrup, eds., *Psychiatric Diagnosis: A World Perspective,* pp. 11–23. New York: Springer-Verlag.

Frances, A. J., Widiger, T. A., First, M. B., Pincus, H. A., Tilly, S., Miele, G., and Davis, W. W . 1991. DSM-IV: Toward a more empirical diagnostic system. *Canadian Psychology* 32:171–73.

Frances, A. J., Widiger, T. A., and Pincus, H. A. 1989. The development of DSM-IV. *Archives of General Psychiatry* 46:373–75.

Frankfurt, H. 1976. Identification and externality. In A. O. Rorty, ed., *The Identity of Persons,* pp. 239–51. Berkeley: University of California Press.

———. 1987. Identification and wholeheartedness. In F. Schoeman, ed., *Responsibility, Character, and the Emotions: New Essays in Moral Psychology,* pp. 27–45. New York: Cambridge University Press.

————. 1988. *The Importance of What We Care About*. New York: Cambridge University Press.

Freedman, A. M., Brotman, R., Silverman, I., and Hutson, D., eds. 1986. *Issues in Psychiatric Classification: Science, Practice, and Social Policy*. New York: Human Sciences Press.

Freedman, J., and Combs, G. 1996. *Narrative Therapy: the Social Construction of Preferred Realities*. New York: W. W. Norton.

Frye v. United States, 293 F. 1013 (D.C. Cir. 1923).

Fulford, K. W. M. 1989. *Moral Theory and Medical Practice*. Cambridge: Cambridge University Press (reprinted 1991 and 1995; 2d ed. forthcoming).

————. 1991. The concept of disease. In S. Bloch and B. Chodoff, eds., *Psychiatric Ethics*, 2d ed. Oxford: Oxford University Press.

————.1993. Value, action, mental illness, and the law. In S. Shute, J. Gardner, and J. Horder, eds., *Action and Value in Criminal Law*, pp. 279–310. Oxford: Oxford University Press.

————. 1994. Closet logics: Hidden conceptual elements in the DSM and ICD classifications of mental disorders. In J. Z. Sadler, O. P. Wiggins, and M. A. Schwartz, eds., *Philosophical Perspectives on Psychiatric Diagnostic Classification*, pp. 211–32. Baltimore: Johns Hopkins University Press.

————. 1999. From culturally sensitive to culturally competent: A seminar in philosophy and practice skills. In K. Bhui and D. Olajide, eds., *Mental Health Service Provision for a Multi-cultural Society*, pp. 21–42. London: W. B. Saunders.

————. 2000a. Philosophy meets psychiatry in the twentieth century: Four looks back and a brief look forward. In P. Louhiala and S. Stenman, eds., *Philosophy Meets Medicine*, pp. 114–31. Helsinki: Helsinki University Press.

————. 2000b. Teleology without tears: Naturalism, neo-naturalism, and evaluationism in the analysis of function statements in biology (and a bet on the twenty-first century). *Philosophy, Psychiatry, and Psychology* 7 (1): 77–94.

————. Forthcoming. Philosophy into practice: The case for ordinary language philosophy. In L. Nordenfelt, ed., *Health, Science, and Ordinary Language*, chap. 2. Amsterdam: Rodopi.

Fulford, K. W. M., and Bloch, S. 2000. Psychiatric ethics: Codes, concepts, and clinical practice skills. In M. G. Gelder, J. López-Ibor, and N. Andreasen, eds., *New Oxford Textbook of Psychiatry*, pp. 27–32. Oxford: Oxford University Press.

Fulker, D. W., and Cardon, L. R. 1993. What can twin studies tell us about the structure and correlates of cognitive abilities? In T. J. Bouchard Jr. and P. Propping, eds., *Twins as a Tool of Behavioral Genetics*, pp. 33–52. Chichester: John Wiley.

Gadamer, H. G. 1975. *Truth and Method*. Trans. G. Barden and J. Cumming. New York: Continuum Press.

Galeano, E. 1976. In defense of the word: Leaving Buenos Aries 1976. In R. Simmonson and S. Walker, eds., *Multicultural Literacy*, pp. 113–25. St. Paul, MN: Greywolf Press.

Garfield, S. L. 1986. Problems in diagnostic classification. In T. Millon and G. L.

Klerman, eds., *Contemporary Directions in Psychopathology: Toward the DSM-IV,* pp. 99–113. New York: Guilford Press.

Gasking, D. 1955. Causation and recipes. *Mind* 6:479–87.

Gelder, M. G. 2000. *New Oxford Textbook of Psychiatry.* Oxford: Oxford University Press.

Genero, N., and Cantor, N. 1987. Exemplar prototypes and clinical diagnosis: Toward a cognitive economy. *Journal of Social and Clinical Psychology* 5:59–78.

Gershon, E. S., and Cloninger, C. R., eds. 1994. *Genetic Approaches to Mental Disorders.* Washington, DC: American Psychiatric Press.

Giddens, A. 1984. *The Constitution of Society: Outline of a Theory of Structuration.* Berkeley: University of California Press.

Gilbert, W. 1992. A vision of the grail. In D. Kevles and L. Hood, eds., *Code of Codes,* pp. 83–97. Cambridge: Harvard University Press.

Glymour, C. 1986. Comment: Statistics and metaphysics. *Journal of the American Statistical Association* 81:964–66.

Goldstein, W. 1993. Psychotherapy with borderline patients: An introduction. *American Journal of Psychotherapy* 47:172–83.

Goodman, A. 1994. Pragmatic assessment and multithcorctical classification: Addictive disorder as a case example. In J. Z. Sadler, O. P. Wiggins, and M. A. Schwartz, eds., *Philosophical Perspectives on Psychiatric Diagnostic Classification,* pp. 295–311. Baltimore: Johns Hopkins University Press.

Goodwin, C. 1996. Professional vision. *American Anthropologist* 96 (3): 606–33.

Goodwin, D. W., and Guze, S. 1994. *Psychiatric Diagnosis.* New York: Oxford University Press.

———. 1996. *Psychiatric Diagnosis,* 5th ed. New York: Oxford University Press.

Gorenstein, E. E. 1992. *The Science of Mental Illness.* New York: Academic Press.

Gorovitz, S., and MacIntyre, A. 1976. Toward a theory of medical fallibility. *Journal of Medicine and Philosophy* 1:51–71.

Gottesman, I. I. 1994. Schizophrenia Epigenesis: Past, present, and future. *Acta Psychiatrica Scandanavica,* Supplement, 90 (384): 26–33.

———. 1997. Twins—en route to QTLs for cognition. *Science* 276:1522–23.

Gottesman, I. I., and Bertelsen, A. 1989a. Confirming unexpressed genotypes for schizophrenia: Risks in the offspring of Fischer's Danish identical and fraternal discordant twins. *Archives of General Psychiatry* 46:867–72.

———. 1989b. Dual mating studies in psychiatry: Offspring of inpatients with examples from reactive (psychogenic) psychoses. *International Review of Psychiatry* 1:287–96.

Gottesman, I. I., and Carey, G. 1983. Extracting meaning and direction from twin data. *Psychiatric Developments* 1:398–404.

Gottesman, I. I., Goldsmith, H. H., and Carey, G. 1997. A developmental *and* a genetic perspective on aggression. In N. L. Segal, G. E. Weisfeld, and C. C. Weisfeld, eds., *Genetic, Cultural, and Evolutionary Perspectives on Human Development,* pp. 485–91. Washington, DC: American Psychological Association.

Gottesman, I. I., and Shields, J. 1972. *Schizophrenia and Genetics: A Twin Study Vantage Point.* New York: Academic Press (second printing, 1978).

Gottfredson, L. S. 1997. Mainstream science on intelligence: An editorial with 52 signatories, history, and bibliography. *Intelligence* 24:13–23.

Graham, G., and Stephens, G. L., eds. 1994. *Philosophical Psychopathology.* Cambridge: MIT Press.

Green, B. A. 1993. Lethal fiction: The meaning of "counsel" in the Sixth Amendment. *Iowa Law Review* 78:433–516.

Greenberg, S. A., and Shuman, D. W. 1997. Irreconcilable conflict between therapeutic and forensic roles. *Professional Psychology: Research and Practice* 28:50–57.

Greenblatt, S. 1980. Limits of knowledge and knowledge of limits: An essay on clinical judgment. *Journal of Medicine and Philosophy* 5:22–29.

Griffiths, A. P., ed. 1994. *Philosophy, Psychology, and Psychiatry.* Cambridge: Cambridge University Press.

Grinnell, F. 1992. *The Scientific Attitude.* 2d ed. New York: Guilford Press.

Grove, W. M. 1987. The reliability of psychiatric diagnosis. In C. B. Last and M. Hersen, eds., *Issues in Diagnostic Research,* pp. 99–119. New York: Plenum Press.

Grove, W. M., Andreasen, N. C., McDonald-Scott, P., Keller, M. B., and Shapiro, R. W. 1981. Reliability studies of psychiatric diagnosis: Theory and practice. *Archives of General Psychiatry* 38:408–13.

Guarnaccia, P. J., and Rogler, L. H. 1999. Research on culture-bound syndromes: New directions. *American Journal of Psychiatry* 156:1322–27.

Gunderson, J. G. 1984. *Borderline Personality Disorders.* Washington, DC: American Psychiatric Press.

———. 1989. Borderline personality disorder. In H. Kaplan and B. Sadock, eds., *Comprehensive Textbook of Psychiatry,* 5th ed., pp. 1387–95. Baltimore: Williams and Wilkins.

Guze, S. B. 1982. Comments on Blashfield's article. *Schizophrenia Bulletin* 8:6–7.

———. 1992. Diagnosis in psychiatry: Philosophical and conceptual issues. In D. Kupfer, ed., *Reflections on Modern Psychiatry,* pp. 1–8. Washington, DC: American Psychiatric Press.

Habermas, J. 1968. *Knowledge and Human Interest.* Boston: Beacon Press.

Hacking, I. 1986. The invention of split personalities. In A. Donagan, A. Perovich, and M. Wedin, eds., *Human Nature and Natural Knowledge,* pp. 351–94. Dordrecht, the Netherlands: D. Reidel Publishing.

———. 1995. The looping-effects of human kinds. In D. Sperber, D. Premack, and A. J. Premack, eds., *Causal Cognition,* pp. 351–94. Oxford: Clarendon Press; New York: Oxford University Press.

Hahn, B. 1998. Systemic lupus erythematosus. In A. Fauci, E. Braunwald, J. D. Wilson, J. B. Martin, S. L. Hauser, D. L. Longo, D. L. Kasper, and K. Isselbacher, eds., *Harrison's Principles of Internal Medicine,* 14th ed., pp. 1874–80. New York: McGraw-Hill.

Haines, J. L. 1991. The genetics of Alzheimer disease: A teasing problem. *American Journal of Human Genetics* 48 (6): 1021–25.

Hak, T. 1992. Psychiatric records as transformations of other texts. In G. Watson and R. M. Seiler, eds., *Text and Context: Contributions to Ethnomethodology,* pp. 138–55. Newbury Park, CA: Sage.

Hak, T., and de Boer, F. 1995. Professional interpretation of patient's talk in the initial interview. In J. Siegfried, ed., *Therapeutic and Everyday Discourse as Behavior Change: Towards a Micro-analysis in Psychotherapy Process Research,* pp. 341–64. Norwood, NJ: Ablex.

Hamilton, J. A., and Gallant, S. 1993. Premenstrual syndromes: A health psychology critique of biomedically-oriented research. In R. J. Gatchel and E. B. Blanchard, eds., *Psychophysiological Disorders,* pp. 383–438. Washington, DC: American Psychological Association.

Hanson, N. R. 1958. *Patterns of Discovery.* Cambridge: Cambridge University Press.

Hare, R. M. 1952. *The Language of Morals.* Oxford: Oxford University Press.

———. 1981. *Moral Thinking: Its Levels, Method, and Point.* Oxford: Clarendon Press.

Harré, R. 1985. Situational rhetoric and self-presentation. In J. P. Forgas, ed., *Language and Social Situations,* pp. 175–86. New York: Springer-Verlag.

Hart, H. L. A., and Honoré, A. M. 1985. *Causation in the Law.* New York: Oxford University Press.

Hawking, S. W. 1988. *A Brief History of Time: From the Big Bang to Black Holes.* New York: Bantam Books.

Hempel, C. G. 1961. Introduction to problems of taxonomy. In J. Zubin, ed., *Field Studies in the Mental Disorders,* pp. 3–22. New York: Grune and Stratton.

———. 1965. Fundamentals of taxonomy. *Aspects of Scientific Explanation.* New York: Free Press. Reprinted in J. Z. Sadler, O. P. Wiggins, and M. A. Schwartz, eds., 1994. *Philosophical Perspectives on Psychiatric Diagnostic Classification,* pp. 315–31. Baltimore: Johns Hopkins University Press.

Hesse, M. 1980. *Revolutions and Reconstructions in the Philosophy of Science.* Bloomington: Indiana University Press.

Hester, S., and Eglin, P., eds. 1997. *Culture in Action: Studies in Membership Categorization Analysis.* Lanham, MD: University Press of America.

Heyman, G. M. 1996. Resolving the contradictions of addiction. *Behavioral and Brain Sciences* 19 (4): 561–610.

Hickmann, M. 1993. The boundaries of reported speech in narrative discourse. In J. Lucy, ed., *Reflexive Language: Reported Speech and Metapragmatics,* pp. 63–89. Cambridge: Cambridge University Press.

Himmelhoch, J., Mezzich, J., and Ganguli, M. 1991. Controversies in psychiatry: The usefulness of DSM-III. *Psychiatric Annals* 21 (10): 621–31.

Hinton, L., and Kleinman, A. 1993. Cultural issues and international psychiatric diagnosis. In J. A. Costa e Silva and C. Nadelson, eds., *International Review of Psychiatry,* pp. 111–33. Washington, DC: American Psychiatric Press.

Hoerl, C., special issue ed. Forthcoming. Philosophy of mind, neuroscience, and schizophrenia. *Philosophy, Psychiatry, and Psychology.*

Holden, C. 1986. Proposed new psychiatric diagnoses raise charges of gender bias. *Science* 231:327–28.

Holland, P. W. 1986. Statistics and causal influence. *Journal of the American Statistical Association* 81:945–60.

hooks, bell. 1990. *Yearning: Race, Gender, and Cultural Politics.* Boston: South End Press.

Howson, C., and Urbach, P. 1989. *Scientific Reasoning: The Bayesian Approach.* LaSalle, IL: Open Court.

Hume, D. 1962. Of personal identity. In D. G. C. Macnabb, ed., *A Treatise of Human Nature,* bk. 1, pt. 1, sec. 6, pp. 164–71. Glasgow: Fontana/Collins.

Hunter, K. 1989. A science of individuals: Medicine and casuistry. *Journal of Medicine and Philosophy* 14:193–212.

Huntington's Disease Collaborative Research Group. 1993. A novel gene containing a trinucleotide that is expanded and unstable on Huntington's disease chromosomes. *Cell* 72:971–983.

Hyman, S. E. 1997. Letters to the Editor: Serious Mental Illness, Not Happiness Therapy. *Wall Street Journal,* November 11, p. A19.

Jablensky, A. 1988. Methodological issues in psychiatric classification. *British Journal of Psychiatry* 152 (1): 15–20.

———. 1993. Impact of the new diagnostic systems on psychiatric epidemiology. In J. A. Costa e Silva and C. Nadelson, eds., *International Review of Psychiatry,* pp. 13–44. Washington, DC: American Psychiatric Press.

Jackson, M. C. 1997. Benign schizotypy? The case of spiritual experience. In G. S. Claridge, ed., *Schizotypy: Relations to Illness and Health.* Oxford: Oxford University Press.

Jackson, M. C., and Fulford, K. W. M. 1997. Spiritual experience and psychopathology. *Philosophy, Psychiatry, and Psychology* 4 (1): 41–66.

Jamison, K. R. 1993. *Touched with Fire: Manic-Depressive Illness and the Artistic Temperament.* New York: Free Press.

———. 1995. *An Unquiet Mind: A Memoir of Moods and Madness.* New York: Vintage Books.

Jaspers, K. 1913. Causal and meaningful connexions between life history and psychosis. In S. R. Hirsch and M. Shepherd, eds., 1974, *Themes and Variations in European Psychiatry,* chap. 5. Bristol: John Wright and Sons.

Jenkins, R., Smeton, N., and Shepherd, M. 1988. Classification of mental illness in primary care. *Psychological Medicine,* Supplement, 12:1–59.

Jonas, H. 1984. *The Imperative of Responsibility: In Search of an Ethics for the Technological Age.* Chicago: University of Chicago Press.

Kagan, J. 1994. *Galen's Prophecy: Temperament in Human Nature.* New York: Basic Books.

Kant, I. 1933. *Critique of Pure Reason.* Trans. N. K. Smith. London: Macmillan.

————. 1987. *Critique of Judgment.* Trans. W. S. Pluhar. Indianapolis: Hackett Publishing.

Kaplan, M. 1983. A woman's view of DSM-III. *American Psychologist* 38:785–92.

Kass, F., Spitzer, R. L., and Williams, J. B. 1983. An empirical study of the issue of sex bias in the diagnostic criteria of DSM-III Axis II personality disorders. *American Psychologist* 38:799–801.

Kendell, R. E. 1975. *The Role of Diagnosis in Psychiatry.* Oxford: Blackwell Scientific Publications.

————. 1982a. The choice of diagnostic criteria for biological research. *Archives of General Psychiatry* 39:1334–39.

————. 1982b. Comments on Blashfield's article. *Schizophrenia Bulletin* 8:11–12.

————. 1986. What are mental disorders? In A. M. Freeman, R. Brotman, I. Silverman, and D. Hulson, eds., *Issues in Psychiatric Classification: Science, Practice, and Social Policy,* pp. 23–45. New York: Human Sciences Press.

————. 1988. Book Review: American Psychiatric Association: *Diagnostic and Statistical Manual of Mental Disorders, 3rd ed, revised (DSM-III-R) American Journal of Psychiatry* 145: 1301–2.

————. 1989. Clinical validity. *Psychological Medicine* 19:45–55.

————. 1991. Relationship between the DSM-IV and the ICD-10. *Journal of Abnormal Psychology* 100 (3): 297–301.

Kendler, K. S. 1988. The familial aggregation of schizophrenia and schizophrenia spectrum disorders: An evaluation of conflicting results. *Archives of General Psychiatry* 45:377–83.

————. 1990. Toward a scientific psychiatric nosology: Strengths and limitations. *Archives of General Psychiatry* 47:969–73.

————. 1991. Mood-incongruent psychotic affective illness. *Archives of General Psychiatry* 48:362–69.

————. 2000. Schizophrenia: Genetics. In B. J. Sardock and V. A. Sadock, eds., *Kaplan and Sadock's Comprehensive Textbook of Psychiatry,* 7th ed., 1:1147–58. Baltimore: Williams and Wilkins.

Kendler, K. S., and Gardner, C. O. 1997. The risk for psychiatric disorders in relatives of schizophrenic and control probands: A comparison of three independent studies. *Psychological Medicine* 27:411–19.

Kendler, K. S., Karkowski-Shuman, L., O'Neill, F. A., Straub, R. E., MacLean, C. J., and Walsh, D. 1997. Resemblance of psychotic symptoms and syndromes in affected sibling pairs from the Irish study of high-density schizophrenia families: Evidence for possible etiologic heterogeneity. *American Journal of Psychiatry* 154:191–98.

Kendler, K. S., Kessler, R. C., Neale, M. C., Heath, A. C., and Eaves, L .J. 1993. The prediction of major depression in women: Toward an integrated etiological model. *American Journal of Psychiatry* 150:1139–48.

Kendler, K. S., Kessler, R. C., Walters, E. E., MacLean, C., Neale, M. C., Heath, A. C., and Eaves, L. J. 1995. Stressful life events, genetic liability, and onset of an episode of major depression in women. *Archives of General Psychiatry* 152:833–42.

Kendler, K. S., McGuire, M., Gruenberg, A. M., O'Hare, A., Spellman, M., and Walsh, D. 1993. The Roscommon family study. I. Methods, diagnosis of probands, and risk of schizophrenia in relatives. *Archives of General Psychiatry* 50:527–40.

Kendler, K. S., McGuire, M., Gruenberg, A. M., and Walsh, D. 1994. Outcome and family study of the subtypes of schizophrenia in the west of Ireland. *American Journal of Psychiatry* 151:849–56.

Kendler, K. S., Neale, M. C., Kessler, R. C., Heath, A. C., and Eaves, L. J. 1992. Major depression and generalized anxiety disorder: Same genes (partly) different environments? *Archives of General Psychiatry* 49:716–22.

Kessler, R. C. 1999. The World Health Organization International Consortium in Psychiatric Epidemiology: Initial work and future directions—the NAPE lecture. *Acta Psychiatrica Scandanavica* 99:2–9.

King, M. L. 1963. Letter from the Birmingham Jail. In A. Joy, ed., *We Are America*, pp. 480–89. New York: Harcourt Brace.

Kirk, S. A., and Kutchins, H. 1992. *The Selling of DSM. The Rhetoric of Science in Psychiatry.* New York: Aldine DeGruyter.

———. 1994. Is bad writing a mental disorder? *New York Times,* June 20, p. A17.

Kirmayer, L. J. 1994. Is the concept of mental disorder culturally relative? In S. A. Kirk and S. D. Einbinder, eds., *Controversial Issues in Mental Health*, pp. 2–9. Boston: Allyn & Bacon.

Kleinman, A. 1988. *Rethinking Psychiatry: From Cultural Category to Personal Experience.* New York: Free Press.

———. 1996. How is culture important for DSM-IV? In J. E. Mezzich, A. Kleinman, H. Fabrega, and D. L. Parron, eds., *Culture and Psychiatric Diagnosis: A DSM-IV Perspective*, pp. 15–25. Washington, DC: American Psychiatric Press.

Klerman, G. L., Vaillant, G. E., Spitzer, R. L., and Michels, R. 1984. A debate on DSM-III. *American Journal of Psychiatry* 141 (4): 539–53.

Kohut, H. 1977. *The Restoration of the Self.* New York: International Universities Press.

Kopelman, L. M. 1994. Normal grief: Good or bad? Health or disease? *Philosophy, Psychiatry, and Psychology* 1 (4): 209–20.

Kovel, J. 1982. Book Review: *Diagnostic and Statistical Manual of Mental Disorders, Edition III. Einstein Quarterly Journal of Biology and Medicine* 1 (2): 103–4.

Kranzler, H. R., Babor, T. F., and Moore, P. 1997. Alcohol use disorders. In A. Tasman, J. Kay, and J. A. Lieberman, eds., *Psychiatry,* 1:755–78. Philadelphia: W. B. Saunders.

Kräupl-Taylor, F. 1980. The concepts of disease. *Psychological Medicine* 10:419–24.

Kraus, A. 1994. Phenomenological and criteriological diagnosis: Different or complementary? In J. Z. Sadler, O. P. Wiggins, and M. A. Schwartz, eds., *Philosoph-*

ical Perspectives on Psychiatric Diagnostic Classification, pp. 148–60. Baltimore: Johns Hopkins University Press.

Kriesman, J., and Strauss, H. 1989. *I Hate You, Don't Leave Me: Understanding the Borderline Personality.* New York: Avon Books.

Kuhn, T. S. 1962. The structure of scientific revolutions [2d ed.]. *International Encyclopedia of Unified Science.* Vol. 2, no. 2. Chicago: University of Chicago Press.

———. 1970. *The Structure of Scientific Revolutions.* 2d ed. Chicago: University of Chicago Press.

———. 1977. Objectivity, value judgment, and theory choice. In T. S. Kuhn, *The Essential Tension,* pp. 320–29. Chicago: University of Chicago Press.

Kutchins, H. 1987. DSM-III and social work malpractice. *Social Work* 32 (3): 205–11.

Labov, W., and Fanschel, D. 1977. *Therapeutic Discourse: Psychotherapy as Conversation.* New York: Academic Press.

Laing, R. D. 1959. *The Divided Self.* London: Tavistock.

Laing, R. D., and Esterson, A. 1964. *Sanity, Madness, and the Family.* London: Tavistock.

Lander, E. S., and Schork, N. J. 1994. Genetic dissection of complex traits. *Science* 265:2037–48.

Lane, H. 1992. The mask of benevolence: Disabling the dear community. New York: Knopf.

Larkin, J., and Caplan, P. J. 1992. The gatekeeping process of the DSM. *Canadian Journal of Community Mental Health* 11:17–28.

Latour, B. 1987. *Science in Action: How to Follow Scientists and Engineers through Society.* Cambridge: Harvard University Press.

Le Couteur, A., Bailey, A., Goode, S., Pickels, A., Robertson, S., Gottesman, I. I., and Rutter, M. 1996. A broader phenotype of autism: The clinical spectrum in twins. *Journal of Child Psychology and Psychiatry* 37:785–801.

Lendon, C. L., Ashall, F., and Goate, A. M. 1997. Exploring the etiology of Alzheimer disease using molecular genetics. *JAMA* 277:825–31.

Lennox, J. G. 1995. Health as an objective value. *Journal of Medicine and Philosophy* 20:499–511.

Lewis, D. 1973. Causation. *Journal of Philosophy* 70:556–57.

Lieberman, J. A., and Rush, A. J. 1996. Redefining the role of psychiatry in medicine. *American Journal of Psychiatry* 153:1388–97.

Lijam, N., Paylor, R., McDonald, M. P., Crawley, J. N., Deng, C., Herrup, K., Stevens, K. E., Maccaferri, G., McBain, C. J., Sussman, D. J., and Wynshaw-Boris, A. 1997. Social interaction and sensorimotor gating abnormalities in mice lacking *Dvll. Cell* 90 (5): 895–905.

Lilienfeld, S. O., and Marino, L. 1995. Mental disorder as a Roschian concept: A critique of Wakefield's "harmful dysfunction" analysis. *Journal of Abnormal Psychology* 104:411–20.

———. 1999. Essentialism revisited: Evolutionary theory and the concept of mental disorder. *Journal of Abnormal Psychology* 108:400–411.

Linde, A. 1991. *Particle Physics and Inflationary Cosmology.* New York: Harwood Academy Publishers.

Linehan, M. 1993. *Cognitive-Behavioral Treatment of Borderline Personality Disorder.* New York: Guilford Press.

Linell, P. 1998. Discourse across professional boundaries. *Text* 18 (2): 211–39.

Livesley, W. J., Schroeder, M. L., Jackson, D. N., and Jang, K. L. 1994. Categorical distinctions in the study of personality disorder: Implications for classification. *Journal of Abnormal Psychology* 103:6–17.

Lock, M. 1987. DSM-III as a culture-bound construct: Commentary on culture-bound syndromes and international disease classifications. *Culture, Medicine, and Psychiatry* 11:35–42.

Loehlin, J. C. 1992. *Latent Variable Models: An Introduction to Factor, Path, and Structural Analysis,* 2d ed. Hillsdale, NJ: Erlbaum.

Longino, H. E. 1990. *Science as Social Knowledge: Values and Objectivity in Scientific Inquiry.* Princeton: Princeton University Press.

Ludwig, A. M. 1975. The psychiatrist as physician. *Journal of the American Medical Association* 234 (6): 603–4.

Lukoff, D., Lu, F., and Turner, R. 1992. Toward a more culturally sensitive DSM-IV: Psychoreligious and psychospiritual problems. *Journal of Nervous and Mental Disease* 180 (11): 673–82.

Lyle, O. E., and Gottesman, I. I. 1979. Subtle cognitive deficits as 15- to 20-year precursors of Huntington's disease. *Advances in Neurology* 23:227–38.

Lyons, M. J., True, W. R., Eisen, S. A., Goldberg, J., Meyer, J. M., Faraone, S. V., Eaves, L. J., and Tsuang, M. T. 1995. Differential heritability of adult and juvenile antisocial traits. *Archives of General Psychiatry* 52:906–15.

Mace, C. J. 1992. Hysterical conversion: A history and critique. *British Journal of Psychiatry* 161:369–89.

Mackie, J. 1974. *The Cement of the Universe.* New York: Oxford University Press.

Margolis, J. 1994. Taxonomic puzzles. In J. Z. Sadler, O. P. Wiggins, and M. A. Schwartz, eds., *Philosophical Perspectives on Psychiatric Diagnostic Classification,* pp. 104–28. Baltimore: Johns Hopkins University Press.

Marneros, A., and Tsuang, M. T., eds. 1986. *Schizoaffective Psychoses.* Berlin: Springer-Verlag.

Marshall, M. 1994. How should we measure need? Concept and practice in the development of a standardized assessment schedule. *Philosophy, Psychiatry, and Psychology* 1 (1): 27–36.

Marx, J. 1998. New gene tied to common form of Alzheimer's. *Science* 281:507–9.

Maser, J. D., Kaelber, C., and Weise, R. E. 1991. International use and attitudes toward DSM-III and DSM-III-R: Growing consensus in psychiatric classification. *Journal of Abnormal Psychology* 100 (3): 271–79.

May, W. F. 1997. Money and the medical profession. *Kennedy Institute of Ethics Journal* 7 (1): 1–14.

McCarthy, L. P. 1991. A psychiatrist using DSM-III: The influence of a charter document in psychiatry. In C. Bazerman and J. Paradis, eds., *Textual Dynamics of the Professions: Historical and Contemporary Studies of Writing in Professional Communities,* pp. 358–78. Madison: University of Wisconsin Press.

McCarthy, L. P., and Gerring, J. P. 1994. Revising psychiatry's charter document: DSM-IV. *Written Communication* 11 (2): 147–92.

McDermott, R. 1993. The acquisition of a child by a learning disability. In S. Chaiklin and J. Lave, eds., *Understanding Practice: Perspectives on Activity and Context,* pp. 269–305. Cambridge: Cambridge University Press.

McGuffin, P., Farmer, A., and Gottesman, I. I. 1987. Is there really a split in schizophrenia? *British Journal of Psychiatry* 150:581–92.

McGuffin, P., Farmer, A., and Harvey, I. 1991. A polydiagnostic application of operational criteria in studies of psychotic illness. *Archives of General Psychiatry* 48:764–70.

McGuffin, P., Owen, M., O'Donovan, M., Thapar, A., and Gottesman, I. I. 1994. *Seminars in Psychiatric Genetics.* London: Gaskell Press; Washington, DC: American Psychiatric Press.

McGuire, M. T. 1986. Phenomenological classification systems: The case of DSM-III. *Perspectives in Biology and Medicine* 30:135–47.

McHugh, P. R., and Slavney, P. R. 1983. *The Perspectives of Psychiatry.* Baltimore: Johns Hopkins University Press.

McKegney, P. 1982. DSM-III: A definite advance, but the struggle continues. *General Hospital Psychiatry* 4:281–82.

McWhinney, I. 1978. Medical knowledge and the rise of technology. *Journal of Medicine and Philosophy* 3:293–304.

Meehl, P. E. 1954. *Clinical versus Statistical Prediction: A Theoretical Analysis and Review of the Evidence.* Minneapolis: University of Minnesota Press.

———. 1977. Specific etiology and other forms of strong influence: Some quantitative meanings. *Journal of Medicine and Philosophy* 2:33–53.

———. 1978. Sir Karl, Sir Ronald, and the slow progress of soft psychology. *Journal of Consulting and Clinical Psychology* 46:806–34.

———. 1986. Diagnostic taxa as open concepts: Metatheoretical and statistical questions about reliability and construct validity in the grand strategy of nosological revision. In T. Millon and G. L. Klerman, eds., *Contemporary Directions in Psychopathology: Toward the DSM-IV,* pp. 215–31. New York: Guilford Press.

Mehan, H. 1993. Beneath the skin and between the ears: A case study in the politics of representation. In S. Chaiklin and J. Lave, eds., *Understanding Practice: Perspectives on Activity and Context,* pp. 241–68. Cambridge: Cambridge University Press.

Menninger, K. 1963. *The Vital Balance: The Life Process in Mental Health and Illness.* New York: Viking.

Merleau-Ponty, M. 1954. *Phenomenology of Perception.* Trans. C. Smith. London: Routledge & Kegan Paul. Reprint, 1962.

Metzger, W. P. 1975. What is a profession? *Seminar Reports, Program of General and*

Continuing Education in the Humanities 3 (1): 1–12 (New York: Columbia University, September 18, 1975).

Mezzich, J. E., Fabrega, H., and Kleinman, A. 1992. Cultural validity and DSM-IV. *Journal of Nervous and Mental Disease* 180 (1): 4.

Mezzich, J. E., Kleinman, A., Fabrega, H., and Parron, D. L., eds. 1996. *Culture and Psychiatric Diagnosis: A DSM-IV Perspective.* Washington, DC: American Psychiatric Press.

Micale, M. 1995. *Approaching Hysteria: Disease and Its Interpretations.* Princeton: Princeton University Press.

Miller, P. 1986. Critiques of psychiatry and critical sociologies of madness. In N. Rose and P. Miller, eds., *The Power of Psychiatry,* pp. 12–42. Cambridge: Polity Press.

Miller, R. 1990. Why the standard view is standard: People, not machines, understand patients' problems. *Journal of Medicine and Philosophy* 15:581–92.

Millon, T. 1983. The DSM-III: An insider's perspective. *American Psychologist* 38 (July): 804–14.

———. 1986a. On the past and future of the DSM-III: Personal recollections and projections. In T. Millon and G. Klerman, eds., *Contemporary Directions in Psychopathology: Toward the DSM-IV,* pp. 29–72. New York: Guilford Press.

———. 1986b. A theoretical derivation of pathological personalities. In T. Millon and G. Klerman, eds., *Contemporary Directions in Psychopathology: Towards the DSM-IV,* pp. 639–70. New York: Guilford Press.

———. 1991. Classification in psychopathology: Rationale, alternatives, and standards. *Journal of Abnormal Psychology* 100 (3): 245–61.

Mirowski, J. 1990. Subjective boundaries and combinations in psychiatric diagnoses. *Journal of Mind and Behavior* 11 (3–4): 407–24, 161–78.

Mirowski, J., and Ross, C. E. 1989. Psychiatric diagnosis as reified measurement. *Journal of Health and Social Behavior* 30 (March): 11–25.

Mirra, S. S., Heyman, A., McKeel, D., Sumi, S. M., Crain, B. J., Brownlee, L. M., Vogel, F. S., Hughes, J. P., van Belle, G., and Berg, L. 1991. The consortium to establish a registry for Alzheimer's disease (CERAD). Part II. Standardization of the neuropathologic assessment of Alzheimer's disease. *Neurology* 41 (4): 479–86.

Mishara, A. L. 1994. A phenomenological critique of commonsensical assumptions in DSM-III-R: The avoidance of the patient's subjectivity. In J. Z. Sadler, O. P. Wiggins, and M. A. Schwartz, eds., *Philosophical Perspectives on Psychiatric Diagnostic Classification.* Baltimore: Johns Hopkins University Press.

Mishler, E. G. 1984. *The Discourse of Medicine: Dialectics of Medical Interviews.* Norwood, NJ: Ablex.

———. 1986. *Research Interviewing: Context and Narrative.* Cambridge: Harvard University Press.

Mitchell, S. A. 1993. *Hope and Dread in Psychoanalysis.* New York: Basic Books.

Moldin, S. O., and Gottesman, I. I. 1997. Genes, experience, and chance in schizophrenia: Positioning for the twenty-first century. *Schizophrenia Bulletin* 23 (4): 547–61.

Moore, A., Hope, T., and Fulford, K. W. M. 1994. Mild mania and well-being. *Philosophy, Psychiatry, and Psychology* 1(3): 177–78.

Moore, M. S. 1975. Some myths about "mental illness." *Archives of General Psychiatry* 32:1483–97.

Morey, L. C. 1991. Classification of mental disorder as a collection of hypothetical constructs. *Journal of Abnormal Psychology* 100:289–93.

Mulaik, S. A. 1987. Toward a conception of causality applicable to experimentation and causal modeling. *Child Development* 58:18–32.

Munson, R. 1981. Why medicine cannot be a science. *Journal of Medicine and Philosophy* 2:183–208.

Nagel, T. 1979. *Mortal Questions*. Cambridge: Cambridge University Press.

Nathan, P. E. 1994. DSM-IV: Empirical, accessible, not yet ideal. *Journal of Clinical Psychology* 50:103–10.

Nathan, P. E., and Langenbucher, J. W. 1999. Psychopathology: Description and classification. *Annual Review of Psychology* 50:79–107.

National Health Service (UK). 1995. UK's National Health Service Working Group on "The Genetics of Common Diseases."

National Institute of Mental Health. 1996. *The National Institute of Mental Health Schizophrenia Genetics Initiative*. At http://nimh.sratech.com (frequently updated).

Nelson-Gray, R. O. 1991. *DSM-IV*: Empirical guidelines from psychometrics. *Journal of Abnormal Psychology* 100 (3): 308–15.

Nicoll, J. A., Roberts, G. W., and Graham, D. I. 1996. Amyloid beta-protein: APOE genotype and head injury. *Annals of the New York Academy of Sciences* 777:271–75.

Nie, N. H., Hull, C., Jenkins, J., Steinbrenner, K., and Bent, D. 1975. *Statistical Package for the Social Sciences*. New York: McGraw-Hill.

Nordenfelt, L. 1994. Mild mania and the theory of health. *Philosophy, Psychiatry, and Psychology* 1 (3): 179–84.

———. 1996. Talking about health: A philosophical dialogue. Unpublished manuscript.

Nuckolls, C. W. 1992a. Reckless driving, casual sex, and shoplifting: What psychiatric categories, culture, and history reveal about each other. *Social Science and Medicine* 35 (1): 1–2.

———. 1992b. Toward a cultural history of the personality disorders. *Social Science and Medicine* 35 (1): 37–47.

O'Donovan, M. C., and Owen, M. J. 1996. Dynamic mutations and psychiatric genetics. *Psychological Medicine* 26:1–6.

Onstad, S., Skre, I., Torgersen, S., and Kringlen, E. 1991. Twin concordance for DSM-III-R schizophrenia. *Acta Psychiatrica Scandinavica* 83:395–401.

Osborn, A. S. 1935. Reasons and reasoning in expert testimony. *Law and Contemporary Problems* 2:488–94.

Parry-Jones, W. 1972. *The Trade in Lunacy.* London: Routledge & Kegan Paul.

Peele, S. 1990. *The Diseasing of America: Addiction Treatment out of Control.* Lexington, MA: Lexington Books.

Peele, S., and Brodsky, A., with Arnold, M. 1991. *The Truth about Addiction and Recovery: The Life Process Program for Outgrowing Destructive Habits.* New York: Fireside.

Peirce, C. S., 1965. *Collected Papers.* Ed. C. Hartshorne and P. Weis. Cambridge: Harvard University Press, Belknap Press.

Pellegrino, E. D. 1979. Toward a reconstruction of medical morality: The primacy of the act of profession and the fact of illness. *Journal of Medicine and Philosophy* 4 (1): 32–56.

———. 1990. The medical profession as a moral community. *Bulletin of the New York Academy of Medicine* 66 (3): 221–32.

Pellegrino, E., and Thomasma, D. 1981. *A Philosophical Basis of Medical Practice: Toward a Philosophy and Ethic of the Healing Professions.* New York: Oxford University Press.

Peltonen, L. 1995. All out for chromosome 6. *Nature* 378:665–66.

Pericak-Vance, M. A., Bebout, J. L., Gaskell, P. C., Jr., Yamaoka, L. H., Hung, W. Y., Alberts, M. J., Walker, A. P., Bartlett, R. J., Haynes, C. A., Welsh, K. A., Earl, N. L., Heyman, A., Clark, C. M., and Roses, A. D. 1991. Linkage studies in familial Alzheimer disease: Evidence for chromosome 19 linkage. *American Journal of Human Genetics* 48 (6): 1034–50.

Perley, M. J., and Guze, S. B. 1962. Hysteria: The stability and usefulness of clinical criteria. *New England Journal of Medicine* 266:421–26.

Perr, I. N. 1984. Medical and legal problems in psychiatric coding under the DSM and ICD systems. *American Journal of Psychiatry* 141:3, 418–20.

Perry, J., and Vailliant, G. 1989. Personality disorders. In H. Kaplan and B. Sadock, eds., *Comprehensive Textbook of Psychiatry,* 5th ed., pp. 1352–65. Baltimore: Williams and Wilkins.

Petitot, J., Varela, F., Pachoud, B., and Roy, J-M., eds. 2000. *Naturalizing Phenomenology: Issues in Contemporary Phenomenology and Cognitive Science.* Cambridge: Cambridge University Press.

Pfohl, B., and Andreasen, N. C. 1978. Development of classification systems in psychiatry. *Comprehensive Psychiatry* 19 (3): 197–207.

Philpott, M. J. 1998. A phenomenology of dyslexia: The lived-body, ambiguity, and the breakdown of expression. *Philosophy, Psychiatry, and Psychology* 5 (1): 1–20.

Pincus, H. A., Frances, A., Davis, W. W., First, M. B., and Widiger, T. A. 1992. DSM-IV and new diagnostic categories: Holding the line on proliferation. *American Journal of Psychiatry* 149:112–17.

Plomin, R., Owen, M., and McGuffin, P. 1994. The genetic basis of complex human behaviors. *Science* 264:1733–39.

Plutchik, R. 1980. A general psychoevolutionary theory of emotion. In R. Plutchik and H. Kellerman, eds., *Emotion: Theory, Research, and Experience,* pp. 3–33. San Diego, CA: Academic Press.

Pokorski, R. J. 1997. Insurance underwriting in the genetic era. *American Journal of Human Genetics* 60:205–16.

Poland, J., Von Eckardt, B., and Spaulding, W. 1994. Problems with the DSM approach to classifying psychopathology. In G. Graham and G. L. Stephens, eds., *Philosophical Psychopathology,* pp. 235–60. Cambridge: MIT Press.

Polanyi, M. 1962. *Personal Knowledge: Towards a Post-critical Philosophy.* Chicago: University of Chicago Press.

Popper, K. R. 1963. *Conjectures and Refutations.* New York: Harper & Row.

———. 1972. *Objective Knowledge.* Oxford: Oxford University Press.

———. 1994. *The Myth of the Framework: In Defense of Science and Rationality.* London: Routledge.

Proctor, R. N. 1991. *Value-Free Science? Purity and Power in Modern Knowledge.* Cambridge: Harvard University Press.

Putnam, H. 1981. Fact and value. In *Reason, Truth, and History,* pp. 127–49. New York: Cambridge University Press.

———. 1990a. Beyond the fact/value dichotomy. In *Realism with a Human Face,* pp. 135–41. Cambridge: Harvard University Press.

———. 1990b. The place of facts in a world of values. In *Realism with a Human Face,* pp. 142–62. Cambridge: Harvard University Press.

Radden, J. 1985. *Madness and Reason.* London: George Allan & Unwin.

———. 1994. Recent criticisms of psychiatric nosology: A review. *Philosophy, Psychiatry, and Psychology* 1 (3): 193–200.

———. 1996a. Commentary on Lloyd Fields. *Philosophy, Psychiatry, and Psychology* 3 (4): 287–89.

———. 1996b. *Divided Minds and Successive Selves: Ethical Issues in Disorders of Identity and Personality.* Cambridge: MIT Press.

Ramirez, A. 1996. You were right in saying some people make you sick. *New York Times,* Sunday, December 15, p. E2.

Ravotas, D., and Berkenkotter, C. 1998. Voices in the text: The uses of reported speech in a psychotherapist's notes and initial assessments. *Text* 18:211–39.

Reynolds, J. F., Meir, D. C., and Fisher, P. C. 1995. *Writing and Reading Mental Health Records.* Mahwah, NJ: Erlbaum.

Reznek, L. 1987. *The Nature of Disease.* London: Routledge & Kegan Paul.

Richer, D. 1992. An introduction to deconstructionist psychology. In S. Kvale, ed., *Psychology and Postmodernism,* pp. 110–18. London: Sage.

Richters, J. E., and Cicchetti, D. 1993. Mark Twain meets DSM-III-R: Conduct disorder, development, and the concept of harmful dysfunction. *Development and Psychopathology* 5:5–29.

Ritchie, K. 1989. The little woman meets son of DSM-III. *Journal of Medicine and Philosophy* 14:695–708.

Robertson, D. 1996. Ethical theory, ethnography, and differences between doctors and nurses in approaches to patient care. *Journal of Medical Ethics* 22:292–99.

Robins, E., and Guze, S. B. 1970. Establishment of diagnostic validity in psychiatric illness: Its application in schizophrenia. *American Journal of Psychiatry* 126:983–87.

Rogler, L. H. 1996. Framing research on culture in psychiatric diagnosis: The case of the DSM-IV. *Psychiatry* 59:145–55.

———. 1997. Making sense of historical changes in the *Diagnostic and Statistical Manual of Mental Disorders*: Five propositions. *Journal of Health and Social Behavior* 38:9–20.

———. 1999. Methodological sources of cultural insensitivity in mental health research. *American Psychologist* 54:424–33.

Rorer, L. G. 1991. Some myths of science in psychology. In W. M. Grove and D. Cicchetti, eds., *Thinking Clearly about Psychology*, 1:61–87. Minneapolis, MN: University of Minnesota Press.

Rose, S. 1995. The rise of neurogenetic determinism. *Nature* 373:380–82.

Rosenthal, D., ed. 1963. *The Genain Quadruplets*. New York: Basic Books.

Roses, A. D. 1996. Apolipoprotein E Alleles as risk factors in Alzheimer's disease. *Annual Review of Medicine* 47:387–400.

———. 1997. Genetic testing for Alzheimer disease: Practical and ethical issues. *Archives of Neurology* 54 (10): 1226–29.

———. 1998a. Alzheimer diseases: A model of gene mutations and susceptibility polymorphisms for complex psychiatric diseases. *American Journal of Medical Genetics* 81:49–57.

———. 1998b. A new paradigm for clinical evaluation of dementia: Alzheimer disease and apolipoprotein E genotypes. In S. G. Post and P. J. Whitehouse, eds., *Genetic Testing for Alzheimer Disease: Ethical and Clinical Issues*, pp. 37–64. Baltimore: Johns Hopkins University Press.

Ross, R., Frances, A. J., and Widiger, T. A. 1995. Gender issues in DSM-IV. In J. M. Oldham and M .B. Riba, eds., *Review of Psychiatry*, 14:205–26. Washington, DC: American Psychiatric Press.

Rosser, S. V. 1992. Is there androcentric bias in psychiatric diagnosis? *Journal of Medicine and Philosophy* 17 (2): 215–32.

Roth, M., and Kroll, J. 1986. *The Reality of Mental Illness*. Cambridge: Cambridge University Press.

Rothblum, E. D., Solomon, L. J., and Albee, G. W. 1986. A sociopolitical perspective of DSM-III. In T. Millon and G. L. Klerman, eds., *Contemporary Directions in Psychopathology: Towards the DSM-IV*, pp. 167–89. New York: Guilford Press.

Rothstein, M. A., ed. 1997. *Genetic Secrets: Protecting Privacy and Confidentiality in the Genetic Era*. New Haven: Yale University Press.

Rousseau, J-J. 1978. *On the Social Contract*. Ed. R. Masters and trans. J. Masters. New York: St. Martin's Press.

Rubin, D. B. 1978. Bayesian inference for causal effects: The role of randomizations. *Annals of Statistics* 6:34–58.

———. 1986. Comment: Which ifs have causal answers. *Journal of the American Statistical Association* 81:961–62.

Rubinsztein, D. C., et al. 1996. Phenotypic characterization of individuals with 30–40 CAG repeats in the Huntington disease gene (HD) reveals HD cases with 36 repeats and apparently normal elderly individuals with 36–39 repeats. *American Journal of Human Genetics* 59:16–22.

Russell, D. 1994. Psychiatric diagnosis and the interests of women. In J. Z. Sadler, O P. Wiggins, and M. A. Schwartz, eds., *Philosophical Perspectives on Psychiatric Diagnostic Classification*, pp. 246–58. Baltimore: Johns Hopkins University Press.

Sabat, S. R., and Harré, R. 1997. The Alzheimer's disease sufferer as semiotic subject. *Philosophy, Psychiatry, and Psychology* 4 (2): 145–60.

Sabshin, M. 1993. APA official actions: Report of the medical director. *American Journal of Psychiatry* 150 (10): 1591–1601.

Sackett, D. L. 1997. Evidence-based medicine. *Seminars in Perinatology* 21:3–5.

Sacks, H. 1972. On the analyzability of stories by children. In J. J. Gumperz and D. Hymes, eds., *Directions in Sociolinguistics: The Ethnography of Communication*, pp. 325–45. Oxford: Blackwell.

———. 1995. *Lectures on Conversation*. Oxford: Blackwell.

Sadler, J. Z. 1996a. Epistemic value commitments in the debate over categorical vs. dimensional personality diagnosis. *Philosophy, Psychiatry, and Psychology* 3:203–22.

———. 1996b. Rationales, values, and DSM-IV: The case of "medication-induced movement disorders." *Comprehensive Psychiatry* 37:441–51.

———. 1997. Recognizing values: A descriptive/causal method for medical/scientific discourses. *Journal of Medicine and Philosophy* 22:541–65.

Sadler, J. Z., and Agich, G. J. 1996. Disease, functions, values, and psychiatric classification. *Philosophy, Psychiatry, and Psychology* 2:219–31.

Sadler, J. Z., and Hulgus, Y. F. 1990. Knowing, valuing, acting: Clues to revising the biopsychosocial model. *Comprehensive Psychiatry* 31 (3): 185–95.

———. 1994. Enriching the psychosocial content of a multiaxial nosology. In J. Z. Sadler, O. P. Wiggins, and M. A. Schwartz, eds., *Philosophical Perspectives on Psychiatric Diagnostic Classification*, pp. 261–78. Baltimore: Johns Hopkins University Press.

Sadler, J. Z., Hulgus, Y. F., and Agich, G. J. 1994. On values in recent American psychiatric classification. *Journal of Medicine and Philosophy* 19:261–77.

Sadler, J. Z., Wiggins, O. P., and Schwartz, M. A. 1994a. Introduction. In J. Z. Sadler, O. P. Wiggins, and M. A. Schwartz, eds., *Philosophical Perspectives on Psychiatric Diagnostic Classification*, pp. 1–15. Baltimore: Johns Hopkins University Press.

———, eds. 1994b. *Philosophical Perspectives on Psychiatric Diagnostic Classification*. Baltimore: Johns Hopkins University Press.

Sales, B. D., and Shuman, D. W. 1993. Reclaiming the integrity of science in expert witnessing. *Ethics and Behavior* 3:223–29.

Salmon, W. 1989. Four decades of scientific explanation. In W. C. Salmon and P. Kitcher, eds., *Scientific Explanation*, pp. 3–96. Minneapolis: University of Minnesota Press.

Sartorius, N. 1988. International perspectives of psychiatric classification. *British Journal of Psychiatry* 152:9–14.

Saunders, A. M., Strittmatter, W. J., Schmechel, D., George-Hyslop, P. H., Pericak-Vance, M. A., Joo, S. H, Rosi, B. I., Gusella, J. F., Crapper-McLachlan, D. R., Alberts, M. J., Hulette, C., Carain, B., Goldgaber, D., and Roses, A. D. 1993. Association of apolipoprotein e allele epsilon 4 with late-onset familial and sporadic Alzheimer's disease. *Neurology* 43 (8): 1467–72.

Scadding, J. G. 1967. Diagnosis: The clinician and the computer. *Lancet* 3:877–82.

Schacht, T. E. 1985. DSM-III and the politics of truth. *American Psychologist* 40:513–21.

Schacht, T. E., and Nathan, P. E. 1977. But is it good for the psychologists? Appraisal and status of DSM-III. *American Psychologist* 32:1017–25.

Schaffner, K. F. 1992. Philosophy of method. In J. Lederberg, ed., *Encyclopedia of Microbiology*, 3:111–20. San Diego, CA: Academic Press.

———. 1993a. Clinical trials and causation: Bayesian and non-Bayesian perspectives. *Statistics in Medicine* 12:1477–94.

———. 1993b. *Discovery and Explanation in Biology and Medicine*. Chicago: University of Chicago Press.

———. 1998. Genes, behavior, and developmental emergentism: One process, indivisible? *Philosophy of Science* 65:209–52.

Schaffner, K. F., and Wachbroit, R. 1994. Il cancero come malitta genetics: Problemi sociali ed ethici. *L'arco di Giano: Rivista di medical humanities* 6 (settembre–dicembre): 13–29.

Scheff, T. J. 1984. *Being Mentally Ill: A Sociological Theory*. New York: Aldine de Gruyer.

Schwab, S. G., et al. 1995. Evaluation of a susceptibility gene for schizophrenia on chromosome 6p by multipoint affected sib-pair linkage analysis. *Nature Genetics* 11 (3): 325–27.

Schwartz, M. A., and Wiggins, O. P. 1986. Logical empiricism and psychiatric classification. *Comprehensive Psychiatry* 27 (2): 101–14.

———. 1987. Diagnosis and ideal types: A contribution to psychiatric classification. *Comprehensive Psychiatry* 28:277–91.

Schwartz, M. A., Wiggins, O. P., and Norko, M. 1989. Prototypes, ideal types, and personality disorders: The return to classical psychiatry. *Journal of Personality Disorders* 3:1–9.

Sedgwick, P. 1973. Illness—mental and otherwise. *Hastings Center Studies* 1 (3): 19–40.

———. 1982a. Illness—mental and otherwise. In R. B. Edwards, ed., *Psychiatry and Ethics*, pp. 49–60. Buffalo: Prometheus Books.

———. 1982b. *Psycho Politics*. New York: Harper & Row.

Seedhouse, D. 1994. The trouble with well-being. *Philosophy, Psychiatry, and Psychology* 1 (3): 185–91.

Sengupta, P., Colbert, H., and Bargmann, C. 1994. The *C. Elegans* gene *odr-7* encodes an olfactory-specific member of the nuclear receptor superfamily. *Cell* 79:971–80.

Shanteau, J. 1992. Competence in experts: The role of task characteristics. *Organizational Behavior and Human Decision Process* 53:252–66.

Sharfstein, S. S. 1987. Third-party payments, cost containment, and DSM-III. In G. L. Tischler, ed., *Diagnosis and Classification in Psychiatry: A Critical Appraisal of DSM-III*, pp. 530–38. Cambridge: Cambridge University Press.

Sherrington, C. 1946. *The Endeavor of Jean Fernel*. Cambridge: Cambridge University Press.

Shields, J., Heston, L. L., and Gottesman, I. I. 1975. Schizophrenia and the schizoid: The problem for genetic analysis. In R. R. Fieve, D. Rosenthal, and H. Brill, eds., *Genetic Research in Psychiatry*, pp. 167–97. Baltimore: Johns Hopkins University Press.

Shorter, E. 1997. *A History of Psychiatry: From the Era of the Asylum to the Age of Prozac*. New York: John Wiley.

Showalter, E. 1985. *The Female Malady: Women, Madness, and English Culture, 1830–1980*. New York: Pantheon.

Shuman, D. W. 1989. The diagnostic and statistical manual of mental disorders in the courts. *Bulletin of the American Academy of Psychiatry and Law* 17:25–32.

———. 1994. *Psychiatric and Psychological Evidence*. 2d ed. Colorado Springs: Shepherds/McGraw-Hill.

———. 1995. Persistent reexperiences in psychiatry and the law. In R. Simon, ed., *Post-traumatic Stress Disorder in Litigation: Guidelines for Forensic Assessment*, pp. 1–11. Washington, DC: American Psychiatric Press.

Shuman, D. W., Champagne, A., and Whitaker, E. 1996. Assessing the believability of expert witnesses: Science in the jurybox. *Jurimetrics Journal* 37:23–33.

Silverman, D. 1987. *Social Relations in the Clinic*. London: Sage.

Simola, S. K. 1992. Differences among sexist, nonsexist, and feminist family therapies. *Professional Psychology: Research and Practice* 23:397–403.

Sing, C. F., Haviland, M. B., and Reilly, S. L. 1996. Genetic architecture of common multifactorial diseases. In G. Cardew, ed., *Variation in the Human Genome*, pp. 211–32. Chichester: John Wiley.

Skinner, H. A. 1986. Construct validation approach to psychiatric classification. In T. Millon and G. Klerman, eds., *Contemporary Directions in Psychopathology: Toward the DSM-IV*, pp. 307–30. New York: Guilford Press.

Smith, D., and Kraft, W. A.. 1983. DSM-III: Do psychologists really want an alternative? *American Psychologist* 38:777–85.

Soyland, A. J. 1994. Functions of the psychiatric case-summary. *Text* 14:113–40.

———. 1995. Analyzing therapeutic professional discourse. In. J. Siegfried, ed., *Therapeutic and Everyday Discourse as Behavior Change: Towards a Micro-analysis in Psychotherapy Process Research*, pp. 277–300. Norwood, NJ: Ablex.

Spence, S. A. 1996. Free will in the light of neuropsychiatry. *Philosophy, Psychiatry, and Psychology* 3 (2): 75–90.

Spirtes, P., Glymour, C., and Scheines, R. 1993. *Causation, Prediction, and Search.* New York: Springer-Verlag.

Spitzer, R. L. 1981. The diagnostic status of homosexuality in DSM-III: A reformulation of the issues. *American Journal of Psychiatry* 138 (2): 210–15.

———. 1985. DSM-III and the politics-science dichotomy syndrome: A response to Thomas E. Schacht's "DSM-III and the politics of truth." *American Psychologist* 40:522–26.

Spitzer, R. L., and Endicott, J. 1978. Medical and mental disorder: Proposed definition and criteria. In R. L. Spitzer and D. F. Klein, eds., *Critical Issues in Psychiatric Diagnosis*, pp. 15–39. New York: Raven Press.

Spitzer, R .L., Endicott, J., and Robins, E. 1978. Research diagnostic criteria: Rationale and reliability. *Archives of General Psychiatry* 35:773–82.

Spivak, G. 1987. *In Other Worlds: Essays in Cultural Politics.* New York: Routledge.

State v. Hungerford, 1995 WL 378571 (N.H. Super. Ct. May 23, 1995).

Stengel, E. 1959. Classification of mental disorders. *Bulletin of the World Health Organization* 21:601–63.

Stern, J., Murphy, M., and Bass, C. 1993. Attitudes of British psychiatrists to the diagnosis of somatisation disorder. *British Journal of Psychiatry* 162:463–66.

Stone, M. 1993. Paradoxes in the management of suicidality in borderline patients. *American Journal of Psychotherapy* 47:255–72.

Strain, E. C., and Griffiths, R. R. 1997. Caffeine use disorders. In A. Tasman, J. Kay, and J. A. Lieberman, eds., *Psychiatry*, 1:779–94. Philadelphia: W. B. Saunders.

Straub, R. E., MacLean, C. J., O'Neill, F. A., Burke, J., Murphy, B., Duke, F., Shinkwin, R., Webb, B. T., Zhang, J., Walsh, D., and Kendler, K. S. 1995. A potential vulnerability locus for schizophrenia on chromosome 6p24-22: Evidence for genetic heterogeneity. *Nature Genetics* 11:287–93.

Strauss, J. S. 1982. Comments on Blashfield's article. *Schizophrenia Bulletin* 8:8–9.

Strong, T. 1993. DSM-IV and describing problems in family therapy. *Family Process* 32:249–53.

Svensson, T. 1995. *On the Notion of Mental Illness.* Aldershot, England: Ashgate Publishing.

Sydenham, Thomas. 1848. The Works of Thomas Sydenham. Vol. 2. Trans. R. G. Latham. London: Printed for the Sydenham Society.

Szasz, T. S. 1960. The myth of mental illness. *American Psychologist* 15:113–18.

———. 1972. *The Myth of Mental Illness.* London: Paladin.

———. 1974. *The Myth of Mental Illness: Foundations of a Theory of Personal Conduct.* Rev. ed. New York: Harper & Row.

———. 1987. *Insanity: The Idea and Its Consequences.* New York: John Wiley.

Tannen, D. 1989. *Talking Voices: Repetition, Dialogue, and Imagery in Conversational Discourse.* Cambridge: Cambridge University Press.

Tannen, D., and Wallat, C. 1993. Interactive frames and knowledge schemas in interaction: Examples from a medial examination/interview. In D. Tannen, ed., *Framing in Discourse,* pp. 57–113. New York: Oxford University Press.

Task Force on DSM-IV. 1991 (December). *DSM-IV Options Book: Work in Progress.* Washington, DC: American Psychiatric Association.

———. 1993 (March). *DSM-IV Draft Criteria, 3/1/93.* Washington, DC: American Psychiatric Association.

Taylor, C. 1985. *Human Agency and Language: Philosophical Papers I.* Cambridge: Cambridge University Press.

———. 1995. *Philosophic Arguments.* Cambridge: Harvard University Press.

Temkin, O. 1968. The history of classification in the medical sciences. In M. M. Katz, J. O. Cole, and W. E. Barton, eds., *The Role and Methodology of Classification in Psychiatry and Psychopathology,* pp. 11–19. Washington, DC: National Institute of Mental Health.

Thagard, P. 1992. *Conceptual Revolutions.* Princeton: Princeton University Press.

Toulmin, S. 1953. *The Philosophy of Science.* London: Heinemann.

———. 1972a. Conceptual change and the problem of relativity. In M. Kraus, ed., *Critical Essays on the Philosophy of R. G. Collingwood,* pp. 201–21. Oxford: Clarendon Press.

———. 1972b. *Human Understanding.* Vol. 1. Oxford: Oxford University Press.

———. 1976. On the nature of the physician's understanding. *Journal of Medicine and Philosophy* 1:32–50.

Tsuang, M. T., Faraone, S. V., and Lyons, M. J. 1993. Identification of the phenotype in psychiatric genetics. *European Archives of Psychiatry and Clinical Neuroscience* 243:131–42.

Tucker, G. 1998. Putting DSM-IV in perspective. *American Journal of Psychiatry* 155:159–61.

Turner, R., Lukoff, P. D., Barnhouse, R. T., and Lu, F. G. 1995. Religious or spiritual problem: A culturally sensitive diagnostic category in the DSM-IV. *Journal of Nervous and Mental Disease* 183 (7): 435–44.

U.S. Department of Health and Human Services (DHHS). 1997. *ICD-9-CM, International Classification of Diseases, 9th Revision, Clinical Modification.* 6th ed. CD-ROM. Washington, DC: U.S. Government Printing Office.

Van Staden, C. W. 1999. Linguistic changes during recovery: A philosophical and empirical study of first person pronoun usage and semantic positions of patients as expressed in psychotherapy and mental illness. Ph.D. thesis, Department of Philosophy, University of Warwick, Coventry, United Kingdom.

Veatch, R .M. 1973. The medical model: Its nature and problems. *Hastings Center Studies* 1:59–76.

Veith, I. 1957. Psychiatric nosology: From Hippocrates to Kraepelin. *American Journal of Psychiatry* 114:385–91.

Vincent, J. B., Kalsi, G., Klempan, T., Tatuch, Y., Sherrington, R. P., Breschel, T., McInnins, M. G., Brynjolfsson, J., Petursson, H., Gurling, H. M. D., Gottesman, I. I., Torrey, E. F., Petronis, A., and Kennedy, J. L. 1998. No evidence of CAG or GAA repeats in schizophrenia families and monozygotic twins. *Human Genetics* 103:41–47.

Virchow, R. 1958. *Disease, Life, and Man: Selected Essays by Rudolph Virchow.* Trans. Lelland J. Rather. Stanford: Stanford University Press.

von Wright, G. H. 1971. *Explanation and Understanding.* Ithaca, NY: Cornell University Press.

Wakefield, J. C. 1992a. The concept of mental disorder: On the boundary between biological facts and social values. *American Psychologist* 47:373–88.

———. 1992b. Disorder as harmful dysfunction: A conceptual critique of DSM-III-R's definition of mental disorder. *Psychological Review* 99:232–47.

———. 1993. Limits of operationalization: A critique of Spitzer and Endicott's (1978) proposed operational criteria for mental disorder. *Journal of Abnormal Psychology* 102:160–72.

———. 1994. Is the concept of mental disorder culturally relative? In S. A. Kirk and S. D. Einbinder, eds., *Controversial Issues in Mental Health,* pp. 11–17. Boston: Allyn & Bacon.

———. 1995. Dysfunction as a value-free concept: A reply to Sadler and Agich. *Philosophy, Psychiatry, and Psychology* 2:233–46.

———. 1996. DSM-IV: Are we making diagnostic progress? *Contemporary Psychology* 41:646–52.

———. 1997a. The concept of mental disorder: On the boundary between biological facts and social values. In R. Edwards, ed., *Ethics in Psychiatry,* pp. 63–97. York: Prometheus Books.

———. 1997b. Diagnosing DSM-IV, Part 1: DSM-IV and the concept of mental disorder. *Behavior Research and Therapy* 35:633–50.

———. 1997c. Diagnosing DSM-IV, Part 2: Eysenck (1986) and the essentialist fallacy. *Behavior Research and Therapy* 35:651–66.

———. 1999. Evolutionary versus prototype analyses of the concept of disorder. *Journal of Abnormal Psychology* 108 (3): 374–99.

———. 2000. Aristotle as sociobiologist: The "function of a human being" argument, black box essentialism, and the concept of mental disorder. *Philosophy, Psychiatry, and Psychology* 7 (1): 17–44.

Walker, L. E. A. 1987. Inadequacies of the masochistic personality disorder diagnosis for women. *Journal of Personality Disorders* 1:183–89.

———. 1989. Psychology and the violence against women. *American Psychologist* 44:695–702.

————. 1994. Are personality disorders gender biased? In S. A. Kirk and S. D. Einbinder, eds., *Controversial Issues in Mental Health*, pp. 22–29. New York: Allyn
& Bacon.

Wallace, E. R. 1994. Psychiatry and its nosology: A historico-philosophical
overview. In J. Z. Sadler, O. P. Wiggins, and M. A. Schwartz, eds., *Philosophical
Perspectives on Psychiatric Diagnostic Classification*, pp. 16–86. Baltimore: Johns
Hopkins University Press.

Walters, L., and Palmer, J. 1997. *The Ethics of Human Gene Therapy*. New York: Oxford University Press.

Warnock, G. J. 1971. *The Object of Morality*. London: Methuen.

Watson, D., Clark, L. A., and Harkness, A. 1994. Structures of personality and their
relevance to psychopathology. *Journal of Abnormal Psychology* 103:18–31.

Weimer, W. B. 1979. *Notes on the Methodology of Scientific Research*. Hillsdale, NJ:
Erlbaum.

Westermeyer, J. 1996. Culture and the diagnostic classification of substance-related
disorders. In J. E. Mezzich, A. Kleinman, H. Fabrega, and D. L. Parron, eds., *Culture and Psychiatric Diagnosis: A DSM-IV Perspective*, pp. 81–90. Washington,
DC: American Psychiatric Press.

White, B., and Epston, D. 1990. *Narrative Means to Therapeutic Ends*. New York: W.
W. Norton.

Widdershoven-Heerding, I. 1987. Medicine as a form of practical understanding.
Theoretical Medicine 8:1179–85.

Widiger, T. A. 1993a. Issues in the validation of the personality disorders. In L. J.
Chapman, J. R. Chapman, and D. C. Fowles, eds., *Progress in Experimental Personality and Psychopathology Research*, pp. 117–36. New York: Springer.

————. 1993b. Validation strategies for the personality disorders. *Journal of Personality Disorders*, Supplement, 1:34–43.

————. 1997. Mental disorders as discrete clinical conditions: Dimensional versus
categorical classification. In S. M. Turner and M. Hersen, eds., *Adult Psychopathology and Diagnosis*, 3d ed., pp. 3–23. New York: John Wiley.

————. 1997. The construct of mental disorder. *Clinical Psychology: Science and
Practice* 4:262–66.

Widiger, T. A., and Axelrod, S. R. 1995. Recent developments in the clinical assessment of personality disorders. *European Journal of Psychological Assessment*
11:213–21.

Widiger, T. A., Frances, A. J., Pincus, H. A., and Davis, W. W. 1990. DSM-IV literature reviews: Rationale, process, and limitations. *Journal of Psychopathology and
Behavioral Assessment* 12:189–202.

Widiger, T. A., Frances, A. J., Pincus, H. A., Davis, W. W., and First, M. B. 1991. Toward an empirical classification for DSM-IV. *Journal of Abnormal Psychology*
100:280–88.

Widiger, T. A., Frances A. J., Pincus H. A., First, M. B., Ross, R., and Davis, W. 1994.
DSM-IV Sourcebook. Vol. 1. Washington, DC: American Psychiatric Press.

Widiger, T. A., Frances, A. J., Pincus, H. A., Ross, R., First, M. B., Davis, W., and Kline, M. 1998. *DSM-IV Sourcebook*. Vol. 4. Washington, DC: American Psychiatric Association.

Widiger, T. A., and Nietzel, M. T. 1984. Kaplan's view of DSM-III: The data revisited. *American Psychologist* 39:1319–20.

Widiger, T. A., and Spitzer, R. L. 1991. Sex bias in the diagnosis of personality disorders: Conceptual and methodological issues. *Clinical Psychology Review* 11:1–22.

Widiger, T. A., and Trull, T. J. 1991. Diagnosis and clinical assessment. *Annual Review of Psychology* 42:109–33.

———— 1993. The scholarly development of DSM-IV. In J. A. Costa e Silva and C. C. Nadelson, eds., *International Review of Psychiatry*, 1:59–78. Washington, DC: American Psychiatric Press.

Wiggins, O. P., and Schwartz, M. A. 1994. The limits of psychiatric knowledge and the problem of classification. In J. Z. Sadler, O. P. Wiggins, and M. A. Schwartz, eds., *Philosophical Perspectives on Psychiatric Diagnostic Classification*, pp. 89–103. Baltimore: Johns Hopkins University Press.

Wiggins, O. P., Schwartz, M. A., and Northoff, G. 1990. Towards a Husserlian phenomenology of the initial stages of schizophrenia. In M. Spitzer and B. A. Maher, eds., *Philosophy and Psychopathology*. New York: Springer-Verlag.

Williams, B. 1985. *Ethics and the Limits of Philosophy*. Cambridge: Harvard University Press.

Williams, J. B. W., and Spitzer, R. L. 1983. The issue of sex bias in DSM-III: A critique of "A Woman's View of DSM-III" by Marcie Kaplan. *American Psychologist* 38:793–98.

Williams, J. B. W., Spitzer, R. L., and Skodol, A. E. 1985. DSM-III in residency training: Results of a national survey. *American Journal of Psychiatry* 142 (6): 755–58.

Wilson, M. 1993. DSM-III and the transformation of American psychiatry: A history. *American Journal of Psychiatry* 150 (3): 399–410.

Wing, J. K., Cooper, J. E., and Sartorius, N. 1974. *Measurement and Classification of Psychiatric Symptoms*. Cambridge: Cambridge University Press.

Winnicott, D. 1965. Ego distortion in terms of true and false self. In *The Maturational Process and the Facilitating Environment*, pp. 140–52. New York: International Universities Press.

Woodruff, R. A. 1967. Hysteria: An evaluation of objective diagnostic criteria by the study of women with chronic medical illnesses. *British Journal of Psychiatry* 114:1115–19.

Woody, G. E., and McNicholas, L. F. 1997. Opioid-related disorders. In A. Tasman, J. Kay, and J. A. Lieberman, eds., *Psychiatry*, 1:867–80. Philadelphia: W. B. Saunders.

World Health Organization. 1948. *Manual of the International Statistical Classification of Disease, Injuries, and Causes of Death*. 6th ed. Geneva: World Health Organization.

————. 1955. *Manual of the International Statistical Classification of Disease, Injuries, and Causes of Death*. 7th ed. Geneva: World Health Organization.

————. 1967. *Manual of the International Statistical Classification of Disease, Injuries, and Causes of Death*. 8th ed. Geneva: World Health Organization.

————. 1973. Report of *The International Pilot Study of Schizophrenia*. Geneva: World Health Organization.

————. 1977. *Manual of the International Statistical Classification of Disease, Injuries, and Causes of Death*. 9th ed. Geneva: World Health Organization.

————. 1992a. *ICD-10: International Statistical Classification of Diseases and Related Health Problems*. 3 vols. Geneva: World Health Organization.

————. 1992b. *The ICD-10 Classification of Mental and Behavioral Disorders: Clinical Descriptions and Diagnostic Guidelines*. Geneva: World Health Organization.

————. 1993. *The ICD-10 Classification of Mental and Behavioral Disorders: Diagnostic Criteria for Research*. Geneva: World Health Organization.

Wright, I., Sloman, A., and Beaudoin, L. 1996. Towards a design-based analysis of emotional episodes. *Philosophy, Psychiatry, and Psychology* 3 (2): 101–26.

Wylie, M. S. 1995. Diagnosing for dollars? *Family Therapy Networker* (June): 23–33.

Younkin, S. G., Tanzi, R. E., and Christen, Y., eds. 1998. *Presenilins and Alzheimer's Disease*. Berlin: Springer-Verlag.

Yutzy, S. H., Cloninger, C. R., Guze, S. B., Pribor, E. F., Martin, R. L., Kathol, R. G., Smith, G. R. and Strain, J. J. 1995. DSM-IV field trial: Testing a new proposal for somatization disorder. *American Journal of Psychiatry* 152:97–101.

Zaner, R. 1990. Medicine and dialogue. *Journal of Medicine and Philosophy* 15:303–25.

Zilboorg, G., and Henry, G. W. 1941. *A History of Medical Psychology*. New York: W. W. Norton.

Zimmerman, M. 1988. Why are we rushing to publish DSM-IV? *Archives of General Psychiatry* 45:1135–38.

Zubin, J. 1977. But is it good for science? *Clinical Psychologist* 31:5–7.

Zuger, A. 1997. New way of doctoring: By the book. *New York Times, Science Times*, December 16, sec. F, p. 1.

Index

accountability: of the DSMs, 5; of medicine, 14; professional, 252; as a value, 310–311, 318, 320, 322
accountability thesis, 5
accuracy, 142, 157, 205, 225–226, 234, 263
action, 4, 7, 205; client, 265; in definition of values, 301–302; by the DSM leadership, 309–311; failure of, 106, 177, 185; involuntary, 184–185, 187, 190–192, 194–195; legal, 335; mental function, 343, 347–348, 351–352; of phronēsis, 81–83; political, 320; preventative, 207; professional, 64, 87, 100; public, 310
activity theory, 275
actuarial decision making, 225–226
acute stress disorder, 18
addiction, 5, 191, 194–196
adding categories, principles behind, 17
Adjustment Disorder, 264
affected pedigree method, 283
aggregation, 139, 273, 277, 280
Agich, George J., 96, 105–108, 112, 304, 314; on normativism, 114–120, 122–123, 125–127
alcoholism, 188, 193–196
American Health Information Management Association, 11

American Psychiatric Association: amicus brief, 221; approval process, 20, 307–308, 310, 317, 319, 321; collaboration with other organizations, 11, 12; on homosexuality, 4; meeting with feminists, 52; practice guidelines, 15; as professional organization, 5, 302, 307; profits, 40, 305, 309; relationship to DSM-IV, 32–33, 200, 207, 212
American Psychological Association, 33
Americans with Disabilities Act, 196, 211
anti-etiological position, 272
antineuroscience stance, 291
antipsychiatrists as a critical group, 115, 118, 120–123, 149, 329
Antisocial Personality Disorder: cultural expectations and, 140; definition, 136–138; evaluation and, 144, 192; incapacity and, 179; inference in, 19; involuntariness and, 194n; remorse and, 145; social norms and, 119; treatment of, 107
Anxiety Disorders, 18, 299
APA. See American Psychiatric Association
APOE4, 284, 292
apolitical, as a value, 25, 26, 33, 246

causal statements, 289n
causal stimulus, 361
causation, probabilistic, 289n
character: antisocial, 179–181; change of, 191; as domain of behavior, 132, 187; free expression of, 186; Kretschmer, 72; out of, 191; rhetorical, 253; traits, 179, 231; weakness of, 189
citizenship, 312, 320
classification: abandonment of, 209; arbitrary elements, 192; atheoretical, 167, 175, 177; black boxed, 253; changes in DSM, 17–21; defensible values of, 165; development of, 23, 341; of disease, 100–101; ethic of, 304; evaluative rigor of, 5–7; evidence-based, 9, 21–22; functions of, 232, 234, 268, 272; genetic susceptibility and, 272, 300; happiness, 185; heterogeneity of, 346, 350; history of, 11–12, 98–99, 180, 327–328; ideal types and, 94–95; idiographic, 88; importance of values in, 7–8, 114–124; involuntariness and, 184, 188–190, 192; labeling and, 214; mutuality and, 240; naturalism and 65; objectivity and, 45–54, 123; overpowering desires, 193; patients and, 229–30; of people, 239; politics and, 246; pragmatic aspects of, 102–105, 108–112, 304; psychotherapy and, 251; relation to clinical thinking, 74–75; role in practice and research, 200, 216, 303, 341; role of expertise in, 308; scientific credentials and, 200; Soviet Union and, 151–152; success of, 315–316; symptom-based, 343, 351, 357; system aspects of, 56–58; theory-ladenness of, 117; things *vs.* humans, 124; training and, 213; validity of, 117–118; value-based view of, 121–124
clinical judgment, 19, 21, 79–80, 99, 142, 202, 337, 346–349, 361
clinical picture, 13, 73, 254, 257–259, 264
clinical relevance, 6
clinical significance, 28, 135–136, 144, 166, 185, 244, 293, 343, 346–353, 361, 362
cognitive abilities, 131, 141

cognitive aspects of pain, 173
cognitive claims, 106
cognitive components of emotions, 171
cognitive disorder, 22
cognitive functioning, 293, 353
cognitive impairment, 284, 293–294
cognitive processes, 334
cognitive science, 59
cognitive skills, 178
cognitive systems, 353
cognitive treatment, 233
Collingwood, R. G., 59, 275
committee: advisory, 40; appointments to, 307, 310; critical review for DSM-IV, 38; DSM-III, 5; input to, 310; interests of, 315; membership, 311; politics and, 309; revision process, 53. *See also* Task Force for DSMs
common pathway, 283, 286, 293
communalism, as a value, 312
comorbidity, 13, 189, 300
compact discipline, 60
compatibility, as a value, 11, 21, 113, 310, 315, 320
compromise, 33, 52, 53, 57, 244
conceptual analysis, 112, 276
conceptual change, 58–61, 65, 66, 72, 74, 75, 361
conceptual framework, 10, 20, 107, 360
conceptual innovation, 74
conceptual validity, 148, 149, 152, 153, 163
conceptualism, 64, 65
concordance rates, 295, 297
Conduct Disorder, 150, 162, 163, 335, 362
conflict: in application of criteria, 202; in classifying Alzheimer disease, 283; concordance and, 314; diversity and, 308; ethical, 8; resolution of, 8; self-defeating personality disorder and, 121; social/interpersonal, 159, 186; theoretical and scientific, 96, 111, 306; of validators, 37
Connolly, William, 311–314
consensus: clear definition and, 140; compact discipline and, 60; compromise and, 52–53; concordance and, 318; expert, 15, 113, 118, 288; genetic di-